Interdisciplinary Medicine

Interdisciplinary Medicine

Editor

Camelia Cristina Diaconu

MDPI • Basel • Beijing • Wuhan • Barcelona • Belgrade • Manchester • Tokyo • Cluj • Tianjin

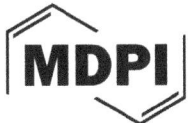

Editor
Camelia Cristina Diaconu
University of Medicine and Pharmacy "Carol Davila"
Bucharest, Romania

Editorial Office
MDPI
St. Alban-Anlage 66
4052 Basel, Switzerland

This is a reprint of articles from the Special Issue published online in the open access journal *Medicina* (ISSN 1648-9144) (available at: https://www.mdpi.com/journal/medicina/special_issues/Interdisciplinary_Medicine).

For citation purposes, cite each article independently as indicated on the article page online and as indicated below:

LastName, A.A.; LastName, B.B.; LastName, C.C. Article Title. *Journal Name* **Year**, *Volume Number*, Page Range.

ISBN 978-3-0365-2329-3 (Hbk)
ISBN 978-3-0365-2330-9 (PDF)

© 2021 by the authors. Articles in this book are Open Access and distributed under the Creative Commons Attribution (CC BY) license, which allows users to download, copy and build upon published articles, as long as the author and publisher are properly credited, which ensures maximum dissemination and a wider impact of our publications.

The book as a whole is distributed by MDPI under the terms and conditions of the Creative Commons license CC BY-NC-ND.

Contents

About the Editor ix

Camelia Cristina Diaconu
Interdisciplinary Medicine
Reprinted from: *Medicina* **2021**, *57*, 427, doi:10.3390/medicina57050427 1

Yu-Wei Fang and Chieh-Yu Liu
Determining Risk Factors Associated with Depression and Anxiety in Young Lung Cancer Patients: A Novel Optimization Algorithm
Reprinted from: *Medicina* **2021**, *57*, 340, doi:10.3390/medicina57040340 3

Dragos Serban, Bogdan Socea, Simona Andreea Balasescu, Cristinel Dumitru Badiu, Corneliu Tudor, Ana Maria Dascalu, Geta Vancea, Radu Iulian Spataru, Alexandru Dan Sabau, Dan Sabau and Ciprian Tanasescu
Safety of Laparoscopic Cholecystectomy for Acute Cholecystitis in the Elderly: A Multivariate Analysis of Risk Factors for Intra and Postoperative Complications
Reprinted from: *Medicina* **2021**, *57*, 230, doi:10.3390/medicina57030230 15

Klaudiusz Nadolny, Magdalena Wierzbik-Strońska, Jerzy R. Ładny, Beniamin O. Grabarek, Oliwia Warmusz, Dariusz Boroń and Aleksander Ostenda
Emergency Medical Teams Interventions due to Cardiovascular Diseases in 2018: Polish Regional Observational Study
Reprinted from: *Medicina* **2021**, *57*, 139, doi:10.3390/medicina57020139 31

Gina Gheorghe, Madalina Ilie, Simona Bungau, Anca Mihaela Pantea Stoian, Nicolae Bacalbasa and Camelia Cristina Diaconu
Is There a Relationship between COVID-19 and Hyponatremia?
Reprinted from: *Medicina* **2021**, *57*, 55, doi:10.3390/medicina57010055 37

Spătaru Radu-Iulian, Avino Adelaida, Iozsa Dan-Alexandru, Ivanov Monica, Serban Dragos, Tomescu Luminiţa Florentina and Cirstoveanu Cătălin
Caudal Duplication Syndrome Systematic Review—A Need for Better Multidisciplinary Surgical Approach and Follow-Up
Reprinted from: *Medicina* **2020**, *56*, 650, doi:10.3390/medicina56120650 45

Cornel Savu, Alexandru Melinte, Vasile Grigorie, Laura Iliescu, Camelia Diaconu, Mihai Dimitriu, Bogdan Socea, Ovidiu Stiru, Valentin Varlas, Carmen Savu, Irina Balescu and Nicolae Bacalbasa
Primary Pleural Hydatidosis—A Rare Occurrence: A Case Report and Literature Review
Reprinted from: *Medicina* **2020**, *56*, 567, doi:10.3390/medicina56110567 55

Anca A. Simionescu, Alexandra Horobeț, Lucian Belaşcu and Dragoş Mircea Median
Real-World Data Analysis of Pregnancy-Associated Breast Cancer at a Tertiary-Level Hospital in Romania
Reprinted from: *Medicina* **2020**, *56*, 522, doi:10.3390/medicina56100522 63

Natalia Darii Plopa, Nicolae Gica, Marie Gerard, Marie-Cécile Nollevaux, Milenko Pavlovic and Emil Anton
A Very Rare Case of Colosalpingeal Fistula Secondary to Diverticulitis: An Overview of Development, Clinical Features and Management
Reprinted from: *Medicina* **2020**, *56*, 477, doi:10.3390/medicina56090477 77

Natalia Zdanowska, Agnieszka Owczarczyk-Saczonek, Joanna Czerwińska, Jacek J. Nowakowski, Anna Kozera-Żywczyk, Witold Owczarek, Wojciech Zdanowski and Waldemar Placek
Methotrexate and Adalimumab Decrease the Serum Levels of Cardiovascular Disease Biomarkers (VCAM-1 and E-Selectin) in Plaque Psoriasis
Reprinted from: *Medicina* **2020**, *56*, 473, doi:10.3390/medicina56090473 83

Vlad Padureanu, Octavian Dragoescu, Victor Emanuel Stoenescu, Rodica Padureanu, Ionica Pirici, Radu Cristian Cimpeanu, Dop Dalia, Alexandru Radu Mihailovici and Paul Tomescu
Management of a Patient with Tuberous Sclerosis with Urological Clinical Manifestations
Reprinted from: *Medicina* **2020**, *56*, 369, doi:10.3390/medicina56080369 93

Arin Sava, Andra Piciu, Sergiu Pasca, Alexandru Mester and Ciprian Tomuleasa
Topical Corticosteroids a Viable Solution for Oral Graft versus Host Disease? A Systematic Insight on Randomized Clinical Trials
Reprinted from: *Medicina* **2020**, *56*, 349, doi:10.3390/medicina56070349 101

Adelaida Avino, Laura Răducu, Adrian Tulin, Daniela-Elena Gheoca-Mutu, Andra-Elena Balcangiu-Stroescu, Cristina-Nicoleta Marina and Cristian-Radu Jecan
Vaginal Reconstruction in Patients with Mayer–Rokitansky–Küster–Hauser Syndrome—One Centre Experience
Reprinted from: *Medicina* **2020**, *56*, 327, doi:10.3390/medicina56070327 111

Petruța Tarciuc, Ana Maria Alexandra Stanescu, Camelia Cristina Diaconu, Luminita Paduraru, Alina Duduciuc and Smaranda Diaconescu
Patterns and Factors Associated with Self-Medication among the Pediatric Population in Romania
Reprinted from: *Medicina* **2020**, *56*, 312, doi:10.3390/medicina56060312 121

Bianca Hanganu, Magdalena Iorga, Iulia-Diana Muraru and Beatrice Gabriela Ioan
Reasons for and Facilitating Factors of Medical Malpractice Complaints. What Can Be Done to Prevent Them?
Reprinted from: *Medicina* **2020**, *56*, 259, doi:10.3390/medicina56060259 133

Gener Ismail, Bogdan Obrișcă, Roxana Jurubiță, Andreea Andronesi, Bogdan Sorohan and Mihai Hârza
Inherited Risk Factors of Thromboembolic Events in Patients with Primary Nephrotic Syndrome
Reprinted from: *Medicina* **2020**, *56*, 242, doi:10.3390/medicina56050242 149

Krasimir Kostov and Alexander Blazhev
Use of Glycated Hemoglobin (A1c) as a Biomarker for Vascular Risk in Type 2 Diabetes: Its Relationship with Matrix Metalloproteinases-2, -9 and the Metabolism of Collagen IV and Elastin
Reprinted from: *Medicina* **2020**, *56*, 231, doi:10.3390/medicina56050231 159

Bogdan Marian Sorohan, Andreea Andronesi, Gener Ismail, Roxana Jurubita, Bogdan Obrisca, Cătălin Baston and Mihai Harza
Clinical Predictors of Preeclampsia in Pregnant Women with Chronic Kidney Disease
Reprinted from: *Medicina* **2020**, *56*, 213, doi:10.3390/medicina56050213 175

Irina Balescu, Nona Bejinariu, Simona Slaniceanu, Mircea Gongu, Brandusa Masoud, Smaranditta Lacau, George Tie, Maria Ciocirlan, Nicolae Bacalbasa and Catalin Copaescu
Krukenberg Tumor in Association with Ureteral Stenosis Due to Peritoneal Carcinomatosis from Pulmonary Adenocarcinoma: A Case Report
Reprinted from: *Medicina* **2020**, *56*, 187, doi:10.3390/medicina56040187 183

Cornel Savu, Alexandru Melinte, Radu Posea, Niculae Galie, Irina Balescu, Camelia Diaconu, Dragos Cretoiu, Simona Dima, Alexandru Filipescu, Cristian Balalau and Nicolae Bacalbasa
Pleural Solitary Fibrous Tumors—A Retrospective Study on 45 Patients
Reprinted from: *Medicina* **2020**, *56*, 185, doi:10.3390/medicina56040185 195

Nicolae Bacalbasa, Irina Cecilia Balescu, Camelia Diaconu, Simona Dima, Laura Iliescu, Mihaela Vilcu, Alexandru Filipescu, Ioana Halmaciu, Dragos Cretoiu and Iulian Brezean
Synchronous Cervical Adenocarcinoma and Ovarian Serous Adenocarcinoma—A Case Report and Literature Review
Reprinted from: *Medicina* **2020**, *56*, 152, doi:10.3390/medicina56040152 209

Nicolae Bacalbasa, Irina Balescu, Mihaela Vilcu, Simona Dima, Camelia Diaconu, Laura Iliescu, Alexandru Filipescu, Mihai Dimitriu and Iulian Brezean
The Risk of Para-Aortic Lymph Node Metastases in Apparent Early Stage Ovarian Cancer
Reprinted from: *Medicina* **2020**, *56*, 108, doi:10.3390/medicina56030108 217

Waqas Sami, Khalid M Alabdulwahhab, Mohd Rashid Ab Hamid, Tariq A. Alasbali, Fahd Al Alwadani and Mohammad Shakil Ahmad
Dietary Attitude of Adults with Type 2 Diabetes Mellitus in the Kingdom of Saudi Arabia: A Cross-Sectional Study
Reprinted from: *Medicina* **2020**, *56*, 91, doi:10.3390/medicina56020091 225

Călin Bogdan Chibelean, Răzvan-Cosmin Petca, Dan Cristian Radu and Aida Petca
State of the Art in Fertility Preservation for Female Patients Prior to Oncologic Therapies
Reprinted from: *Medicina* **2020**, *56*, 89, doi:10.3390/medicina56020089 235

Adelaida Avino, Laura Răducu, Lăcrămioara Aurelia Brînduşe, Cristian-Radu Jecan and Ioan Lascăr
Timing between Breast Reconstruction and Oncologic Mastectomy—One Center Experience
Reprinted from: *Medicina* **2020**, *56*, 86, doi:10.3390/medicina56020086 247

Laura Răducu, Adelaida Avino, Raluca Purnichescu Purtan, Andra-Elena Balcangiu-Stroescu, Daniela Gabriela Bălan, Delia Timofte, Dorin Ionescu and Cristian-Radu Jecan
Quality of Life in Patients with Surgically Removed Skin Tumors
Reprinted from: *Medicina* **2020**, *56*, 66, doi:10.3390/medicina56020066 255

Nicolae Bacalbasa, Irina Balescu, Mihaela Vilcu, Simona Dima, Camelia Diaconu, Laura Iliescu, Alexandru Filipescu and Iulian Brezean
Total Exenteration En Bloc with a Nephrectomy for Locally Advanced Cervical Cancer Invading a Pelvic Kidney—A Case Report and Literature Review
Reprinted from: *Medicina* **2020**, *56*, 33, doi:10.3390/medicina56010033 263

About the Editor

Camelia Cristina Diaconu, FESC, FACC, FACP; "Carol Davila" University of Medicine and Pharmacy, Internal Medicine Department, Clinical Emergency Hospital of Bucharest, Romania; President of the Balkan Medical Union. E-mail: drcameliadiaconu@gmail.com; Research Interests: heart failure; arterial hypertension; comorbidities; interdisciplinary issues; ultrasonography; arterial diseases; dyslipidemia management; diabetes. More than 200 full-text articles indexed in Clarivate Analytics (ISI Web of Science), approx. 300 full-text articles indexed in other international databases. Member of the editorial board of 25 scientific journals.

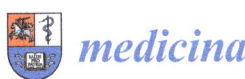

Editorial

Interdisciplinary Medicine

Camelia Cristina Diaconu [1,2]

1. Department 5, "Carol Davila" University of Medicine and Pharmacy, 050474 Bucharest, Romania; drcameliadiaconu@gmail.com
2. Clinical Emergency Hospital of Bucharest, 105402 Bucharest, Romania

Motto:

"Coming together is a beginning, working together is success, keeping together is progress"

Henry Ford.

Dear Colleagues,

Medicine of the 21st century requires multidisciplinary problem solving, for the best diagnostic and therapeutic results, to improve the healthcare of our patients.

The rapidly changing field of medicine and healthcare is increasingly adopting scientific and technological innovations, making interdisciplinary collaborations especially important. In this context, medical disciplines are becoming increasingly interlinked with other specialties and fields. A more interdisciplinary approach to the patient is needed, especially for complex patients with numerous comorbidities, most of them usually elderly and fragile. The greatest challenges to human health lie at the intersection of different medical fields. An interdisciplinary medical team is more and more necessary, with the rapid expansion of medical knowledge. Healthcare professionals need to acquire new skills regarding patient care delivery, which facilitate a better interaction between them. Healthcare is a team project and collaboration among practitioners is the key to optimal patient outcomes. Each member of the healthcare team has different and specific knowledge and skills, allowing them to contribute to a better case management. An effective interdisciplinary team may decrease the costs associated with healthcare, improve patient satisfaction, and decrease the number of medical errors and morbimortality, ultimately leading to prolonged survival of our patients and a better quality of life.

Given the importance of interdisciplinarity in the field of medicine and research, the journal *Medicina* published a very successful Special Issue on this subject, "Interdisciplinary Medicine". The articles included in this Special Issue demonstrate that every patient is a team project. Reviews and original articles dealing with interdisciplinary medical issues, as well as articles providing an up-to-date overview of the diagnostic protocols and individualized treatments for patients with multiple comorbidities, were published. The broad international distribution of the authors, with different backgrounds, demonstrates that healthcare challenges are similar in different countries. I invite you to read the articles of "Interdisciplinary Medicine", to understand the new directions in the field of healthcare and the challenges associated with them.

Funding: This research received no external funding.

Conflicts of Interest: The author declares no conflict of interest.

Citation: Diaconu, C.C. Interdisciplinary Medicine. *Medicina* **2021**, *57*, 427. https://doi.org/10.3390/medicina57050427

Received: 24 April 2021
Accepted: 26 April 2021
Published: 28 April 2021

Publisher's Note: MDPI stays neutral with regard to jurisdictional claims in published maps and institutional affiliations.

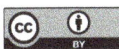

Copyright: © 2021 by the author. Licensee MDPI, Basel, Switzerland. This article is an open access article distributed under the terms and conditions of the Creative Commons Attribution (CC BY) license (https://creativecommons.org/licenses/by/4.0/).

Article

Determining Risk Factors Associated with Depression and Anxiety in Young Lung Cancer Patients: A Novel Optimization Algorithm

Yu-Wei Fang [1,2] and Chieh-Yu Liu [3,4,*]

1. Department of Nephrology, Shin Kong Memorial Wu Ho-Su Hospital, Taipei 111, Taiwan; M005916@ms.skh.org.tw
2. Department of Medicine, Fu-Jen Catholic University, New Taipei 242, Taiwan
3. Biostatistical Consulting Lab, Department of Speech Language Pathology and Audiology, National Taipei University of Nursing and Health Sciences, Taipei 112, Taiwan
4. Department of Teaching and Research, Taipei City Hospital, Taipei 106, Taiwan
* Correspondence: chiehyu@ntunhs.edu.tw; Tel.: +886-2-28227101 (ext. 6205/3312)

Abstract: *Background and Objectives*: Identifying risk factors associated with psychiatrist-confirmed anxiety and depression among young lung cancer patients is very difficult because the incidence and prevalence rates are obviously lower than in middle-aged or elderly patients. Due to the nature of these rare events, logistic regression may not successfully identify risk factors. Therefore, this study aimed to propose a novel algorithm for solving this problem. *Materials and Methods*: A total of 1022 young lung cancer patients (aged 20–39 years) were selected from the National Health Insurance Research Database in Taiwan. A novel algorithm that incorporated a *k*-means clustering method with *v*-fold cross-validation into multiple correspondence analyses was proposed to optimally determine the risk factors associated with the depression and anxiety of young lung cancer patients. *Results*: Five clusters were optimally determined by the novel algorithm proposed in this study. *Conclusions*: The novel Multiple Correspondence Analysis–*k*-means (MCA–*k*-means) clustering algorithm in this study successfully identified risk factors associated with anxiety and depression, which are considered rare events in young patients with lung cancer. The clinical implications of this study suggest that psychiatrists need to be involved at the early stage of initial diagnose with lung cancer for young patients and provide adequate prescriptions of antipsychotic medications for young patients with lung cancer.

Keywords: young lung cancer; depression; anxiety; multiple correspondence analysis; k-means clustering

1. Introduction

Lung cancer is a very aggressive malignant disease; people who smoke or are exposed to polluted environments or with genetic mutation may be at significantly higher risk of lung cancer [1–3]. Published studies have shown that Asian women who never smoke still have a higher risk of lung cancer compared with women in European countries or the United States [4,5]. Based on a worldwide report issued by the International Agency for Research on Cancer in 2018, for both males and females, lung cancer had become the most prevalent cancer globally (with incidence rate of 11.6% of all cancers) and had been ranked as the leading cause of cancer death (death rate of 18.4% of the total cancer deaths). The economic burden of treatments and care for lung cancer has also globally increased in recent years [6,7]. Published studies have showed that lung cancer is significantly associated with older age (70 years old being the average age of initial diagnosis) [7,8], but very low incidence rate in young people aged 20–40 years around the world [8]. In recent decades, due to the dramatic improvements of clinical treatments and screening techniques for lung cancer, the survival of newly diagnosed lung cancer patients has been significantly prolonged [9,10] and the incidence rate in young patients with lung cancer also increased [1,5,8]. Published studies also showed that young patients with lung cancer had better treatment outcomes of receiving surgery, chemotherapy, or radiotherapy and have relatively longer relapse-free survival, which indicates that young lung cancer patients are more likely to have prolonged survival [11–13].

Therefore, young patients with lung cancer are a noteworthy group of patients, because they have obviously lower incidence rate and prevalence rate than middle-age or elder people and they may have longer survival time. Liu et al. (2019) [14] used a retrospective review of patients with lung cancer in one hospital in China from January 2010 to June 2017, the prevalence of lung cancer in young adults aged between 18 and 35 years old was 1.37%; and Rich et al. (2015) [15] also used a retrospective cohort review using a validated national audit dataset and the results showed that the prevalence of lung cancer in young adults aged between 18 and 39 years was 0.5%. The overall incidence and prevalence in elder age groups (>50 years old) was increasing in recent decade, however, the incidence and prevalence of lung cancer in young adults (<40 years old) can be still regarded as relatively low in nowadays global cancer epidemiology. Recent studies showed that young lung cancer survivors are also at a high risk of psychiatric diseases, such as anxiety and depression in the following years of survival [16–18]. However, most of the published studies used self-reported scales or questionnaires to measure anxiety and depression instead of using diagnoses by psychiatrists; therefore, the so-called depression or anxiety in published studies can solely regarded as depression symptoms or anxiety symptoms. For example, Yan et al. [17] showed that the anxiety and depression prevalence rates of lung cancer patients were 43.5% and 57.1% by using the Hospital Anxiety and Depression Scale (HADS), which look high proportions in lung cancer patients. In addition, if young lung cancer patients who may have prolonged survival and are at high risk of psychiatrist-confirmed depression and anxiety, they will consume considerable medical resources due to the additional treatments for psychiatric diseases [6,19]. Nevertheless, there is still a lack of literature investigating risk factors associated with psychiatrist-confirmed depression and anxiety in young lung cancer patients. This study was aimed to develop a novel algorithm for identifying risk factors for psychiatrist-confirmed anxiety and depression in young lung cancer patients aged 20–39 years old by using the population-based database (National Health Insurance Research Database (NHIRD) in Taiwan), which can assist clinicians or young patients with lung cancer in preventing anxiety and depression at early stages.

2. Materials and Methods

2.1. Study Design and Study Database

This study design of this research adopted the secondary analysis of longitudinal data from NHIRD. The study database used here was retrieved from the NHIRD in Taiwan. Since the National Health Insurance (NHI) program was launched on 1 March 1995, the NHI program provided healthcare service coverage to more than 99% of the population by 2017 [20]. The NHIRD includes medical reimbursement records for outpatient and inpatient healthcare services, hospital or clinic visits, dental service visits and traditional Chinese medicine service visits. All of the reimbursement records for diagnostic and medical-related procedures for diseases are based on the international classification of diseases (ICD)—ninth and tenth revisions (after 1 January 2016 [21]) of the clinical modification (CM, or ICD-9-CM and ICD-10-CM, respectively)—and on a procedure coding system for all medical service claims.

2.2. Ethics Statement

The ethical review of this study was approved by the Institutional Review Board of the School of Nursing, National Taipei University of Nursing and Health Sciences (approval number: IRB# CN-IRB-2011-063). The date of approval was 23 October 2011. The encryption and protection of the personal information from the NHIRD were performed by the National Health Insurance Administration in Taiwan by using a complex double encryption procedure. In addition, because the present study was a secondary data analysis, written informed consent forms were not required from the recruited or selected patients. This study was also registered at Open Science Framework (OSF, reference osf.io/fkhm8 (accessed on 15 March 2021)).

2.3. Study Population and Possible Risk Factors Selection

The ICD-9-CM codes that were used to define patients with depression were 296.2X–296.3X, 300.4 and 311.X and the ICD-9-CM codes used to define patients with anxiety were 300.XX, 291.89 and 292.89. In Taiwan, if cancer patients are suspected of having depression or anxiety, they are refereed by the oncologists to psychiatrists, which is recorded as the first National Health Insurance (NHI) outpatient visit. After the referral, the cancer patients receive some psychological tests by clinical psychologists and the cancer patients are diagnosed by psychiatrists again to determine if they need anti-depressant or anti-anxiety medications; this is recorded as the second NHI psychiatric visit. After a period of time, the cancer patients need to be confirmed again by psychiatrists; therefore, to confirm that a cancer patient has depression or anxiety usually needs at least three outpatient visits and the prescription of anti-depressant or anti-anxiety drugs. In this study, young lung cancer patients that were aged 20–39 years and who were newly diagnosed with lung cancer (ICD-9-CM code = 162.XX) between 1 January 2001, and 31 December 2007, were retrieved from the NHIRD. Young lung cancer patients who died or withdrew from the NHI program during the study period were excluded. Young patients with lung cancer who had been diagnosed with baseline psychiatric diseases, such as depressive disorder (ICD-9-CM codes: 296.2X–296.3X, 300.4 and 311.X), anxiety states (ICD-9-CM codes: 300.XX, 291.89 and 292.89), bipolar disorders (ICD-9-CM codes: 296.0, 296.1, 296.4, 296.5, 296.6, 296.7, 296.8, 296.80 and 296.89), or alcohol-induced mental disorders (ICD-9-CM codes: V113, 9800, 2650, 2651, 3575, 4255, 3050, 291, 303 and 571.0–571.3) between 1 January and 31 December in 2001 were also excluded. In order to avoid selecting false-positive patients with depression and anxiety, young lung cancer patients with at least three consecutive corresponding diagnoses were eligible to be coded as having depression and anxiety.

The possible risk factors associated with depression and anxiety among lung cancer patient were determined based on Park et al. [19], who investigated if hypertension, diabetes mellitus, history of tuberculosis, liver disease (liver cancer and liver cirrhosis), end-stage renal disease, coronary artery disease (including heart failure), stroke (ischemic stroke and hemorrhage stroke) and Chronic obstructive pulmonary disease (COPD) are risk factors associated with anxiety and depression after surgical treatment for lung cancer; and Clarke and Currie [20], who took into account heart disease, stroke, cancer, diabetes mellitus, rheumatoid arthritis and asthma as the possible risk factors associated with depression and anxiety in cancer patients. Therefore, in this study, we took into account diabetes mellitus (DM), hypertension, asthma, liver cirrhosis, COPD, autoimmune diseases (including rheumatoid arthritis, systemic lupus erythematosus and aplastic anemia), cerebral diseases (including ischemic stroke, hemorrhage stroke and transient ischemic attack (TIA)), heart failure, hepatitis B virus (HBV), renal diseases and osteoporosis.

2.4. Combining Multiple Correspondence Analysis and the K-Means Clustering Algorithm with v-Fold Cross-Validation (MCA–k-Means Clustering Algorithm)

The raw data matrix was first transformed into a matrix with solely index variables (i.e., encoded as 0 or 1) through multiple correspondence analysis (MCA) [21,22], which was the data preprocessing procedure for the raw data matrix. The index variables indicate the levels of all of the categorical variables in this study. The MCA then converted all index variables into multi-dimensional Euclidean coordinates. The multi-dimensional Euclidean coordinate matrix derived from the MCA could be considered a high-dimensional dataset that could be carried into the further optimal clustering algorithm. In order to determine the optimal clustering in the high-dimensional dataset obtained from the MCA, the k-means clustering algorithm with v-fold cross-validation was applied to obtain the optimal clustering. The algorithm is described in detailed in the following:

2.4.1. Step 1. Multiple Correspondence Analysis

Let $M_{I \times K}$ be the raw data matrix with I subjects and k categorical variables.

(1) Transform the raw data matrix into a Burt matrix:
- If a categorical variable is binary, then place it in the Burt matrix as an original variable matrix.
- If a categorical variable has more than two levels (i.e., $J_k > 2$ levels), then convert this variable into an index variable (containing only 0 and 1); this forms an indicator matrix $I \times J_k$ where each column contains index variables coded with 0 or 1.
- Place all index variable columns together to form the indicator matrix $X_{I \times J}$.
- Calculate the Burt matrix as $(X_{I \times J})' \cdot X_{I \times J}$.

(2) Calculate the column and row coordinates as follows:
- The total orders of $M_{I \times K}$ (N) are observed and the probability matrix is defined as $P = N - 1X$.
- Define r as the vector of the row totals of P (i.e., $r = P1$, where 1 is a unit vector of ones) and define c as the vector of the column totals of P. Then, $Dc = diag\{c\}$ and $Dr = diag\{r\}$.
- Calculate the Euclidean coordinates by using a singular value decomposition method as follows:

$$D_r^{-\frac{1}{2}}\left(Z - rc^T\right)D_c^{-\frac{1}{2}} = P\Delta Q^T$$

where Δ and $\Lambda = \Delta^2$ are the diagonal matrix of singular values and the matrix containing eigenvalues, respectively. Therefore, the row and column coordinate matrices (F and G, respectively) are calculated as follows:

$$F = D_r^{-\frac{1}{2}} P\Delta$$

$$G = D_c^{-\frac{1}{2}} Q\Delta$$

(3) The number of dimensions is determined using an inertia value as follows:
- The inertia value is calculated based on a Pearson chi-squared (χ^2) value from the rows and columns to identify their coordinate centers as follows:

$$d_r = diag\left\{FF^T\right\} \text{ and } d_c = diag\left\{GG^T\right\}.$$

- If a subset of F or G is selected, then the inertia values for the row and column coordinates are calculated as:

$$Inertia_r = \frac{diag\left\{F'F'^T\right\}}{N} \text{ and } Inertia_c = \frac{diag\left\{G'G'^T\right\}}{N},$$

where F' and G' are subsets of F and G.

2.4.2. Step 2. K-Means Clustering with v-Fold Cross-Validation

The k-means clustering algorithm with v-fold cross-validation was applied to analyze the F and G that were obtained from the MCA [23,24]. The algorithm is as follows:

(1) Determination of the range of numbers of clusters for the k-means clustering algorithm: In this study, the number was set from $k = 2$ to n, where $n \leq 10$;
(2) Determination of the initial cluster centers: The initial cluster centers were selected at random;
(3) Iteration scheme: Assigning all index variables to their nearest cluster centers. The Euclidean distance was used as the distance measurement in the iterative classification scheme;

(4) To determine the optimal clustering, v-fold cross-validation was applied to estimate the optimal number of clusters and the optimal clustering. The details of the v-fold cross-validation are as follows:
   (a) Divide **F** or **G** into v folds (denoted F_i or G_i, I = 1, ..., v), in this study, we set $v = 5$;
   (b) For i = 1 to v, take F_i or G_i as the testing set and $\{F\}\backslash F_i$ or $\{G\}\backslash G_i$ as the training sets;
   (c) Compute the mean Euclidean distances, which are called the clustering costs in this study, within each cluster of training sets, set these as the new cluster centers and replace the cluster centers of the previous step;
   (d) Compute the mean Euclidean distances of each index variable (or the level of all of the categorical variables) of the testing set from the new cluster centers derived from the training sets;
(5) Iterate from (1);
(6) If $k = j$, which indicates the minimum mean Euclidean distances (i.e., minimal clustering cost) of each index variable of the testing set, j would be the optimum number of clusters.
(7) Clustering stopping rule: If $|\overline{D}_{j+1} - \overline{D}_j| < 0.01$, then stop further dividing and clustering.
(8) Regarding the determination of number of clusters, we adopted the method proposed by Wang [25], the optimal algorithm will iterate in order to classify factors into different numbers of clusters, calculate the cluster cost (in this study, we used the mean sum of squares within clusters as the cluster cost measurement) and compare the sums of squares between clusters. If the sum of squares of k clusters did not show statistically significant difference from $k + 1$ clusters, the optimal number of clusters is determined as k.

The MY Structured Query Language (MySQL) was used for selection, linkage, processing and cleaning of the dataset from the NHIRD. The algorithm we proposed in this study was implemented with STATISTICA Data Miner ver. 10.0 (StatSoft, Inc., Tulsa, OK, USA).

3. Results

In the present study, 1022 young lung cancer patients aged 20–39 years were studied and their demographic information is shown in Table 1. The study sample comprised 520 male (50.9%) and 502 female patients (49.1%); 154 of the patients were aged 20–29 years old (15.1%) and 868 patients were aged 30–39 years old (84.9%).

Table 1. Demographic information of the study sample ($n = 1022$).

Variable	n	(%)
Sex		
Female	502	49.1
Male	520	50.9
Age		
20–29 y	154	15.1
30–39 y	868	84.9
Charlson comorbidity index (CCI)		
CCI = 0	870	85.1
CCI = 1	91	8.9
CCI ≥ 2	61	6
Diabetes mellitus (DM)		
Yes	23	2.3
No	999	97.7

Table 1. Cont.

Variable		n	(%)
Hypertension			
	Yes	23	2.3
	No	999	97.7
Asthma			
	Yes	16	1.6
	No	1006	98.4
Liver cirrhosis			
	Yes	9	0.9
	No	1013	99.1
Chronic obstructive pulmonary disease (COPD)			
	Yes	51	5
	No	971	95
Autoimmune diseases			
	Yes	8	0.8
	No	1014	99.2
Cerebral diseases			
	Yes	11	1.1
	No	1011	98.9
Heart failure			
	Yes	2	0.2
	No	1020	99.8
Hepatitis B virus (HBV)			
	Yes	34	3.3
	No	988	96.7
Renal diseases			
	Yes	6	0.6
	No	1016	99.4
Osteoporosis			
	Yes	16	1.6
	No	1006	98.4
Depression			
	Yes	25	2.4
	No	997	97.6
Anxiety			
	Yes	15	1.5
	No	1007	98.5

As a result of the k-means clustering of **F** and **G**, which were Euclidean coordinate matrixes derived from the multiple correspondence analysis (MCA) and by using v-fold cross-validation, the clustering costs of different numbers used for the k-means clustering algorithm are shown in Figure 1. According to the results shown in Figure 1, on the basis of the clustering cost, there was no statistically significant difference between using five clusters or six clusters. Based on the principal of parsimony of clustering, the optimum number of clusters was determined to be five. Table 2 presents the clustering results that comprise these five clusters. Table 2 indicates that anxiety was clustered with osteoporosis and depression was clustered with the lack of diabetes mellitus (DM), Charlson comorbidity index (CCI) = 0 and female sex.

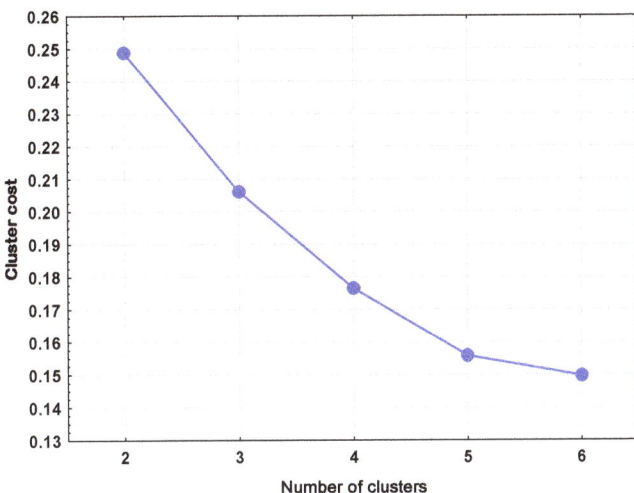

Figure 1. Cluster costs of different numbers of clusters resulting from k-means clustering combined with v-fold cross-validation.

Table 2. Results of the multiple correspondence analysis (MCA) and k-means algorithm with v-fold cross-validation.

Variable	Final Classification
Autoimmune disease = Yes	1
Cerebral disease = Yes	1
Heart failure = Yes	1
Osteoporosis = Yes	2
Anxiety = Yes	2
Depression = Yes	3
DM = No	3
Age: 20–29 y	3
Age: 30–39 y	3
CCI = 0	3
Sex = Female	3
DM = Yes	4
Hypertension = Yes	4
Asthma = Yes	4
Liver cirrhosis = Yes	4
COPD = Yes	4
HBV = Yes	4
CCI $\geq$ 2	4
Depression = No	5
Hypertension = No	5
Asthma = No	5
Liver cirrhosis = No	5
COPD = No	5
Autoimmune disease = No	5
Cerebral disease = No	5
Heart failure = No	5
HBV = No	5
Osteoporosis = No	5
Anxiety = No	5
CCI = 1	5
Sex = Male	5

Note: DM = Diabetes mellitus; CCI = Charlson comorbidity index; COPD = Chronic obstructive pulmonary disease; HBV = Hepatitis B virus.

In addition, in the present study, a control arm statistical analysis was also performed using a multiple logistic regression model, which is the most widely used method for investigating risk factors associated with diseases. Table 3a shows the results of score tests of both dependent variables—depression and anxiety—for each independent variable. In Table 3a, no statistical significance was observed for any of the independent variables with these two dependent variables, indicating that using a stepwise variable selection strategy (forward or backward variable selection) cannot be used to find any statistically significant predictors. Furthermore, Table 3b shows the results of the multiple logistic regression model (without variable selection procedures), which also indicated that there were no statistically significant predictors (except for constant terms for both dependent variables).

Table 3. (a) Score test results for each variable of the logistic regression model. (b) Results of multiple logistic regression models for depression and anxiety.

(a)

Variable	DV = Depression		DV = Anxiety	
	Score	p-Value	Score	p-Value
Sex: Male vs. Female	0.485	0.486	0.108	0.742
Age: 30–39 vs. 20–29 years	0.017	0.895	0.036	0.85
CCI = 1 vs. CCI = 0	2.505	0.113	0.368	0.544
CCI ≥ 2 vs. CCI = 0	1.661	0.197	0.966	0.326
DM: Yes vs. No	0.59	0.442	0.35	0.554
Hypertension: Yes vs. No	0.357	0.55	0.35	0.554
Asthma: Yes vs. No	0.408	0.523	2.571	0.109
Liver cirrhosis: Yes vs. No	0.228	0.633	0.135	0.713
COPD: Yes vs. No	0.053	0.818	0.09	0.764
Autoimmune: Yes vs. No	0.202	0.653	0.12	0.729
Cerebral diseases: Yes vs. No	0.279	0.597	0.166	0.684
Heart failure: Yes vs. No	0.05	0.823	0.03	0.863
HBV: Yes vs. No	1.74	0.187	0.524	0.469
Renal diseases: Yes vs. No	0.151	0.697	0.09	0.764
Osteoporosis: Yes vs. No	0.408	0.523	2.571	0.109

(b)

Variable	DV = Depression				DV = Anxiety			
	Beta	S.E.	Odds Ratio (OR)	p-value	Beta	S.E.	Odds Ratio (OR)	p-value
Sex: Male vs. Female	−0.352	0.418	0.703	0.399	−0.122	0.530	0.885	0.818
Age: 30–39 vs. 20–29 years	−0.010	0.561	0.990	0.986	0.038	0.781	1.038	0.961
CCI = 1 vs. CCI = 0	−17.329	4055.844	<0.001	0.997	0.302	0.872	1.353	0.729
CCI ≥ 2 vs. CCI = 0	1.377	0.829	3.964	0.097	−15.014	4327.707	<0.001	0.997
DM: Yes vs. No	−18.980	7844.428	<0.001	0.998	−14.048	6665.142	<0.001	0.998
Hypertension: Yes vs. No	1.217	1.092	3.377	0.265	−16.095	7460.922	<0.001	0.998
Asthma: Yes vs. No	−17.069	8269.606	<0.001	0.998	18.338	6580.883	92,044,936.212	0.998
Liver cirrhosis: Yes vs. No	−16.960	11,705.571	<0.001	0.999	−16.057	11,754.148	<0.001	0.999
COPD: Yes vs. No	−0.177	1.116	0.838	0.874	−16.910	6580.883	<0.001	0.998
Autoimmune: Yes vs. No	−17.528	12,892.859	<0.001	0.999	−17.150	13,490.401	<0.001	0.999
Cerebral diseases: Yes vs. No	−17.579	11,033.665	<0.001	0.999	−16.307	11,052.028	<0.001	0.999
Heart failure: Yes vs. No	−18.191	25,475.907	<0.001	0.999	−16.436	26,494.679	<0.001	1.000
HBV: Yes vs. No	0.225	0.962	1.252	0.815	−16.248	6243.383	<0.001	0.998
Renal diseases: Yes vs. No	−18.808	16,186.569	<0.001	0.999	−14.876	14,129.940	<0.001	0.999
Osteoporosis: Yes vs. No	−17.344	9805.003	<0.001	0.999	1.507	1.131	4.511	0.183
Constant	−3.468	0.561	0.031	<0.001	−4.152	0.778	0.016	<0.001

Note: S.E. = Standard Error; DM = Diabetes mellitus; CCI = Charlson comorbidity index; COPD = Chronic obstructive pulmonary disease; HBV = Hepatitis B virus.

4. Discussion

The objective of this study aimed to develop a novel algorithm for identifying risk factors for anxiety and depression in young lung cancer patients aged 20–39 years by using the population-based database (National Health Insurance Research Database (NHIRD) in Taiwan), which are regarded rare events and very limited number of methods were proposed to solve this problem. A novel algorithm was proposed in this study which integrated v-fold cross-validation into MCA–k-means clustering for solving the problem of determining risk factors associated with rare events.

Compared with the results of a univariate analysis using traditional multiple logistic regression analysis, which is a widely used method for determining risk factors associated with diseases (see Table 3), the results showed that none of the risk factors were statistically significantly associated with anxiety and depression, respectively, in young patients with lung cancer. Moreover, some parameter estimates were very unreliable because of their large standard errors (even bigger than the parameter estimates). In Table 3a, for the depression outcome variable, CCI = 1 vs. CCI = 0, DM, asthma, liver cirrhosis, autoimmune diseases, cerebral diseases, heart failure, renal diseases and osteoporosis indicated that parameter estimates were unreliable and exhibited extremely low odds ratios (ORs); for the anxiety outcome variable, CCI $\geq$ 2 vs. CCI = 0, DM, hypertension, asthma, liver cirrhosis, chronic obstructive pulmonary disease (COPD), autoimmune diseases, cerebral diseases, heart failure, hepatitis B (HBV) and renal diseases also indicated that the parameter estimates were unreliable and exhibited extremely low odds ratios (ORs), or an extremely high OR for asthma. Previous studies have indicated that parameter estimation methods such as maximum likelihood estimation provide biased or inestimable estimates for rare events [26,27]. According to King and Zeng (2001) [28], logistic regression would sharply underestimate the probability of rare events. For resolving the problems, some methods have been proposed, but there is still a lack of optimal methods and agreements on how to better estimate the coefficient of logistic regression for rare event data. In this study, not only were the dependent variables (depression and anxiety) rare events, but so were the independent variables, which may have resulted in many zeros in the database and the estimation of the standard error may have been biased. The novel algorithm proposed in this study can be considered to be a good approach for resolving rare event problems. In addition, compared with the results using self-reported questionnaire or inventory, such as Yan et al. [17], which used binary logistic regression analysis and the results showed that the risk factors of both anxiety and depression were lack of surgery and age; however, binary logistic regression did not successfully identify statistically significant risk factors in this study and the difference can be resulted from different operational definitions of depression and anxiety. Both kinds of studies using self-reported questionnaires or ICD-9-CM codes by psychiatrist-confirmed diagnoses provide different contributions to the clinical practices. Studies using self-reported questionnaires or inventory to measure depression and anxiety are more likely to look for factors associated with the self-perceived depression symptom and anxiety symptoms, which may be easier to express by patients themselves and some behavior interventions may be suggested, such as exercise, focus group consultant or health promotion life adjustment. However, the results of the current study using ICD-9-CM codes of depression and anxiety which are confirmed by psychiatrists, what young patients with lung cancer need are not only behavior interventions, but also the prescriptions of antidepressant drugs or anti-anxiety drugs, or the psychiatric hospitalization.

The advantages of the MCA–k-means clustering algorithm proposed in this study are: (1) the adoption of the clustering-based method to determine risk factors associated with rare events, which may avoid the parameter estimation problems encountered when using conventional logistic regression models; (2) the algorithm can take more than one dependent variable ($\geq$2) into account simultaneously, especially for easily confused diseases, for example, anxiety and depression in this study. In comparison with a logistic regression model, it deals with only one dependent variable at a time. (3) The algorithm determines the optimum number of clusters by using the v-fold cross-validation algorithm; through the repeated random sub-sampling scheme, all observations were used for both the training and validation sets and each observation was used for validation exactly once, which can help determine the optimum number of clusters with less influence from rare event data, such as the dataset used in this study.

Regarding the final clustering results of this study (see Table 2), the results indicated that anxiety was clustered with osteoporosis and depression was clustered with the lack of DM, CCI = 0 and female sex in young patients with lung cancer. These factors were optimally clustered with anxiety and depression. The results obtained in this study are validated by other studies that have indicated that patients with anxiety and osteoporosis easily encounter more complications than those with several other disease groups [29–31]. The results of this study indicate that young patients with lung cancer and osteoporosis are also at a high risk for the onset of anxiety. In addition, young female lung cancer patients were also at a higher risk of the onset of depression. Previously published studies have shown that female cancer patients are at significantly higher risk of depression than males [29,32,33]. In this study, the clustering results also supported that young female lung cancer patients were at a higher risk of the onset of depression.

This study still had some limitations. First, although the National Health Insurance (NHI) program in Taiwan covers more than 98% of the Taiwanese population [34–36], the NHIRD does not provide information about some potential confounding factors, such as smoking, alcohol consumption, exercise habits, diet and lifestyle, which may also influence the association with the risk of anxiety and depression. Second, some young lung cancer patients who experience anxiety and depression may not consult psychiatrists; they usually express their concerns about their cancer diseases to their oncologists and the oncologists may easily neglect or ignore their patients' anxiety and depression symptoms. Thus, cancer patients may search for religious help or may isolate themselves from people or medical professionals; therefore, the number of patients with anxiety and depression may be underestimated. Third, because the young patients with lung cancer enrolled in this study were primarily of the Chinese or Han ethnicities, the results derived from the novel algorithm proposed here require further examination and validation for generalization to other ethnicities. Furthermore, according to Lu et al. (2019) [37], in recent decades, the overall incidence of lung cancer initially increased and then gradually decreased. The surgical rate and radiotherapy rate for lung cancer showed a general downward trend, while the chemotherapy rate experienced a significantly increasing trend [30]. Although the five-year relative survival rate has increased over the years, it has remained very low for the last 20 years [31]. Therefore, this study, which used a nationwide database from 2001 to 2007, can still provide useful findings for clinicians.

5. Conclusions

The novel MCA–k-means clustering algorithm in this study successfully identified risk factors associated with anxiety and depression, which are considered rare events in young patients with lung cancer. The clinical implications of this study suggest that psychiatrists need to be involved at the early stage of initial diagnose with lung cancer for young patients and provide adequate prescriptions of antipsychotic medications for young patients with lung cancer.

Author Contributions: Drafting of the article: Y.-W.F.; critical revision of the article for important intellectual content: Y.-W.F. and C.-Y.L.; final approval of the article: C.-Y.L.; statistical expertise: C.-Y.L. All authors have read and agreed to the published version of the manuscript.

Funding: This study was supported by an industry–academia collaboration grant whose grant number is DSLPA-PC-107-003.

Institutional Review Board Statement: The study was conducted according to the guidelines of the Declaration of Helsinki and it was approved by the Institutional Review Board of the School of Nursing, National Taipei University of Nursing and Health Sciences (approval number: IRB# CN-IRB-2011-063).

Informed Consent Statement: Patient consent was waived because the encryption and protection of the personal information from the NHIRD were performed by the National Health Insurance Administration in Taiwan by using a complex double-encryption procedure. As this present study was a secondary data analysis, written informed consent forms were not required from the recruited or selected patients.

Data Availability Statement: The study dataset (NHIRD) was not publicly archived; to access it, an application from the Bureau of National Health Insurance in Taiwan is needed. The application website is: https://www.nhi.gov.tw (the access date was 10 December 2012).

Acknowledgments: The authors of this study are very grateful to the National Health Insurance Administration for providing the National Health Insurance claim database and to the Health Data Value-Added Center of the Ministry of Health and Welfare of Taiwan for maintaining the National Health Insurance Research Database (NHIRD).

Conflicts of Interest: The funders had no role in the design of the study; in the collection, analyses, or interpretation of data; in the writing of the manuscript, or in the decision to publish the results.

References

1. Cheng, T.-Y.D.; Cramb, S.M.; Baade, P.D.; Youlden, D.R.; Nwogu, C.; Reid, M.E. The international epidemiology of lung cancer: Latest trends, disparities, and tumor characteristics. *J. Thorac. Oncol.* **2016**, *11*, 1653–1671. [CrossRef] [PubMed]
2. Cho, J.H.; Zhou, W.; Choi, Y.-L.; Sun, J.-M.; Choi, H.; Kim, T.-E.; Dolled-Filhart, M.; Emancipator, K.; Rutkowski, M.A.; Kim, J. Retrospective molecular epidemiology study of PD-L1 expression in patients with EGFR-Mutant non-small cell lung cancer. *Cancer Res. Treat.* **2018**, *50*, 95–102. [CrossRef]
3. Christiani, D.C. Smoking and the molecular epidemiology of lung cancer. *Clin. Chest Med.* **2000**, *21*, 87–93. [CrossRef]
4. Ha, S.Y.; Choi, S.-J.; Cho, J.H.; Choi, H.J.; Lee, J.; Jung, K.; Irwin, D.; Liu, X.; Lira, M.E.; Mao, M.; et al. Lung cancer in never-smoker Asian females is driven by oncogenic mutations, most often involving EGFR. *Oncotarget* **2015**, *6*, 5465–5474. [CrossRef] [PubMed]
5. Bray, F.; Ferlay, J.; Soerjomataram, I.; Siegel, R.L.; Torre, L.A.; Jemal, A. Global cancer statistics 2018: GLOBOCAN estimates of incidence and mortality worldwide for 36 cancers in 185 countries. *CA Cancer J. Clin.* **2018**, *68*, 394–424. [CrossRef]
6. Enstone, A.; Greaney, M.; Povsic, M.; Wyn, R.; Penrod, J.R.; Yuan, Y. The economic burden of small cell lung cancer: A systematic review of the literature. *Pharm. Open* **2017**, *2*, 139–152. [CrossRef]
7. De Groot, P.M.; Wu, C.C.; Carter, B.W.; Munden, R.F. The epidemiology of lung cancer. *Transl. Lung Cancer Res.* **2018**, *7*, 220–233. [CrossRef]
8. van der Meer, D.J.; Karim-Kos, H.E.; van der Mark, M.; Aben, K.K.H.; Bijlsma, R.M.; Rijneveld, A.W.; van der Graaf, W.T.A.; Husson, O. Incidence, survival, and mortality trends of cancers diagnosed in adolescents and young adults (15–39 Years): A population-based study in The Netherlands 1990–2016. *Cancers* **2020**, *18*, 3421. [CrossRef]
9. Sacco, P.C.; Maione, P.; Guida, C.; Gridelli, C. The combination of new immunotherapy and radiotherapy: A new potential treatment for locally advanced non-small cell lung cancer. *Curr. Clin. Pharmacol.* **2017**, *12*, 4–10. [CrossRef]
10. Hirsh, V. New developments in the treatment of advanced squamous cell lung cancer: Focus on afatinib. *OncoTargets Ther.* **2017**, *10*, 2513–2526. [CrossRef]
11. Wang, H.; Zhang, J.; Shi, F.; Zhang, C.; Jiao, Q.; Zhu, H. Better cancer specific survival in young small cell lung cancer patients especially with AJCC stage III. *Oncotarget* **2017**, *8*, 34923–34934. [CrossRef]
12. Arnold, B.N.; Thomas, D.C.; Rosen, J.E.; Salazar, M.C.; Blasberg, J.D.; Boffa, D.J.; Detterbeck, F.C.; Kim, A.W. Lung cancer in the very young: Treatment and survival in the national cancer data base. *J. Thorac. Oncol.* **2016**, *11*, 1121–1131. [CrossRef]
13. Liu, M.; Cai, X.; Yu, W.; Lv, C.; Fu, X. Clinical significance of age at diagnosis among young non-small cell lung cancer patients under 40 years old: A population-based study. *Oncotarget* **2015**, *6*, 44963–44970. [CrossRef] [PubMed]
14. Liu, B.; Quan, X.; Xu, C.; Lv, J.; Li, C.; Dong, L.; Liu, M. Lung cancer in young adults aged 35 years or younger: A full-scale analysis and review. *J. Cancer* **2019**, *10*, 3553–3559. [CrossRef] [PubMed]
15. Rich, A.L.; Khakwani, A.; Free, C.M.; Tata, L.J.; Stanley, R.A.; Peake, M.D.; Hubbard, R.B.; Baldwin, D.R. Non-small cell lung cancer in young adults: Presentation and survival in the English National Lung Cancer Audit: QJM. *Int. J. Med.* **2015**, *108*, 891–897. [CrossRef] [PubMed]
16. Arrieta, Ó.; Angulo, L.P.; Núñez-Valencia, C.; Dorantes-Gallareta, Y.; Macedo, E.O.; Martínez-López, D.; Alvarado, S.; Corona-Cruz, J.-F.; Oñate-Ocaña, L.F. Association of depression and anxiety on quality of life, treatment adherence, and prognosis in patients with advanced non-small cell lung cancer. *Ann. Surg. Oncol.* **2012**, *20*, 1941–1948. [CrossRef]
17. Yan, X.; Chen, X.; Li, M.; Zhang, P. Prevalence and risk factors of anxiety and depression in Chinese patients with lung cancer: A cross-sectional study. *Cancer Manag. Res.* **2019**, *11*, 4347–4356. [CrossRef]
18. Johnson, C.G.; Brodsky, J.L.; Cataldo, J.K. Lung cancer stigma, anxiety, depression, and quality of life. *J. Psychosoc. Oncol.* **2014**, *32*, 59–73. [CrossRef]
19. Park, S.; Kang, C.H.; Hwang, Y.; Seong, Y.W.; Lee, H.J.; Park, I.K.; Kim, Y.T. Risk factors for postoperative anxiety and depression after surgical treatment for lung cancer. *Eur. J. Cardiothorac. Surg.* **2016**, *49*, e16–e21. [CrossRef]
20. Ting, C.-T.; Kuo, C.-J.; Hu, H.-Y.; Lee, Y.-L.; Tsai, T.-H. Prescription frequency and patterns of Chinese herbal medicine for liver cancer patients in Taiwan: A cross-sectional analysis of the National Health Insurance Research Database. *BMC Complement. Altern. Med.* **2017**, *17*, 1–11. [CrossRef]
21. Jung, J.Y.; Lee, J.M.; Kim, M.S.; Shim, Y.M.; Zo, J.I.; Yun, Y.H. Comparison of fatigue, depression, and anxiety as factors affecting posttreatment health-related quality of life in lung cancer survivors. *Psych. Oncol.* **2018**, *27*, 465–470. [CrossRef]

22. Ambrogi, F.; Biganzoli, E.; Boracchi, P. Multiple correspondence analysis in S-PLUS. *Comput. Methods Programs Biomed.* **2005**, *79*, 161–167. [CrossRef]
23. Shrivastav, M.; Iaizzo, P. Discrimination of ischemia and normal sinus rhythm for cardiac signals using a modified k means clustering algorithm. In Proceedings of the 2007 29th Annual International Conference of the IEEE Engineering in Medicine and Biology Society, Lyon, France, 22–26 August 2007; Institute of Electrical and Electronics Engineers (IEEE): New York, NY, USA, 2007; Volume 2007, pp. 3856–3859.
24. Saatchi, M.; McClure, M.C.; McKay, S.D.; Rolf, M.M.; Kim, J.; Decker, J.E.; Taxis, T.M.; Chapple, R.H.; Ramey, H.R.; Northcutt, S.L.; et al. Accuracies of genomic breeding values in American Angus beef cattle using K-means clustering for cross-validation. *Genet. Sel. Evol. (GSE)* **2011**, *43*, 40. [CrossRef] [PubMed]
25. Wang, J. Consistent selection of the number of clusters via cross validation. *Biometrika* **2010**, *97*, 893–904. [CrossRef]
26. Hagen, K.B.; Aas, T.; Kvaloy, J.T.; Eriksen, H.R.; Soiland, H.; Lind, R. Fatigue, anxiety and depression overrule the role of oncological treatment in predicting self-reported health complaints in women with breast cancer compared to healthy controls. *Breast* **2016**, *28*, 100–106. [CrossRef] [PubMed]
27. Gorman, J.R.; Su, H.I.; Roberts, S.C.; Dominick, S.A.; Malcarne, V.L. Experiencing reproductive concerns as a female cancer survivor is associated with depression. *Cancer* **2015**, *121*, 935–942. [CrossRef] [PubMed]
28. King, G.; Zeng, L. Logistic Regression in Rare Events Data. *Politi. Anal.* **2001**, *9*, 137–163. [CrossRef]
29. Westphal, C. Logistic regression for extremely rare events: The case of school shootings. *SSRN Electron. J.* **2013**. [CrossRef]
30. Nations, J.A.; Nathan, S.D. Comorbidities of Advanced Lung Disease. *Mt. Sinai J. Med. A J. Transl. Pers. Med.* **2009**, *76*, 53–62. [CrossRef]
31. Sculier, J.P.; Botta, I.; Bucalau, A.M.; Compagnie, M.; Eskenazi, A.; Fischler, R.; Gorham, J.; Mans, L.; Rozen, L.; Speybrouck, S.; et al. Medical anticancer treatment of lung cancer associated with comorbidities: A review. *Lung Cancer* **2015**, *87*, 241–248. [CrossRef] [PubMed]
32. Paal, B.V. *A Comparison of Different Methods for Modelling Rare Events Data*; Universiteit Gent: Brussel, Belgium, 2014.
33. Seib, C.; Porter-Steele, J.; Ng, S.K.; Turner, J.; McGuire, A.; McDonald, N.; Balaam, S.; Yates, P.; McCarthy, A.; Anderson, D. Life stress and symptoms of anxiety and depression in women after cancer: The mediating effect of stress appraisal and coping. *Psychooncology* **2018**, *27*, 1787–1794. [CrossRef] [PubMed]
34. Hong-Jhe, C.; Chin-Yuan, K.; Ming-Shium, T.; Fu-Wei, W.; Ru-Yih, C.; Kuang-Chieh, H.; Hsiang-Ju, P.; Ming-Yueh, C.; Pan-Ming, C.; Chih-Chuan, P. The incidence and risk of osteoporosis in patients with anxiety disorder: A Population-based retrospective cohort study. *Medicine* **2016**, *95*, e4912. [CrossRef] [PubMed]
35. Yeh, M.J.; Chang, H.H. National health insurance in Taiwan. *Health Aff.* **2015**, *34*, 1067. [CrossRef]
36. Shi, Q.; Li, K.J.; Treuer, T.; Wang, B.C.M.; Gaich, C.L.; Lee, C.H.; Wu, W.S.; Furnback, W.; Tang, C.H. Estimating the response and economic burden of rheumatoid arthritis patients treated with biologic disease-modifying antirheumatic drugs in Taiwan using the National Health Insurance Research Database (NHIRD). *PLoS ONE* **2018**, *13*, e0193489. [CrossRef]
37. Lu, T.; Yang, X.; Huang, Y.; Zhao, M.; Li, M.; Ma, K.; Yin, J.; Zhan, C.; Wang, Q. Trends in the incidence, treatment, and survival of patients with lung cancer in the last four decades. *Cancer Manag. Res.* **2019**, *11*, 943–953. [CrossRef]

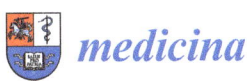

Article

Safety of Laparoscopic Cholecystectomy for Acute Cholecystitis in the Elderly: A Multivariate Analysis of Risk Factors for Intra and Postoperative Complications

Dragos Serban [1,2,*,†], Bogdan Socea [2,3], Simona Andreea Balasescu [1,*,†], Cristinel Dumitru Badiu [2,4], Corneliu Tudor [1], Ana Maria Dascalu [2,†], Geta Vancea [2], Radu Iulian Spataru [2,5,†], Alexandru Dan Sabau [6], Dan Sabau [6] and Ciprian Tanasescu [6,†]

[1] 4th Department of Surgery, University Emergency Hospital Bucharest, 050098 Bucharest, Romania; lulu.tudor@gmail.com
[2] Faculty of Medicine, "Carol Davila" University of Medicine and Pharmacy, 020021 Bucharest, Romania; bogdan.socea@umfcd.ro (B.S.); cristian.d.badiu@gmail.com (C.D.B.); ana.dascalu@umfcd.ro (A.M.D.); getavancea@gmail.com (G.V.); raduspataru@yahoo.com (R.I.S.)
[3] Department of Surgery, "Sf. Pantelimon" Emergency Hospital, 021659 Bucharest, Romania
[4] Department of Surgery, "Bagdasar Arseni" Clinical Emergency Hospital, 041915 Bucharest, Romania
[5] Department of Pediatric Surgery, Emergency Clinic Hospital for Children "Maria S. Curie", 41451 Bucharest, Romania
[6] 3rd Department Surgery, Faculty of Medicine, "Lucian Blaga" University Sibiu, 550169 Sibiu, Romania; alexandru.sabau@ulbsibiu.ro (A.D.S.); dan.sabau@ulbsibiu.ro (D.S.); ciprian.tanasescu@ulbsibiu.ro (C.T.)
* Correspondence: dragos.serban@umfcd.ro (D.S.); simona.a.balasescu@gmail.com (S.A.B.); Tel.: +40-723-300-370 (D.S.); +40-722-204-699 (S.A.B.)
† These authors contributed equally to this work.

Abstract: *Background and Objectives:* This study investigates the impact of age upon the safety and outcomes of laparoscopic cholecystectomy performed for acute cholecystitis, by a multivariate approach. *Materials and Methods:* A 2-year retrospective study was performed on 333 patients admitted for acute cholecystitis who underwent emergency cholecystectomy. The patients included in the study group were divided into four age subgroups: A ≤49 years; B: 50–64 years; C: 65–79 years; D ≥80 years. *Results:* Surgery after 72 h from onset ($p = 0.007$), severe forms, and higher American Society of Anesthesiologists Physical Status Classification and Charlson comorbidity index scores ($p < 0.001$) are well correlated with older age. Both cardiovascular and surgical related complications were significantly higher in patients over 50 years ($p = 0.045$), which also proved to be a turning point for increasing the rate of conversion and open surgery. However, the comparative incidence did not differ significantly between patients aged from 50–64 years, 65–79 years and over 80 years (6.03%, 9.09% and 5.8%, respectively). Laparoscopic cholecystectomy (LC) was the most frequently used surgical approach in the treatment of acute cholecystitis in all age groups, with better outcomes than open cholecystectomy in terms of decreased overall and postoperative hospital stay, reduced surgery related complications, and the incidence of acute cardiovascular events in the early postoperative period ($p < 0.001$). *Conclusions:* The degree of systemic inflammation was the main factor that influenced the adverse outcome of LC in the elderly. Among comorbidities, diabetes was associated with increased surgical and systemic postoperative morbidity, while stroke and chronic renal insufficiency were correlated with a high risk of cardiovascular complications. With adequate perioperative care, the elderly has much to gain from the benefits of a minimally invasive approach, which allows a decreased rate of postoperative complications and a reduced hospital stay.

Keywords: acute cholecystitis; laparoscopic cholecystectomy; elderly; safety

1. Introduction

As the world population is aging, there is an increased surgical demand for elderly people. Geriatric surgery is presently a topic of research, as many surgeons acknowledge there are specific features regarding the type of surgery, the duration and intensity of treatment and the significant complications related to the therapeutic approach at advanced ages. The term of "frailty" is often used to describe a vulnerability, a lack of resilience of the elderly to stress and increased demands upon the function of organs or systems. [1–3] Understanding the specific age-related challenges may help improve perioperative care by a multidisciplinary approach [3–5].

Acute cholecystitis is one of the most frequent conditions requiring abdominal surgery in emergencies in elderly people [6]. The current guidelines recommend surgery as soon as possible because evidenced-based clinical studies confirmed that an early treatment reduces the total hospital stay and does not increase the complication or conversion rates [7–11].

Laparoscopic cholecystectomy has become the "gold standard" due to its undeniable advantages in reducing pain and postoperative complications. Together with the development of anesthesia and intensive care skills and techniques, the safety limit for performing laparoscopy has also increased nowadays towards the age of 80–85 years.

In previously published studies on the results of laparoscopic cholecystectomy in the elderly, the age considered as a threshold differs: some studies consider it to be 65 years [12–14], 70 years [15] or 75 years [16], while several studies refer to outcomes of laparoscopic cholecystectomy in extreme ages, such as over 80 years of age [6,17–21]. Most studies compare the conversion rate and the incidence of postoperative complications in groups of young vs. elderly patients. There are limits in terms of reporting the results, as the effect of age is difficult to be dissociated from the presence of comorbidities, which are obviously more common with aging. Other studies [14,22–24] compared the complications of laparoscopic vs. classical cholecystectomy in elderly patients and found better outcomes with a minimally invasive approach.

This study aims to investigate the impact of age upon the safety and outcomes of laparoscopic cholecystectomy performed for acute cholecystitis, by a multivariate approach. The novelty factor is that age is analyzed in correlation with the anesthetic-surgical systemic risk factors and with the severity of the infectious process. The preoperative variables which correlate best with surgical decisions and postoperative outcomes were analyzed.

2. Materials and Methods

2.1. Study Design

A 2-year retrospective study was performed on the patients admitted in the 4th Department of Surgery, Emergency University Hospital Bucharest for acute cholecystitis who underwent emergency cholecystectomy, between January 2018 and December 2019. Data were collected from observation charts and postoperative notes.

The diagnosis of acute cholecystitis was assessed according to Tokyo Guidelines, based on clinical findings (Murphy sign; right upper quadrant pain, tenderness, palpable mass, fever), laboratory inflammation tests and an ultrasound exam confirming gallstones and thickness of the gallbladder wall. The inclusion criteria for the study consisted of: (I) emergency admission for acute cholecystitis followed by cholecystectomy during the same hospital admission, (II) accurate documentation of the clinical signs, paraclinical data, surgery and complications. Exclusion criteria were: (I) associated pancreatitis or any (II) malignancy.

The preoperative evaluation of the anesthetic-surgical risk was based on the American Society of Anesthesiologists Physical Status Classification (ASA PS). The severity of acute cholecystitis was evaluated according to Tokyo Guidelines criteria (TG13/TG18) (Table 1). Charlson Comorbidity Index (CCI) scores were calculated retrospectively for the patients enrolled in the study based on the comorbidities documented in the observation charts.

Table 1. Tokyo Guidelines (TG13/TG18) severity risk scale [9,25].

Grade III (severe) acute cholecystitis	Acute cholecystitis with organ/system (renal, cardiovascular, hepatic, respiratory, neurologic, hematologic) dysfunction
Grade II (moderate) acute cholecystitis	Acute cholecystitis associated with: 1. WBC * > 18,000/mmc 2. Palpable tender mass in the right upper abdominal quadrant 3. Marked local inflammation 4. Onset > 72 h
Grade I (mild) acute cholecystitis	Acute cholecystitis which does not meet criteria for grade II or III

* WBC—white blood cells.

The management of acute cholecystitis was according to the Tokyo Guidelines 2018 flowchart [25] based on the severity of symptoms, ASA and CCI index. Emergency laparoscopic cholecystectomy was performed as soon as possible to be performed safely, within a time frame of 96 h after the admission. Broad spectrum intravenous antibiotic therapy was used in all cases. In mild cases, we used intravenous ceftriaxone (1 g/12 h), and in medium and severe cases we used a combination of ceftriaxone or piperacillin/tazobactam (4 g + 0.5 g/8 h) and metronidazole (1 g/12 h). The antibiotic therapy was initiated in emergency and continued up to 24–48 h postoperatively, in cases with a favorable outcome. In cases with pyocholecystitis, parietal micro-abscesses, or pericholecystic abscess, bile was sent for a microbiological exam, and antibiotic therapy was adjusted later in correlation with the antibiogram. Low-molecular-weight Heparin for thrombosis prophylaxis was used as a routine pre and postoperatively during the hospital stay, according to body weight and comorbidities, in doses starting from 0.4 mL/day to 1.2 mL/day.

Conversion to open surgery was used as a second option of bailout procedure, after "fundus first", when technical difficulties were encountered and critical view of safety in the Calot triangle was not achieved. Subtotal cholecystectomy was considered a technical solution in difficult cases, and it can be performed either laparoscopically or by open surgery, depending on the surgeon's experience and the local technical conditions. Drainage was used in all these patients.

Patients with ASA $\geq$ 3 and CCI $\geq$ 6 or sepsis underwent fluid rebalance and general supportive care before surgery.

2.2. Data Comparison and Statistical Analysis

The patients included in the study group were divided into 4 age-subgroups: A: $\leq$49 years; B: 50–64 years; C: 65–79 years; D: $\geq$80 years.

The main outcomes were: mortality rate and incidence of major systemic and surgery related complications. Secondly, the rate of laparoscopic cholecystectomies and the rate of conversion were analyzed comparatively in the four age-subgroups. A statistical analysis was performed to assess the association correlations between age and anesthetic-surgical risk, the severity forms of acute cholecystitis and post-operatory outcomes.

Pearson chi square, Fisher's exact test and the Linear-by-Linear association test (Mantel-Haenszel test for trend) were used to evaluate the association between discrete variables, the ANOVA test was used for continuous variables and Fisher's linear discriminant analysis was used for multivariate analysis. IBM SPSS Statistics 22 was applied.

In order to describe the preoperative and intraoperative patients' characteristics which determined the applied surgical procedure (LC = Laparoscopic Cholecystectomy, Conversion or OC = Open Cholecystectomy), we have used the stepwise variant of Fisher's linear discriminant analysis. The Canonical Discriminant Function is displayed in standardized form in order to allow the comparison of the importance of each variable. Cross-validation models were used to evaluate the statistical power of discrimination.

3. Results

3.1. Demographic Data and Preoperative Evaluation

A total of 345 patients, aged between 18 and 91 years, were admitted in emergency with the diagnostic of acute cholecystitis during January 2018 and December 2019. A total of 12 patients (3.47%) did not undergo cholecystectomy during the same hospital admission and were excluded from the statistical analysis. In one case (0.28%), a man aged 87, with severe cardiac insufficiency and sepsis (ASA IV), emergency cholecystostomy was performed. Drainage of the bilious-purulent content of the gallbladder allowed recovery in a case in which general anesthesia was considered not appropriate due to high risk of death. Conservative management was used in 11 cases (3.18%). Four cases refused surgery (aged between 42 and 83 years), while in seven cases cholecystectomy was postponed by the surgeon for various reasons (Table 2).

Table 2. Demographic and clinical data of non-operated patients.

No.	Age	TG 13/18 Severity Form	Reason for Postponed Surgery	Returned for Elective Surgery during the Study Period
1	37	mild	Refused surgery	no
2	39	mild	Associated giant right renal cyst; deferred to urology after conservative management	yes, 4 months later
3	53	moderate	Neglected arterial hypertension *	yes, after one month
4	53	mild	Refused surgery	no
5	57	moderate	Morbid obesity (BMI ** 43)	no
6	61	mild	Ultrasound (US) and Computed tomography (CT) exam raised suspicion of gallbladder carcinoma	yes, for further evaluation and elective oncological surgery
7	64	mild	Morbid obesity (BMI 41)	no
8	69	mild	Refused surgery	yes, 6 months later
9	72	mild	US and CT exam raised suspicion of colon cancer	yes, for further evaluation and elective oncological surgery
10	82	moderate	Increased anesthetic risk due to severe cardiac insufficiency	no
11	86	mild	Refused surgery	no

* hypertension—Blood pressure (BP) of 22 mmHg at admission. As the patient responded to medical therapy for acute cholecystitis, he was referred to a cardiologist and asked to return for elective surgery, under adequate medication. ** BMI – body mass index.

A total of 333 patients (96.54%) underwent emergency cholecystectomy and were further included in the statistical analysis. The distribution of patients follows a multiple peak pattern, suggesting the overlay of multiple populations (Figure 1).

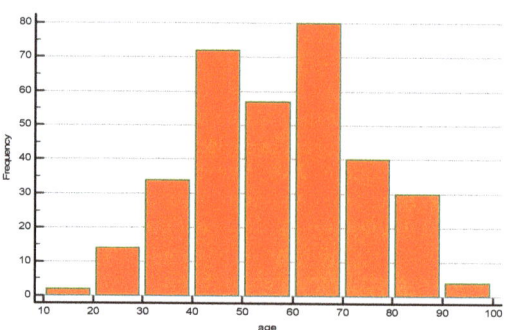

Figure 1. Age distribution of patients with emergency cholecystectomy for acute cholecystitis in the study group (n = 333).

There were no statistically significant differences in terms of gender distribution in the four subgroups (Table 3). Presentation at more than 72 h after onset was considered a sign of severity of the level of local inflammation according to the Tokyo Guidelines. In the study group, there was a upward trend correlated with age and surgery after 72 h from onset, confirmed by the Linear-by-Linear association test ($p = 0.007$).

Table 3. Demographic and preoperative data in the 4 age-subgroups.

Group	A	B	C	D	Total	p Value
Age (years)	≤49	50–64	65–79	≥80	18–91	
Number	122	111	66	34	333	
Onset > 72 h	59.8%	69.4%	75.8%	79.4%	68.2%	$p = 0.007$ [1]
Female (%)	29.5%	29.7%	36.4%	26.5%	30.6%	$p = 0.716$ [2]
Severity forms TG13/TG 18						
Mild	36.10%	27%	22.70%	11.80%	27.90%	
Moderate	61.50%	68.50%	65.20%	70.60%	65.50%	$p < 0.001$ [1]
Severe	2.50%	4.50%	12.10%	17.60%	6.60%	
Leukocytes ≥ 18,000/mmc	2.5%	7.2%	12.1%	14.7%	7.2%	$p = 0.025$ [2]
Fibrinogen > 400 mg/dL	34.4%	48.6%	60.6%	67.6%	47.7%	$p = 0.007$ [1]
Creatinine > 1.2 mg/dL	19%	19.8%	37.9%	50%	26.2%	$p < 0.001$ [1]
Aspartate transaminase (AST), Alanine transaminase (ALT) > 40 UI/L	33.6%	38.7%	28.8%	47.1%	35.7%	$p = 0.268$ [2]
INR(international normalized ratio) > 2	0	2.7%	0	5.9%	1.5%	$p = 0.039$ [2]
Bilirubin > 1.2 mg/dL	11.4%	9.9%	24.2%	29%	15.31%	$p = 0.045$ [2]
Sign of acute cardiac insufficiency at admission ***	2.5%	9.9%	21.2%	44.1%	12.9%	$p < 0.001$ [1]
Neurologic decompensation at admission	0	0	0.015%	0.029%	0.006%	N/A
ASA PS risk						
I	33.60%	18%	6.10%	0	19.50%	
II	54.10%	57.70%	53%	44.10%	54.10%	
III	12.30%	20.70%	37.90%	44.10%	23.40%	$p < 0.001$ [1]
IV	0	2.70%	3%	8.80%	2.40%	
V	0	0.90%	0	2.90%	0.60%	
CCI						
0	88.40%	60.30%	28.70%	20.50%	58.80%	
1	5.70%	14.40%	27.20%	26.50%	15.30%	
2	1.60%	14.10%	21.20%	20.60%	8.40%	
3	5.70%	11.70%	12.10%	8.80%	9.30%	$p < 0.001$ [1]
4	1.60%	3.60%	4.50%	14.70%	5.10%	
5	0	1.80%	3%	0	1.20%	
≥6	0.80%	1.80%	0	8.80%	1.80%	

Footnote: [1] Test of Linear-by-Linear Association; [2] Fisher's exact test; ASA PS: American Society of Anesthesiologists Physical Status Classification; TG13/18: Tokyo Guidelines classification risk; CCI: Charlson Comorbidity Index. *** described according to Common Guide of diagnostic and treatment of Acute Cardiac Insufficiency of European Society of Intensive Therapy and European Society of Cardiology: (i) Aggravated preexisting cardiac insufficiency (edema of the lower limbs, congestion); (ii) Hypertensive Cardiac insufficiency (high BP, tachycardia, signs of vasoconstriction); (iii) Pulmonary acute edema: acute respiratory disfunction, with tachypnea and orthopnea, SaO_2 < 90% before oxygen administration; (iv) Acute coronary syndrome; (v) Cardiogenic shock: hypotension requiring vasopressor medication, signs of organ hypoperfusion, with oliguria.

The moderate forms (TG 13/18) were the most frequent in all age groups. However, the statistical analysis showed a tendency for the mild forms to decrease with age, with a corresponding increase in the severe forms with organ/system decompensation (Figure 2), with statistically significant differences being observed between group A on the one hand and groups C and D on the other hand ($p < 0.001$). The same differences were observed for the leukocytes > 18,000/mmc and fibrinogen > 400 mg/mL.

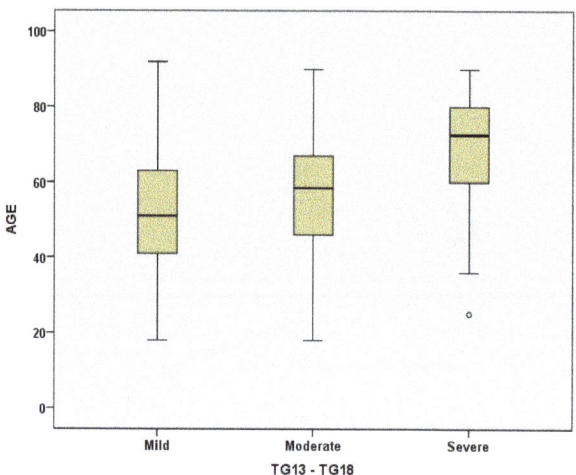

Figure 2. Boxplot representation of age distribution by Tokyo Guidelines TG13/TG18 Classification.

The age of 65 represents a statistically significant demarcation limit in terms of associated comorbidities and anesthetic-surgical risk. CCI correlates well with age (Spearman rho 0.462, $p < 0.001$). In groups C and D compared to groups A and B, there were significantly fewer patients with ASA PS risk I and significantly more patients with ASA PS $\geq$ 3, with the increase in the ASA score with age being confirmed by the Linear-by-Linear association test ($p < 0.001$).

The incidence of signs of acute cardiac insufficiency at admission significantly increased with age, from 2.5% in group A to 44.1% in group D. Similar correlations were found with creatinine levels > 1.2 mg/mL, an expression of a pre-existing age-related limitation of renal function, with decompensation in the context of systemic inflammation and sepsis. There were only five cases with INR > 2. It correlated with chronic anticoagulant therapy for cardiovascular associated comorbidities.

3.2. Surgical Approach and Postoperative Outcomes

As general management, the laparoscopic approach was the first choice for all patients of all ages. Open cholecystectomy was performed only when laparoscopy was not considered safe due to comorbidities or local conditions.

We noted a statistically significant difference between the age distribution for LC compared to OC and conversion: the mean age for LC is 55, while the mean age for OC and conversion is 68 ($p < 0.001$ for ANOVA test). However laparoscopic cholecystectomy was the most frequent procedure in all subgroups, with superior outcomes when compared to open surgery and conversion in terms of hospital stay and surgical and cardiovascular complications ($p < 0.001$).

Furthermore, the linear-by-linear association shows an increase in the conversion rate with age ($p < 0.001$). The frequencies of the conversion rate and the classic surgical approach were significantly higher in patients aged over 50.

Conversion to open was a surgical decision due to elective (lack of advancing in dissection and specimen removal, lack of critical view of safety—20 cases) or emergent causes (incontrollable hemorrhages—four cases; main bile duct lesion—one case, cholecysticduodenal fistula—one case). In the present study, we found no statistically significant differences between conversion and open cholecystectomy in terms of mortality, morbidity and hospital stay. In the case of intraoperative main bile duct lesion, the conversion was imposed by the difficult dissection due to chronic inflammation of the cystic pedicle. The lesion was situated in the proximity of the cystic duct and was classified as minor according to the Mc Mahon Classification (<25% of main bile duct diameter) and was repaired by a T tube insertion. Large papillosphincterotomy was performed by endoscopic retrograde cholangio-pancreatography (ERCP) in the early postoperative period (3 days later) to allow faster recovery.

The classic approach of first intention was used in a total of 12 cases (one in group A, four in group B, five in group C, two in group D). The causes for open surgery were: increased local inflammation (gangrenous gallbladder, biliary peritonitis) in eight cases, the association of the main biliary duct lithiasis with mechanical jaundice ± angiocholitis (two cases) and a history of previous surgical interventions in the upper abdominal region (two cases) (Table 4).

Table 4. Surgical approach and postoperative outcomes in the 4 subgroups.

Group	A (<50 Years) n = 122	B (50–64 Years) n = 101	C (65–79 Years) n = 66	D (>80 Years) n = 34	Total n = 333	p Value
Type of surgery						
LC	119 (97.5%)	99 (89.2%)	51 (77.3%)	26 (76.5%)	295 (88.6%)	
Conversion	2 (1.6%)	8 (7.2%)	10 (15.2%)	6 (17.6%)	26 (7.8%)	$p < 0.001$ [1]
OC	1 (0.8%)	4 (3.6%)	5 (7.6%)	2 (5.9%)	12 (3.6%)	
Drainage in LC	8 (6.72%)	9 (9.09%)	12 (21.05%)	9 (34.6%)	36 (12.2%)	$p < 0.001$ [1]
Hospital days (mean ± SD *)						
Total	4.65 ± 3.03	6.35 ± 3.03	6.53 ± 3.9	7.4 ± 4.4	6 ± 3.35	
LC	4.58 ± 2.21	5.38 ± 2.7	5.83 ± 3.47	5.66 ± 2.53	5.51 ± 2.9	$p < 0.001$ [2]
Conversion	6.8 ± 2.77	9.2 ± 3.52	11.42 ± 4.5	12.2 ± 5.01	9.92 ± 4.15	
OC	9	9 ± 5.56	7.25 ± 3.26	10.8 ± 3.6	9.15+/4.15	
Postoperative hospital days (mean ± SD)						
Total	3.46 ± 2.27	3.75 ± 3.43	4.22 ± 3.53	5.35 ± 4.1	3.63 ± 2.8	
LC	2.49 ± 1.46	2.68 ± 1.7	2.75 ± 1.81	3.83 ± 1.91	3.12 ± 2.22	$p < 0.001$ [2]
Conversion	5.2 ± 2.77	6.72 ± 2.63	9.14 ± 4.45	10 ± 5.33	7.73 ± 3.9	
OC	6	8 ± 3.6	5.75 ± 3.77	10.8 ± 3.6	6.92 ± 2.92	

[1] Fisher's exact test; [2] ANOVA Linearity test; LC: laparoscopic cholecystectomy; OC: open cholecystectomy; Drain insertion was not a routine practice in our clinic for laparoscopic cholecystectomy; * SD—standard deviation.

The cases in which drainage of the subhepatic space was considered necessary were those cases with severe local inflammation, increased intraoperative bleeding or suspected lesion of the bile duct. The fact that the drain was used more often in the elderly is well correlated with the increased incidence of the moderate and severe forms with advanced age. Drainage was used in all cases with open surgery and conversion to open.

The postoperative outcome was favorable in most cases for all age subgroups. No patients required re-surgery in the following 30 days. Surgical related complications were managed conservatory: hemorrhages (seven cases), bile leakage (nine cases), one septic intraperitoneal collection and one main bile duct lesion, classified as minor according to the Mc Mahon Classification solved by ERCP stenting. The procedure consisted of papillosphincterotomy, and a plastic material 7F stent of 10 cm length was introduced in the main bile duct to allow healing. The stent was removed after 3 months, with a favorable outcome. Surgical site infections were less common in laparoscopic cholecystectomy vs. open cholecystectomy and conversion (Table 5), and increased with age.

Table 5. Postoperative complications according to Clavier-Dindo Classification.

Clavier-Dindo Classification	A (<50 Years) n = 122	B (50–64 Years) n = 101	C (65–79 Years) n = 66	D (>80 Years) n = 34	Total n = 333	p Value
I (surgical site infections)						
Total	1 (0.81%)	3 (3.03%)	3 (4.53%)	2 (5.71%)	5 (3.05%)	
LC	1 (0.8%)	2 (2%)	2 (3.92%)	1 (3.85%)	6 (2%)	$p < 0.001$ [1]
conversion	0	1 (12.5%)	1 (10%)	0	2 (7.6%)	
OC	0	0	0	1 (50%)	1 (8.3%)	
II (surgical related complications, treated pharmacological)						
Total	2 (1.6%)	6 (%)	5 (%)	2 (5.8%)	16 (%)	
LC	1 (0.84%)	2 (%)	2 (3.9%)	1 (3.8%)	7 (%)	$p < 042$ [1]
conversion	0	3 (37.5%)	2 (%)	1 (16.6%)	6 (%)	
OC	1 (100%)	1 (25%)	1 (20%)	0	3 (25%)	
III (surgical related complications requiring endoscopic/surgical/Rx approach)						
Total		1 (0.9%)	1 (1.5%)		2 (0.6%)	$p = 1$ [1]
LC	0	1 (1%)	0	0	1 (0.33%)	
conversion		0	1 (10%)		1 (3.84%)	
OC		0	0		0	
IV (requiring intensive care)						
Total	3 (2.4%)	7 (6.3%)	5 (7.57%)	3 (8.8%)	18 (5.4%)	$p < 0.344$ [1]
LC	1 (0.8%)	4 (4.04%)	3 (5.8%)	2 (7.6%)	10 (3.36%)	$p < 0.001$ [2]
conversion	1 (50%)	0	1 (10%)	1 (16.6%)	3 (11.5%)	
OC	1 (100%)	3 (75%)	2 (40%)	0	6 (50%)	
V (Deceased)						
Total	1 (0.81%)	2 (1.8%)	1 (1.51%)	0	4 (1.2%)	
LC	0	1 (1.01%)	0	0	0.33%	$p = 1$ [1]
conversion	1 (50%)	1 (12.5%)	0	0	8.33%	
OC	0	0	1 (20%)	0	7.69%	

[1] Fisher's exact test; [2] ANOVA Linearity test; LC: laparoscopic cholecystectomy.

The rate of surgery related complications was significantly higher in patients over 50 years old ($p = 0.045$), which also proved to be a turning point for an increasing rate of conversion and open surgery. However, the comparative incidence did not differ significantly between patients aged from 50–64 years, 65–79 years and over 80 years. (6.3%, 9.09% and 5.8%, respectively).

The Fisher's linear discriminant analysis was performed to identify the risk factors significantly related to surgical complications. The highest correlation was found with systemic comorbidities: diabetes ($r = 0.813$) and chronic bronchopneumopathy ($r = 0.502$) and CCI ($r = 0.381$, but with no significant increase in discrimination power). Among the local factors, the severity of inflammation and the presence of gangrenous cholecystitis had the most significant predictive power ($r = 0.288$), followed by fibrinogen ($r = 0.348$), and TG13/TG18 severity forms ($r = 0.218$).

Severe cardiovascular complications encountered in the study group were: acute myocardial infarction (nine cases), stroke (seven cases) and malign arterial hypertension (two cases). In total, three out of four causes of death were cardiovascular acute events. Only one patient died of sepsis: a diabetic patient aged 57 with a severe form of acute cholecystitis. The incidence of severe cardiovascular postoperative complications increased with age (ANOVA test for linearity: $p < 0.001$; Mantel-Haenszel test for trend: $p < 0.001$). There were no statistically significant differences between the incidence of cardiovascular complications in groups B, C and D ($p = 0.344$).

3.3. Multivariate Analysis of Risk Factors for Open Surgery and Conversion

In order to describe the preoperative and intraoperative patients' characteristics which determined the applied surgical procedure (LC = Laparoscopic Cholecystectomy, Conversion or OC = Open Cholecystectomy), we have used the stepwise variant of Fisher's linear discriminant analysis. The discrimination between the classes is based on the two Canonical Discriminant Function described in Table 6. The Canonical Discriminant Function is displayed in standardized form in order to allow the comparison of the importance of each variable.

Table 6. Standardized Canonical Discriminant Functions for (LC, OC, Conversion).

	Standardized Canonical Discriminant Function Coefficients	
	Standardized Function	
	F1	F2
Age	0.300	−0.151
Bilirubin	0.127	0.711
Leukocytes	0.426	0.173
Gangrenous cholecystitis	0.637	−0.523
CCI	0.094	0.661

The variables significantly correlated with Standardized Canonical Discriminant Function F1 are gangrenous cholecystitis ($r = 0.807$), leukocytes ($r = 0.650$), fibrinogen, and severity form classified by TG 13/18. The variables significantly correlated with Standardized Canonical Discriminant Function F2 are total bilirubin ($r = 0.637$), CCI ($r = 0.531$) and high aspartate transaminase (AST) and alanine transaminase (ALT) ($r = 0.351$), previous history of stroke ($r = 0.296$), diabetes ($r = 0.223$) and cardiovascular disease ($r = 0.236$). The parameters not included in the definition of F1 and F2 are clinically significant, but they do not add a supplementary increase in the discrimination power.

F1 could be labeled as the score of inflammatory risk (higher values of leukocytes, the presence of severe inflammation and higher age imply high values if F1), and F2 could be labeled as the score of comorbidities (CCI and associated pathologies). Main bile duct complications, such as lithiasis, angiocholitis, and Mirizzi Syndrome (characterized by increased bilirubin), but also increased inflammation with a secondary increase in bilirubin, are also associated with Function 2.

Figure 3 suggests the following simple interpretation: small and moderate values of F1 and F2 (near zero) generally characterize the laparoscopic approach; positive values of F1 (severe inflammation and sepsis) and negative values of F2 generally characterize the open approach; and positive values of F1 and F2 (association with severe inflammation and comorbidities/main bile duct complications) generally characterize conversion.

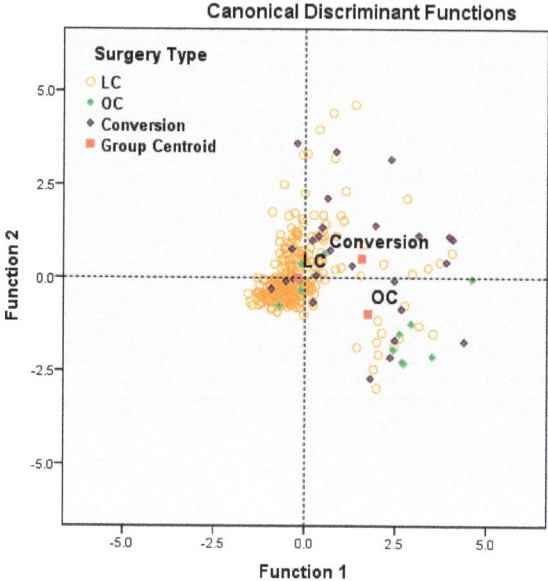

Figure 3. Patient representation ($n = 333$) in the space (F1, F2) of Unstandardized Canonical Discriminant Functions between (LC, OC, Conversion). (Specification: functions at Group Centroids are: (−0.203, −0.004) for LC (laparoscopic cholecystectomy); (1.739, −0.964) for OC (open cholecystectomy) and (1.564, 0.508) for Conversion). Wilks' lambda computed for the two canonical functions are significant (test of the two functions: chi-square (df = 10) 111.08, $p < 0.001$; test of second function: chi-square (df = 4) = 17.05, $p = 0.002$). Cross-validation of the model: 81.4% of cross-validated cases are correctly classified. The relative dispersion of patients with conversion to open surgery indicates that other factors, such as surgical experience or particular intraoperative findings, may be involved.

3.4. Multivariate Analysis of Risk Factors for Adverse Outcome in the Eldery

The incidence of acute cardiovascular events in the early postoperative period increases statistically significantly in patients with ASA ≥ 3, and that of deaths in ASA ≥ 4 ($p = 0.001$). When the correlations between the severe forms of acute cholecystitis and the occurrence of complications were analyzed, statistical analysis showed that severe forms with organ/system dysfunction correlated with the incidence of severe complications and deaths, for all age groups.

Regarding the type of operation, the incidence of cardiovascular complications is significantly higher in the case of the open approach and conversion in comparison with laparoscopic cholecystectomy. However, conversion and open surgery were chosen in severe forms, with necrotic gallbladder, pericholecystic plastron or biliary peritonitis. Multivariate analysis of preoperative and intraoperative risk factors shows that the incidence of severe cardiovascular complications and deaths correlates best with the severity of the septic process and inflammation (gangrenous cholecystitis, fibrinogen > 400 mg/dL and Grade III cholecystitis according to TG13/18 severity forms), and among comorbidities, with a previous history of stroke, chronic renal failure and diabetes (Table 7).

Table 7. The Fisher's linear discriminant analysis for cardiovascular severe complications and mortality.

	Standardized Canonical Discriminant Function Coefficients
	Function
	1
Gangrenous cholecystitis	0.211
Stroke	0.785
Diabetes	0.249
Chronic renal insufficiency	0.264
Fibrinogen > 400 mg/dL	0.348
Grade III Cholecystitis (TG13/TG18 Severity forms)	0.163

4. Discussion

Increased technical experience with laparoscopic cholecystectomy favorably affected outcomes over time [26]. Together with the important achievements in intensive care, more patients, initially considered at risk, can benefit from the important advantages of minimally invasive surgery. The present contraindications for laparoscopic cholecystectomy are few, and they may be classified as absolute (uncorrected coagulopathy, high anesthetic and surgical risk, gallbladder carcinoma) or relative. The latter includes either general conditions (end-stage liver disease) or local findings (previous surgery in the upper abdominal region, calcified gallbladder, cholecysto-enteric fistula, Mirizzi's syndrome) [27]. Age and severe inflammatory forms, such as gangrenous and emphysematous cholecystitis, are no longer considered unsuitable for laparoscopy [28]. In the present study, we analyzed the factors that influence the surgical decision the most. We found that severe local inflammation as well as a high CCI and high values of total bilirubin could favor open surgery or conversion. Other unquantifiable factors such as local anatomy, tissue friability, or surgeon's experience may play a significant role in the decision to convert to open.

Hyperbilirubinemia significantly increases the likelihood of finding common duct stones in patients with acute cholecystitis, but it also occurs in patients with acute cholecystitis without common duct stones. In these cases, the increase in value is mild and it returns to normal values quickly after resolving the septic process. The significance of bilirubin in acute cholecystitis and other intraperitoneal infections was also investigated by other authors [29–36]. Hyperbilirubinemia in acute abdominal infections is caused either by the excessive production of bilirubin or by altered clearance. Both mechanisms lead to bilirubin accumulation and play a role in the hyperbilirubinemia observed in patients with appendicular perforation. Patients in severe sepsis express proinflammatory cytokines, with cholestasis triggered by nitric oxide, by blocking bilirubin conjugation and elimination at the hepatocellular and intraductal level [32]. Common pathogens of the biliary and digestive wall, such as Escherichia coli and Bacteroides fragilis, were supposed to interfere with hepatocyte microcirculation, inducing sinusoidal lesions [35]. In addition, Escherichia coli infection has been shown to induce hemolysis of normal erythrocytes. This results in increased bilirubin loading in infected individuals, a process that promotes hyperbilirubinemia [34–36].

There are concerns about using the laparoscopic approach in patients with respiratory and cardiovascular comorbidities due to the metabolic effects of the induced pneumoperitoneum. This loss of reserve capacity is the single most important factor that decreases the elderly patient's ability to tolerate operations. The proper management of fluid and electrolyte replacement, respiratory management to prevent atelectasis and pneumonia, and monitoring for possible cardiac complications are necessary to minimize the risk of systemic complications in the perioperative period [2,3,37,38].

4.1. Comparative Characterization of the Age-Related Subgroups

The comparative statistical analysis of the four subgroups defined according to age showed that each of them behaves differently and presents specific challenges and outcomes.

Group A, of young patients (<50 years), is a group without significant comorbidities and without significant anesthetic-surgical risk, which generally presents with mild and moderate forms resolvable in a proportion of 97.5% laparoscopically, with a short postoperative stay and without significant complications. In the presence of a septic factor, they can still develop severe cardiovascular acute events and even death. Fluid and electrolyte rebalancing and supportive care were important as an adjuvant to combat septic shock.

Group B (50–64 years) did not differ statistically significantly from group A in terms of anesthetic-surgical risk and CCI score. The severity of the forms of acute cholecystitis was not significantly increased, but there were patients with longer biliary distress with local fibro-inflammatory remodeling, which explains the intraoperative technical difficulties, with an increased conversion rate (7.2% vs. 1.6% in group A) and the classic approach by open cholecystectomy (3.6% vs. 0.8%). During the early postoperative period, these patients were at risk of major cardiovascular complications, especially when diabetes or chronic renal disease are associated.

Group C (65–79 years) was characterized by a statistically significant increase in both the anesthetic-surgical risk (ASA-PS and CCI) compared to group A, but also a significant increase in severe cases according to TG13/TG18 criteria (12.1% vs. 2.5%, $p = 0.001$). Recall that severe forms of acute cholecystitis mean the association of significant local and general inflammation with systemic or organ dysfunction. This result therefore correlated with significant increases in biological markers of inflammation (leukocytosis, fibrinogen) compared to group A. Additionally, the presence of increased CCI and associated comorbidities, especially cardiovascular disease and diabetes, explained the evolution of cholecystitis from moderate to severe, with functional decompensation. In the therapeutic management of these patients, careful preoperative rebalancing was particularly important to prevent major systemic complications and reduce perioperative mortality.

Group D (>80 years) presented the same clinical-therapeutic challenges as group C, but the differences from group A were more marked: late presentation, higher frequency of severe forms of TG 13/18, anesthetic-surgical risk increased by the presence of comorbidities, having as outcomes an increased rate of conversions and major postoperative systemic complications. Thus, the conversion rate increased from 1.6% in group A to 17.6% in group D, and open surgery from 0.8% to 5.9%. However, there were no statistically significant differences in terms of preoperative evaluation and surgery approach and postoperative outcomes between group C (65–79 years) and group D ($\geq$80 years).

Consequently, patients over 50 years of age in the presence of cardiovascular comorbidities or diabetes should be closely monitored in the postoperative period to avoid cardiovascular ischemic incidents and cardiovascular decompensation.

The utility of drain insertion in laparoscopic cholecystectomy is still a subject of debate. In a recent systematic review, Cirrochi et al. [39] found that the incidences of wound infection and abdominal collections are significantly higher in the drain group vs. the no-drain group, while the postoperative recovery and hospital days are shorter in cases without drain. In our clinic, drain insertion was not a routine procedure after laparoscopic cholecystectomy. However, it is still used in cases with severe inflammation, difficult dissection or bleeding in order to prevent intra-abdominal collections in the early postoperative period. An increased incidence of drain insertion with age was well correlated with the severity of acute cholecystitis in the elderly. This could also be an explanation for the increased incidence of postoperative septic complications, such as wound infection and intra-abdominal collections, described by other authors [40–42].

4.2. Safety of Laparoscopic Cholecystectomy in the Elderly

Although laparoscopic cholecystectomy is currently considered to be a routine abdominal procedure with minor risks, a deep understanding of the physiological reserve of elderly patients is also mandatory in surgery, as it can be used to assess the vulnerability of patients with frailty syndrome to complications [1–3,20].

Acute cholecystitis has clinical particularities in aged patients: statistically significant increases in severe forms, as well as the presence of associated comorbidities, with an increased rate of conversion and a higher percentage of postoperative complications. These findings were also encountered in other studies [19–21,24,43–45]. In a crossectional analysis on cholecystectomy in the elderly, Kuy et al. found that older people have more complex forms of disease and that a longer time from admission to surgery is a predictor for poor outcome [43].

In a meta-analysis on 99 studies between 1995 and 2018, Kamarajah et al. [44] found a tenfold increase in mortality in patients aged over 80. One of the major drawbacks they remarked on in their research was that the studies evaluated did not take into account the associated comorbidities and their impact on the final outcomes. In a meta-analysis on 11 studies published between 1993 and 2011, on 101,559 patients aged 65 or older (48,195 treated laparoscopically and 53,364 by open cholecystectomy), Antoniou et al. found that mortality was 1.0% for the laparoscopic approach and 4.4% for the open approach [24].

In the present study, there were 100 patients aged over 65, and 77% of them successfully underwent laparoscopic cholecystectomy, with 0% mortality. In the 23 cases in which laparoscopy could not be performed (direct open surgery and conversion groups), there was only one death (4.34%). In our study, despite an increased conversion and complications rate, there were no deaths in group D (aged over 80). There were no significant differences regarding cardiovascular complications between the four age-groups. Similar findings are also encountered by Shin et al. [38]. With the pre-operative optimization of comorbidities and medications and addressing frailty in a multi-disciplinary team, an experienced surgical staff with good technical equipment are effective in improving postoperative outcomes [16,38]. Moreover, the multivariate analysis showed that severe inflammation (gangrenous cholecystitis) and comorbidities such as diabetes, previous stroke and chronic renal and pulmonary disease, but not age itself, are risk factors for postoperative morbidity. This finding is also communicated by Kim et al. [46,47]. Moreover, Agrusa et al. recommended elective laparoscopic surgery in elderly people with symptomatic gallstone disease before the development of acute cholecystitis and related complications [48].

When comparing open to laparoscopic surgery, most of the studies found better outcomes in terms of mortality and morbidity associated with laparoscopic procedures [15,24,49], while a limited number of studies founded similar results for both methods [22]. These findings confirmed that laparoscopic cholecystectomy is a safe procedure and should be used in the elderly. On the other hand, a proper comparison cannot be performed between the open and laparoscopic approach due to the fact that the open approach does not represent a first line option in our surgical department, regardless of the patient's age. Open surgery (and conversion) was used only in cases in which laparoscopic surgery could not be performed. The severity of the inflammatory process and sepsis might also be associated with increased mortality in the open surgery group.

Laparoscopy is associated with a limited response in serum Il-6 and no change in gut mucosa Il-6 [50]. There is strong evidence that laparoscopy provides a decreased inflammatory response at the peritoneal and intestinal level, with a faster intestinal transit recovery. The reduced inflammatory systemic response associated with laparoscopic surgery may also be important, especially in the elderly, in preventing pulmonary related complications [50].

5. Conclusions

The present study showed that laparoscopic cholecystectomy is the most used surgical approach in the treatment of acute cholecystitis in all age groups, with better outcomes than open cholecystectomy in terms of decreased overall and postoperative hospital stay, reduced surgical related complications and a reduced incidence of acute cardiovascular events in the early postoperative period. On the other hand, patients with a higher ASA grade and severe forms of TG 13/18 were more likely to undergo open surgery.

Laparoscopic cholecystectomy can be safely performed in elderly and extremely elderly people, but the risk of severe postoperative cardiovascular complications is slightly higher. Careful perioperative care of the vascular, hemodynamic and respiratory status should be provided in order to prevent these adverse events in the elderly. The degree of systemic inflammation and sepsis was one of the main factors that influenced the adverse outcome of LC in the elderly. Among comorbidities, diabetes was associated with both increased surgical related and cardiovascular postoperative morbidity, while a previous history of stroke and chronic renal insufficiency are correlated with a high risk of cardiovascular complications. CCI, ASA PS and the incidence of severe forms increase with age, also leading to slightly more complications. However, age alone should not be the contraindication for laparoscopic cholecystectomy. With adequate perioperative care, the elderly have much to gain from the benefits of a minimally invasive approach, which allows a decreased rate of postoperative complications and a reduced hospital stay.

Author Contributions: Conceptualization, S.A.B., B.S. and D.S. (Dragos Serban); methodology, S.A.B., C.T. and A.M.D.; formal analysis C.T., D.S. (Dan Sabau); investigation, S.A.B., G.V., A.M.D., R.I.S.; resources, D.S. (Dragos Serban); data curation R.I.S., C.T. and C.D.B.; writing—original draft preparation, S.A.B., A.M.D., D.S. (Dragos Serban), C.D.B.; writing—review and editing, B.S., C.D.B., G.V., D.S. (Dan Sabau), A.D.S.; visualization, S.A.B., B.S.; supervision, D.S. (Dragos Serban); project administration, D.S. (Dragos Serban). All authors have read and agreed to the published version of the manuscript.

Funding: This research received no external funding.

Institutional Review Board Statement: Ethical review and approval were waived for this study, since this is the retrospective study, and the data were collected from observation charts and postoperative note.

Informed Consent Statement: Patient consent was waived since this is the retrospective study.

Data Availability Statement: Not applicable.

Conflicts of Interest: The authors declare no conflict of interest.

References

1. Parmar, K.L.; Pearce, L.; Farrell, I.; Hewitt, J.; Moug, S. Influence of frailty in older patients undergoing emergency laparotomy: A UK-based observational study. *BMJ Open* **2017**, *7*, e017928. [CrossRef] [PubMed]
2. Lasithiotakis, K.; Petrakis, J.; Venianaki, M.; Georgiades, G.; Koutsomanolis, D.; Andreou, A.; Zoras, O.; Chalkiadakis, G. Frailty predicts outcome of elective laparoscopic cholecystectomy in geriatric patients. *Surg. Endosc.* **2013**, *27*, 1144–1150. [CrossRef] [PubMed]
3. Lorenzon, L.; Costa, G.; Massa, G.; Frezza, B.; Stella, F.; Balducci, G. The impact of frailty syndrome and risk scores on emergency cholecystectomy patients. *Surg. Today* **2017**, *47*, 74–83. [CrossRef] [PubMed]
4. Dubecz, A.; Langer, M.; Stadlhuber, R.J.; Schweigert, M.; Solymosi, N.; Feith, M.; Stein, H.J. Cholecystectomy in the very elderly—Is 90 the new 70? *J. Gastrointest. Surg.* **2012**, *16*, 282–285. [CrossRef]
5. Kenig, J.; Wałęga, P.; Olszewska, U.; Konturek, A.; Nowak, W. Geriatric assessment as a qualification element for elective and emergency cholecystectomy in older patients. *World J. Emerg. Surg.* **2016**, *11*, 36. [CrossRef]
6. Escartín, A.; González, M.; Cuello, E.; Pinillos, A.; Muriel, P.; Merichal, M.; Palacios, V.; Escoll, J.; Gas, C.; Olsina, J.J. Acute Cholecystitis in Very Elderly Patients: Disease Management, Outcomes, and Risk Factors for Complications. *Surg. Res. Pract.* **2019**, *2019*, 9709242. [CrossRef]
7. Agresta, F.; Campanile, F.C.; Vettoretto, N.; Silecchia, G.; Bergamini, C.; Maida, P.; Lombari, P.; Narilli, P.; Marchi, D.; Carrara, A.; et al. Laparoscopic cholecystectomy: Consensus conference-based guidelines. *Langenbecks Arch. Surg.* **2015**, *400*, 429–453. [CrossRef]

8. Campanile, F.C.; Pisano, M.; Coccolini, F.; Catena, F.; Agresta, F.; Ansaloni, L. Acute cholecystitis: WSES position statement. *World J. Emerg. Surg.* **2014**, *9*, 58. [CrossRef]
9. Amirthalingam, V.; Low, J.K.; Woon, W.; Shelat, V. Tokyo Guidelines 2013 may be too restrictive and patients with moderate and severe acute cholecystitis can be managed by early cholecystectomy too. *Surg. Endosc.* **2017**, *31*, 2892–2900. [CrossRef] [PubMed]
10. Wakabayashi, G.; Iwashita, Y.; Hibi, T.; Takada, T.; Strasberg, S.M.; Asbun, H.J.; Endo, I.; Umezawa, A.; Asai, K.; Suzuki, K.; et al. Tokyo Guidelines 2018: Surgical management of acute cholecystitis: Safe steps in laparoscopic cholecystectomy for acute cholecystitis (with videos). *J. Hepatobiliary Pancreat. Sci.* **2018**, *25*, 73–86. [CrossRef] [PubMed]
11. Gurusamy, K.S.; Davidson, C.; Gluud, C.; Davidson, B.R. Early versus delayed laparoscopic cholecystectomy for people with acute cholecystitis. *Cochrane Database Syst. Rev.* **2013**, *6*, CD005440. [CrossRef]
12. Yokoe, M.; Hata, J.; Takada, T.; Strasberg, S.M.; Bun, T.A.Y.; Wakabayashi, G.; Kozaka, K.; Endo, I.; DeZiel, D.J.; Miura, F.; et al. Tokyo Guidelines 2018: Diagnostic criteria and severity grading of acute cholecystitis (with videos). *J. Hepato Biliary Pancreat. Sci.* **2018**, *25*, 41–54. [CrossRef] [PubMed]
13. Annamaneni, R.K.; Moraitis, D.; Cayten, C.G. Laparoscopic cholecystectomy in the elderly. *J. Soc. Laparoendosc. Surg.* **2005**, *9*, 408–410.
14. Tucker, J.J.; Yanagawa, F.; Grim, R.; Bell, T.; Ahuja, V. Laparoscopic cholecystectomy is safe but underused in the elderly. *Am. Surg.* **2011**, *77*, 1014–1020. [CrossRef] [PubMed]
15. Lujan, J.A.; Sanchez-Bueno, F.; Parrilla, P.; Robles, R.; Torralba, J.A.; Gonzalez-Costea, R. Laparoscopic vs. open cholecystectomy in patients aged 65 and older. *Am. Surg.* **1998**, *64*, 654–658.
16. Yetkin, G.; Uludag, M.; Oba, S.; Citgez, B.; Paksoy, I. Laparoscopic cholecystectomy in elderly patients. *J. Soc. Laparoendosc. Surg.* **2009**, *13*, 587–591. [CrossRef]
17. Kirshtein, B.; Bayme, M.; Bolotin, A.; Mizrahi, S.; Lantsberg, L. Laparoscopic cholecystectomy for acute cholecystitis in the elderly: Is it safe? *Surg. Laparosc. Endosc. Percutaneous Tech.* **2008**, *18*, 334–339. [CrossRef]
18. Leardi, S.; De Vita, F.; Pietroletti, R.; Simi, M. Cholecystectomy for gallbladder disease in elderly aged 80 years and over. *Hepatogastroenterology* **2009**, *56*, 303–306.
19. Brunt, L.M.; Quasebarth, M.A.; Dunnegan, D.L.; Soper, N.J. Outcomes analysis of laparoscopic cholecystectomy in the extremely elderly. *Surg. Endosc.* **2001**, *15*, 700–705. [CrossRef]
20. Fukami, Y.; Kurumiya, Y.; Mizuno, K.; Sekoguchi, E.; Kobayashi, S. Cholecystectomy in octogenarians: Be careful. *Updates Surg.* **2014**, *66*, 265–268. [CrossRef] [PubMed]
21. Lee, S.I.; Na, B.G.; Yoo, Y.S.; Mun, S.P.; Choi, N.K. Clinical outcome for laparoscopic cholecystectomy in extremely elderly patients. *Ann. Surg. Treat. Res.* **2015**, *88*, 145–151. [CrossRef]
22. Kwon, A.H.; Matsui, Y. Laparoscopic cholecystectomy in patients aged 80 years and over. *World J. Surg.* **2006**, *30*, 1204–1210. [CrossRef]
23. Pessaux, P.; Regenet, N.; Tuech, J.J.; Rouge, C.; Bergamaschi, R.; Arnaud, J.P. Laparoscopic versus open cholecystectomy: A prospective comparative study in the elderly with acute cholecystitis. *Surg. Laparosc. Endosc. Percutaneous Tech.* **2001**, *11*, 252–255. [CrossRef]
24. Antoniou, S.A.; Antoniou, G.A.; Koch, O.O.; Pointner, R.; Granderath, F.A. Meta-analysis of laparoscopic vs open cholecystectomy in elderly patients. *World J. Gastroenterol. WJG* **2014**, *20*, 17626–17634. [CrossRef]
25. Okamoto, K.; Suzuki, K.; Takada, T.; Strasberg, S.M.; Asbun, H.J.; Endo, I.; Iwashita, Y.; Hibi, T.; Pitt, H.A.; Umezawa, A.; et al. Tokyo Guidelines 2018: Flowchart for the management of acute cholecystitis. *J. Hepatobiliary Pancreat. Sci.* **2018**, *25*, 55–72. [CrossRef]
26. Bingener, J.; Richards, M.L.; Schwesinger, W.H.; Strodel, W.E.; Sirinek, K.R. Laparoscopic cholecystectomy for elderly patients: Gold standard for golden years? *Arch. Surg.* **2003**, *138*, 531–536. [CrossRef] [PubMed]
27. Laparoscopic Cholecystectomy. Available online: https://www.sages.org/wiki/laparoscopic-cholecystectomy (accessed on 1 October 2020).
28. Campanile, F.C.; Carrara, A.; Motter, M.; Ansaloni, L.; Agresta, F. Laparoscopy and Acute Cholecystitis: The Evidence. In *Laparoscopic Cholecystectomy*; Agresta, F., Campanile, F., Vettoretto, N., Eds.; Springer: Cham, Switzerland, 2014.
29. Gillaspie, D.B.; Davis, K.A.; Schuster, K.M. Total bilirubin trend as a predictor of common bile duct stones in acute cholecystitis and symptomatic cholelithiasis. *Am. J. Surg.* **2019**, *217*, 98–102. [CrossRef]
30. Kurzweil, S.M.; Shapiro, M.J.; Andrus, C.H.; Wittgen, C.M.; Herrmann, V.M.; Kaminski, D.L. Hyperbilirubinemia without common bile duct abnormalities and hyperamylasemia without pancreatitis in patients with gallbladder disease. *Arch. Surg.* **1994**, *129*, 829–833. [CrossRef]
31. Anderson, C.E.; Stewart, L. Hyperbilirubinemia and complicated acute cholecystitis: Improving preoperative diagnostic strategies. *J. Am. Coll. Surg.* **2014**, *219* (Suppl. 4), E114. [CrossRef]
32. Delemos, A.S.; Friedman, L.S. Systemic causes of cholestasis. *Clin. Liver Dis.* **2013**, *17*, 301–317. [CrossRef]
33. Sand, M.; Bechara, F.G.; Holland-Letz, T.; Sand, D.; Mehnert, G.; Mann, B. Diagnostic value of hyperbilirubinemia as a predictive factor for appendiceal perforation in acute appendicitis. *Am. J. Surg.* **2009**, *198*, 193–198. [CrossRef] [PubMed]
34. Socea, B.; Carap, A.; Rac-Albu, M.; Constantin, V. The value of serum bilirubin level and of white blood cell count as severity markers for acute appendicitis. *Chirurgia* **2013**, *108*, 829–834. [PubMed]

35. Serban, D.; Branescu, C.M.; Cristian, D.A.; Dascalu, A.M. Bilirubin, Interleukin 6 (IL 6) and Lipopolysaccharide—Binding Protein (LBP)—Biomarkers of Sepsis in Appendicular Peritonitis. *Rev. Chim.* **2020**, *71*, 444–454. [CrossRef]
36. Serban, D.; Branescu, C.; Savlovschi, C.; Tudor, C.; Borcan, R.; Nica, A.; Vancea, G.; Dascalu, A.M. Correlations between serum bilirubin, leukocytosis and anatomo-pathological form in acute appendicitis. *Rom. J. Med. Pract.* **2015**, *10*, 371–379.
37. Evers, B.M.; Townsend, C.M.J.; Thompson, J.C. Organ physiology of aging. *Surg. Clin. N. Am.* **1994**, *74*, 23–39. [CrossRef]
38. Shin, M.S.; Park, S.H. Clinical outcomes of laparoscopic cholecystectomy in elderly patients after preoperative assessment and optimization of comorbidities. *Ann. Hepatobiliary Pancreat. Surg.* **2018**, *22*, 374–379. [CrossRef]
39. Cirocchi, R.; Kwan, S.H.; Popivanov, G.; Ruscelli, P.; Lancia, M.; Gioia, S.; Zago, M.; Chiarugi, M.; Fedeli, P.; Marzaioli, R.; et al. Routine drain or no drain after laparoscopic cholecystectomy for acute cholecystitis. *Surgeon* **2020**. [CrossRef]
40. Saber, A.; Hokkam, E.; Alshayeb, A. Laparoscopy in acute cholecystitis: To drain or not to drain. Journal of Surgery. *Spec. Issue Minim. Invasive Minim. Access Surg.* **2016**, *5*, 28–32.
41. Qiu, J.; Li, M. Nondrainage after laparoscopic cholecystectomy for acute calculous cholecystitis does not increase the postoperative morbidity. *BioMed Res. Int.* **2018**, *2018*, 8436749. [CrossRef]
42. Lucarelli, P.; Picchio, M.; Martellucci, J.; De Angelis, F.; Di Filippo, A.R.; Stipa, F.; Spaziani, E. Drain After Laparoscopic Cholecystectomy for Acute Calculous Cholecystitis. A Pilot Randomized Study. *Indian J. Surg.* **2015**, *77*, 288–292. [CrossRef]
43. Kuy, S.; Sosa, J.A.; Roman, S.A.; Desai, R.; Rosenthal, R.A. Age matters: A study of clinical and economic outcomes following cholecystectomy in elderly Americans. *Am. J. Surg.* **2011**, *201*, 789–796. [CrossRef]
44. Kamarajah, S.K.; Karri, S.; Bundred, J.R.; Evans, R.; Lin, A.; Kew, T.; Ekeozor, C.; Powell, S.L.; Singh, P.; Griffiths, E.A. Perioperative outcomes after laparoscopic cholecystectomy in elderly patients: A systematic review and meta-analysis. *Surg. Endosc.* **2020**, *34*, 4727–4740. [CrossRef]
45. Nikfarjam, M.; Yeo, D.; Perini, M.; Fink, M.A.; Muralidharan, V.; Starkey, G.; Jones, R.M.; Christophi, C. Outcomes of cholecystectomy for treatment of acute cholecystitis in octogenarians. *ANZ J. Surg.* **2014**, *84*, 943–948. [CrossRef]
46. Kim, H.O.; Yun, J.W.; Shin, J.H.; Hwang, S.I.; Cho, Y.K.; Son, B.H.; Yoo, C.H.; Park, Y.L.; Kim, H. Outcome of laparoscopic cholecystectomy is not influenced by chronological age in the elderly. *World J. Gastroenterol.* **2009**, *15*, 722–726. [CrossRef] [PubMed]
47. Lord, A.C.; Hicks, G.; Pearce, B.; Tanno, L.; Pucher, P.H. Safety and outcomes of laparoscopic cholecystectomy in the extremely elderly: A systematic review and meta-analysis. *Acta Chir. Belg.* **2016**, *119*, 349–356. [CrossRef]
48. Agrusa, A.; Romano, G.; Frazzetta, G.; Chianetta, D.; Sorce, V.; Di Buono, G.; Gulotta, G. Role and outcomes of laparoscopic cholecystectomy in the elderly. *Int. J. Surg.* **2014**, *12* (Suppl. 2), S37–S39. [CrossRef] [PubMed]
49. Massie, M.T.; Massie, L.B.; Marrangoni, A.G.; D'Amico, F.J.; Sell, H.W., Jr. Advantages of laparoscopic cholecystectomy in the elderly and in patients with high ASA classifications. *J. Laparoendosc. Surg.* **1993**, *3*, 467–476. [CrossRef]
50. Schietroma, M.; Piccione, F.; Carlei, F.; Clementi, M.; Bianchi, Z.; de Vita, F.; Amicucci, G. Peritonitis from perforated appendicitis: Stress response after laparoscopic or open treatment. *Am. Surg.* **2012**, *78*, 582–590. [CrossRef] [PubMed]

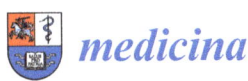

Article

Emergency Medical Teams Interventions due to Cardiovascular Diseases in 2018: Polish Regional Observational Study

Klaudiusz Nadolny [1,2], Magdalena Wierzbik-Strońska [1,*], Jerzy R. Ładny [3], Beniamin O. Grabarek [4,5], Oliwia Warmusz [1], Dariusz Boroń [4,5] and Aleksander Ostenda [1]

1. Faculty of Medicine, University of Technology in Katowice, 40-555 Katowice, Poland; klaudiusznadolny3@gmail.com (K.N.); warmuszoliwia@gmail.com (O.W.); aleksander.ostenda@wst.com.pl (A.O.)
2. Department of Emergency Medical Service, Strategic Planning University of Dabrowa Gornicza, 40-555 Dąbrowa Górnicza, Poland
3. Department of Emergency Medcine, Medical University of Bialystok, 15-295 Białystok, Poland; jerzyladny3@gmail.com
4. Department of Histology, Cytophysiology and Embryology, Faculty of Medicine, University of Technology in Katowice, 41-800 Zabrze, Poland; bgrabarek7@gmail.com (B.O.G.); dariusz@boron.pl (D.B)
5. Department of Gynecology and Obstetrics with Gynecologic Oncology, Ludwik Rydygier Memorial Specialized Hospital, 31-826 Kraków, Poland
* Correspondence: magdalenawierzbikstronska@gmail.com

Abstract: *Background and objectives:* The goal of this work was to assess the interventions for cardiovascular causes (ICD-10: I) and analyze the time between the request for intervention and the arrival of the Medical Emergency Team realized by the Voivodeship Rescue Service in Katowice in the period between 1 January 2018 to 31 December 2018. *Materials and Methods:* Analysis of the characteristics of the interventions was completed based on the information contained on the dispatch order cards and medical emergency services. Statistical analysis was done using the Chi-square test ($p < 0.05$). *Results:* Out of 211,548 cases, 26,672 were associated with cardiovascular diseases. It can be observed that the large majority of interventions took place in urban areas (89.98%; 23,998 cases), whereas only 11.02% took place in rural areas (2674 cases). The most common cause for medical interventions being made by the Medical Emergency Team was primary hypertension—11,649 cases. The average arrival time to urban areas was 9 min and 12 s ± 3 min and 54 s, whereas for rural areas it was 11 min and 57 s ± 4 min and 32 s ($p < 0.05$). *Conclusions:* It can be observed that the Medical Emergency System in Katowice operates accordingly with the intentions of the legislator. The obtained data also indicates that there is a high societal awareness of the residents about the purpose of the Medical Emergency Team.

Keywords: Silesian Voivodeship; gold hour; cardiovascular diseases; Medical Emergency Team

1. Introduction

The process of creating the Emergency Medical Services began in the 1990s from the creation of the Integrated Medical Rescue. However, starting only from 25 July 2001 the first act about the Emergency Medical Services was created [1]. Throughout the following years, the assumptions of the act were revised, which led to the creation of the act currently in place from the 8 September 2006 [2,3]. The creation of a formalized structure in the form of a system based on the interdependencies of the individual components that make it up, such as people, products, and services, which are all connected with the implementation of one common goal was a key undertaking that conditioned the saving of human life. The main goal of the Medical Rescue System is guaranteeing help in sudden situations that directly threaten the life of a person [4,5]. Included in the Emergency Medical Services are Medical Emergency Teams (ambulances; air ambulances; water ambulances) and also Hospital Emergency Wards [6]. The primary task of the Medical Emergency Team is granting help to the victim on site of the incident, and if it is advisable, to also transport the victim to the appropriate reference unit in the shortest time possible [7]. The second, incredibly important units are the Hospital Emergency Wards, which are responsible for carrying out the initial diagnosis as well as treating the person in the necessary range, which is especially important in sudden life-threatening situations [8]. In reference to the Emergency Medical Service system, an incredibly important term is the effectiveness of action, defined as the correct action being done in the correct method, where effectiveness and efficiency are key. It is also worth noting the two critical elements in the functioning of the Emergency Medical Services in Poland [9,10]. One of which is highlighting the role of the medical distributor, who, based on the information they gather from the interview they carried out through telephone communication and also on their own knowledge and subjective instinct decides, whether an intervention by the Medical Emergency Team is or is not necessary [11–13]. A second factor that determines the effectiveness of the system is the time taken between the moment an incident was reported (accident) to the moment the Medical Emergency Team arrives at the incident site. Therefore, a conversion factor is adopted in this regard, that on average every 2 min, a distance of at least 1 km has to be covered [14].

One of the causes of undertaking an intervention by the Medical Emergency Team were reports due to cardiovascular diseases, which are a wide range of diseases according to the International Classification of Diseases—ICD-10 [15]. It is estimated that in Poland, approximately 100 people die each day due to heart failure, which constitutes around 20% of all deaths due to cardiovascular problems. Moreover, an unsettling fact is that one in three male deaths and one in 10 female deaths are due to cardiovascular diseases for people above 64 years of age, which is the group of people most active professionally [16,17].

The goal of this work was to assess the interventions for cardiovascular causes (ICD-10: I) and analyze the time between the request for intervention and the arrival of the Medical Emergency Team realized by the Voivodeship Rescue Service in Katowice in the period between 1 January 2018 to 31 December 2018.

2. Materials and Methods

Firstly, from all the accepted calls by the Voivodeship Ambulance Service, the calls in which the medical dispatcher found it necessary for intervention on-site were selected. For this type of study (survey), approval of the bioethics committee is not required. In the second stage, the analyzed interventions were narrowed down based on identification criteria, according to the International Classification of Diseases, ICD-10. The identifications made using the code I were selected, which covers cardiovascular diseases. Next, the information contained in the "Emergency ambulance dispatch order card" was imported into an Excel calculatory spreadsheet, and afterward, statistical analysis was conducted based on the licensed version of the STATISTICA 13 PL program (StatSoft, Cracow, Poland). The analyzed data was then split based on identification, the intervention site (urban; rural) as well as sex (male; female), and also the way the intervention was completed. In this work, we also present the time that passed from the moment the call was received to the time the Medical Emergency Team arrived at the site. In the statistical analysis, the Chi-square test was used, with the statistical significance threshold adopted at $p < 0.05$.

3. Results

Based on the shared medical documentation, it was determined that interventions made by the Medical Emergency Team due to cardiovascular disease were 12.6% (26,672 cases) of all the completed interventions. The total number of all interventions in 2018 totaled 211,548. It can be observed that the large majority of interventions took place in urban areas (89.98%; 23,998 cases), whereas only 11.02% took place in rural areas (2674 cases). The three most common causes for interventions being made by the Medical Emergency Team included: primary hypertension—11,649 cases; stroke, not specified as hemorrhage or infarction—3740 cases; atrial fibrillation and flutter—2473 cases. In Table 1, the 10 most common causes for the emergency interventions are presented, while less common causes are grouped under "other causes".

Table 1. The characteristics of the injuries to which a trip by a Medical Rescue Team was completed in 2018.

ICD-10 CODE	Name of Disease	Sex	Number of Cases in a Village	Number of Cases in a City	$p < 0.05$
I10	Primary hypertension $n = 11,649$	Female	700	7680	$p = 0.0001$
		Male	350	2905	
I64	Stroke, not specified as hemorrhage or infarction $n = 3740$	Female	201	1780	$p = 0.8850$
		Male	181	1578	
I48	Atrial fibrillation and flutter $n = 2473$	Female	146	1413	$p = 0.1424$
		Male	111	884	
I46	Cardiac arrest $n = 1533$	Female	57	480	$p = 0.7906$
		Male	100	896	
I50	Heart failure $n = 1448$	Female	93	567	$p = 0.032$
		Male	82	706	
I21	Acute myocardial infarction $n = 886$	Female	36	250	$p = 0.4634$
		Male	64	536	
I95	Hypotension $n = 771$	Female	3	427	$p = 0.096$
		Male	7	334	
I49	Other cardiac arrhythmias $n = 653$	Female	29	339	$p = 0.1035$
		Male	29	339	
I47	Paroxysmal tachycardia $n = 625$	Female	35	303	$p = 0.4673$
		Male	35	252	
I20	Unstable angina $n = 431$	Female	36	250	$p = 0.2936$
		Male	64	536	
-	Other causes $n = 2364$	Female	163	1092	$p = 0.0899$
		Male	170	939	

Afterward, how these interventions were concluded by the Medical Emergency Team was assessed. The most common decision was for the patient to be directly transported and received by the hospital emergency department or emergency room (totaling 16,465 cases, which is equal to 61.7% of all total cases). In turn, in the case of 8732 calls (29.18%), help was granted on-site of the intervention, without the need to continue diagnostics and treatment in hospital. The statistical assessment indicated the occurrence of statistical significance (Table 2).

Table 2. Reasons for medical interventions of the Voivodeship Emergency Medical Teams in Katowice in 2018.

Form of Conclusion	Rural	Urban
Other than aforementioned	74 (2.8%)	581 (2.4%)
Medical emergency operations abandoned	46 (1.7%)	528 (2.2%)
The person who was helped was directly transported and received by the hospital organizational unit	11 (0.4%)	177 (0.7%)
The person who was helped was directly transported and received by the hospital emergency department or emergency room	1593 (59.6%)	14,872 (62.1%)
The person who was helped was not transported to the hospital emergency department or emergency room	949 (35.5%)	7783 (32.5%)

In the last part, the time that passed between the call was received and the arrival of the Medical Emergency Team to the intervention site. The average arrival time to urban areas was 9 min and 12 s ± 3 min and 54 s, whereas in rural areas it was 11 min and 57 s ± 4 min and 32 s ($p < 0.05$).

4. Discussion

Cardiovascular diseases constitute the first most common cause of death worldwide; the same tendency was also noted in Poland [18]. Due to this, they form a huge challenge for the Medical Services, Emergency Medical Services as well as for the state, whose primary responsibility is guaranteeing the correct functioning of the system in sudden life-threatening situations [19]. According to the knowledge of the authors, the comparison of the trip characteristics made by the Medical Emergency Team within the territory of the Silesian Voivodeship presented as part of this work is the first of this sort of analysis. This type of analysis seems fully reasonable, as they allow for the assessment of how the organized Emergency Medical Service is used by its users (reporters), and additionally the societal awareness about the purpose of the system itself. Moreover, it also indicates the further decisions made in the given situations, which allows for determining the strengths and weaknesses of the system, and therefore, gives the ability to improve the system further [12,20–22]. Furthermore, such analyses are a valuable resource for developing preventive programs, indicating the target recipient group, and thanks to this, there is the possibility to create a campaign that will be met with a positive societal response [23,24].

Based on the obtained data, it was determined that decidedly, more often cardiovascular diseases were identified in men more than in women. This indicates that risk factors predisposed to the appearance of cardiovascular disease do not differ in a significant way between men and women. Simultaneously, however, it is worth noting that individual factors may have different severity in affecting people of both sexes [25–28]. For example, diabetes contributes 6–7 times more often to the development of ischemic disease in women, whereas only 2–3 times in men [29,30]. The most common reported cardiologic problem was primary hypertension. In 65% of accepted cases, the decision was made that it was necessary to grant further specialist healthcare in the Hospital Emergency Ward. Whereas, in nearly $1/3$ of cases the help was granted on-site. This suggests that the majority of primary hypertension cases could constitute a direct threat to the life and health of a person, and furthermore, shows that the decision and assessment made by the distributor were correct [13]. Indirectly, this may also indicate the ability that the distributor possesses throughout the initial interview, in collecting key information about the health state of the patient, as well as the ability of the person reporting the situation to describe it to ask for help [2,13]. A similar tendency was observed for the second most common cause for calls for the Medical Emergency Team, which is atrial fibrillation and flutter as well as heart failure, which constitutes the third most common cause for interventions being made by the Medical Emergency Team.

However, a key element of the Emergency Medical Service system is also the time taken between accepting a call by the distributor and the arrival of the Medical Emergency Team. According to the act currently in effect about the Emergency Medical Services in regions in which over 10,000 residents are located, the time of arrival for the Medical Emergency Team in urban areas should not be more than 8 min, whereas in rural areas it should not be longer than 15 min [2]. A significant fact also seems to be that in the period the act was being created, it was decided to move towards shortening the maximum allowed time for arrival. First, in the act from 2001, it was decided that a Medical Emergency Team should arrive in urban areas in 20 min and to rural areas in 30 min [1,2]. The changes that were made by the legislator between 2001 and 2006 aimed to use the so-called "golden hour" in the best way possible, as it could decide whether the victim survives or not [31]. The data obtained by us alongside the existing recommendations indicates a shorter than required time for arrival to the victim in urban areas at 9 min and 12 s ± 3 min and 54 s, whereas for rural areas the time taken is 11 min and 57 s ± 4 min and 32 s [2]. It can also be determined that the average arrival time by the Voivodeship Ambulance Service in Katowice is close to the time noted by other teams, such as the Voivodeship Ambulance Service in Lublin which averaged out to be 8.55 ± 5.16 min [20], whereas in the Otwock county the average time was 9.39 ± 6.87 min [32].

5. Conclusions

In conclusion, it can be observed that the Emergency Medical Services in Katowice function according to the intentions of the legislator. The obtained data also indicates a high societal awareness about the correct functioning and purpose of the Medical Emergency Team.

Author Contributions: Conceptualization, K.N., J.R.Ł., and M.W.-S.; methodology, M.W.-S.; validation, J.R.Ł., and D.B.; formal analysis, B.O.G.; investigation, K.N., and M.W.-S.; resources, O.W.; data curation, A.O.; writing—original draft preparation, M.W.-S., D.B., B.O.G.; writing—review and editing, K.N., J.R.Ł.; supervision, K.N.; project administration, A.O. All authors have read and agreed to the published version of the manuscript.

Funding: This research received no external funding.

Institutional Review Board Statement: The data used to support the findings of this study is included in the article. The data will not be shared due to the fact the third-party rights and commercial confidentiality.

Informed Consent Statement: Patient consent was waived due to the retrospective nature of the study and does not bear the characteristics of a medical experiment.

Data Availability Statement: Ethical review and approval were waived for this study, due to the retrospective nature of the study and does not bear the characteristics of a medical experiment (Decision of the Bioethical Committee of the University of Technology in Katowice, no. 5/2020).

Acknowledgments: We would like to thank Oskar Ogloszka for improving our work, checking and correcting the English.

Conflicts of Interest: The authors declare no conflict of interest.

References

1. USTAWA z dnia 25 lipca 2001 r. o państwowym ratownictwie medycznym. *Dz. Ustaw* **2001**, *113*, 1207. Available online: http://isap.sejm.gov.pl/isap.nsf/DocDetails.xsp?id=WDU20011131207&SessionID=1235195837949892B005BFB6DFC73800812D4189 (accessed on 7 November 2020).
2. USTAWA z dnia 8 września 2006 r. o państwowym ratownictwie medycznym. *Dz. Ustaw* **2006**, *191*, 1410. Available online: https://isap.sejm.gov.pl/isap.nsf/DocDetails.xsp?id=WDU20061911410 (accessed on 7 November 2020).
3. Jarosławska-Kolman, K.; Ślęzak, D.; Żuratyński, P.; Krzyżanowski, K.; Kalis, A. System państwowego ratownictwa medycznego w polsce. *Zesz. Nauk. SGSP* **2016**, *60*, 167–183.
4. Goniewicz, M. *Medycyna Katastrof: Problemy Organizacyjno-Diagnostyczne*; Wydawnictwo Wyższej Szkoły Ekonomii i Prawa, Kielce: Kielce, Poland, 2012.
5. Konieczny, J. *Ratownictwo w Polsce: Lata 1990–2010*; Garmond Oficyna Wydawnicza: Poznań, Poland, 2010.
6. Ślęzak, D.; Żuratyński, P.; Krzyżanowski, K.; Kalis, A. Państwowe ratownictwo medyczne w Polsce. *Logistyka* **2015**, *4*, 8419–8426.
7. Guła, P.; Wejnarski, A.; Moryto, R.; Gałązkowski, R.; Karwan, K.; Świeżewski, S. Analiza działań zespołów ratownictwa medycznego w polskim systemie Państwowego Ratownictwa Medycznego. Czy model podziału na zespoły specjalistyczne i podstawowe znajduje uzasadnienie. *Wiad Lek* **2014**, *65*, 468–475.
8. Kisiała, W. Organizacja przestrzenna a zmiany dostępności szpitalnych oddziałów ratunkowych w Polsce. *Zesz. Nauk.* **2014**, *247*, 129–145.
9. Furtak-Niczyporuk, M.; Drop, B. Efektywność organizacji systemu państwowe ratownictwo medyczne. *Studia Ekon.* **2016**, *168*, 53–67.
10. Sagan, A.; Kowalska-Bobko, I.; Mokrzycka, A. The 2015 emergency care reform in Poland: Some improvements, some unmet demands and some looming conflicts. *Health Policy* **2016**, *120*, 1220–1225. [CrossRef]
11. Rozporządzenie Ministra Zdrowia z dnia 21 grudnia 2010 r. w sprawie wojewódzkiego planu działania systemu Państwowe Ratownictwo Medyczne oraz kryteriów kalkulacji kosztów działalności zespołów ratownictwa medycznego. *Dz. Ustaw* **2011**, *3*, 6. Available online: https://isap.sejm.gov.pl/isap.nsf/DocDetails.xsp?id=WDU20110030006 (accessed on 7 November 2020).
12. Michalak, J. Problemy logistyczne w polskim systemie ratownictwa medycznego. *Logistyka* **2014**, *5*, 1977–1984.

13. Chowaniec, C.; Łada, M.; Wajda-Drzewiecka, K.; Skowronek, R.; Drzewiecki, A. Problem odpowiedzialności dyspozytorów medycznych funkcjonujących w systemie ratownictwa medycznego. *Arch. Med. Sadowej. Kryminol.* **2014**, *64*, 34–43. [PubMed]
14. Warczyński, P. *Plan Działania Systemu Państwowe Ratownictwo Medyczne Dla Województwa Mazowieckiego, Tekst Jednolity –Zaktualizowany Według Stanu Na Dzień 31 Grudnia 2014 Roku*; Mazowiecki Urząd Wojewódzki w Warszawie: Warszawa, Poland, 2015.
15. Jetté, N.; Quan, H.; Hemmelgarn, B.; Drosler, S.; Maass, C.; Oec, D.G.; IMECCHI Investigators. The development, evolution, and modifications of ICD-10: Challenges to the international comparability of morbidity data. *Med. Care* **2010**, *48*, 1105–1110.
16. Broda, G.; Rywik, S. Wieloośrodkowe ogólnopolskie badanie stanu zdrowia ludności–projekt WOBASZ. Zdefiniowanie problemu oraz cele badania. *Kardiol. Pol.* **2005**, *63*, 1–4.
17. Cybulska, B. Dlaczego polscy parlamentarzyści powinni wspierać profilaktykę chorób sercowo-naczyniowych? *Kardiolol. Pol.* **2007**, *65*, 5.
18. Majewicz, A.; Marcinkowski, J.T. Epidemiologia chorób układu krążenia. Dlaczego w Polsce jest tak małe zainteresowanie istniejącymi programami profilaktycznymi. *Probl. Hig. Epidemiol.* **2008**, *89*, 322–325.
19. Piwowarski, J.; Rozwadowski, M. System zarządzania kryzysowego jako element bezpieczeństwa narodowego. *Acta Sci. Acad. Ostroviensis Sect. B* **2016**, *7*, 344–368.
20. Aftyka, A.; Rudnicka-Drożak, E. Nieuzasadnione wezwania Zespołów Ratownictwa Medycznego w materiale Wojewódzkiego Pogotowia Ratunkowego SP ZOZ w Lublinie. *Anestezjol. Ratow.* **2013**, *7*, 290–296.
21. Goniewicz, M.; Goniewicz, K. Ewolucja systemu ratownictwa medycznego–od starożytności do czasów współczesnych. The evolution of the emergency medical services system–from ancient to modern times. *EMS* **2016**, *3*, 62.
22. Bem, A. Organizacja i finasowanie ratownictwa medycznego. *Pr. Nauk. Uniw. Ekon. We Wrocławiu* **2013**, *319*, 158–167.
23. Bryła, M.; Maciak, A.; Marcinkowski, J.T.; Maniecka-Bryła, I. Programy profilaktyczne w zakresie chorób układu krążenia przykładem niwelowania nierówności w stanie zdrowia. *Probl. Hig. Epidemiol.* **2009**, *90*, 6–17.
24. Tyszko, P.; Kowalska, J.; Demidowicz, J. Marketing w realizacji programów zdrowotnych. *Fam. Med. Prim. Care Rev.* **2011**, *1*, 95–101.
25. Kapka-Skrzypczak, L.; Biliński, P.; Niedźwiecka, J.; Kulpa, P.; Skowron, J.; Wojtyła, A. Zmiana stylu życia człowieka jako metoda prewencji przewlekłych chorób niezakaźnych. *Probl. Hig. Epidemiol.* **2012**, *93*, 27–31.
26. Monastyrska, E.M.; Beck, O. Psychologiczne aspekty chorób kardiologicznych. *Med. Ogólna Nauki Zdr.* **2014**, *20*, 141–144. [CrossRef]
27. Surma, S.; Szyndler, A.; Narkiewicz, K. Świadomość wybranych czynników ryzyka chorób układu sercowo-naczyniowego w populacji młodych osób. *Chor. Serca. I Naczyń.* **2017**, *14*, 186–193.
28. Kurpas, D.; Steciwko, A. Jakość usług medycznych w podstawowej opiece zdrowotnej. *Adv. Clin. Exp. Med.* **2005**, *14*, 603–608.
29. Sowers, J.R. Diabetes mellitus and cardiovasculardisease in women. *Arch. Intern. Med.* **1998**, *158*, 617–621. [CrossRef]
30. Pośnik-Urbańska, A.; Kawecka-Jaszcz, K. Choroby układu krążenia u kobiet-problem wciąż niedoceniany. *Chor Serca i Naczyń.* **2006**, *3*, 169–174.
31. Brongel, L. Ogólne Zasady Działania Sieci Zintegrowanego Ratownictwa Medycznego. In *Złota Godzina*; Brongel, L., Ed.; Wydawnictwo Medyczne: Kraków, Poland, 2007.
32. Timler, D.; Szarpak, Ł.; Madziała, M. Retrospektywna analiza interwencji zespołów ratownictwa medycznego u osób w wieku powyżej 65 roku życia. *Acta Univ. Łódź Folia Oeconomica* **2013**, *297*, 237–246.

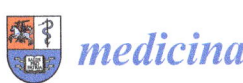

Review

Is There a Relationship between COVID-19 and Hyponatremia?

Gina Gheorghe [1,2,†], Madalina Ilie [1,2], Simona Bungau [3,†], Anca Mihaela Pantea Stoian [4], Nicolae Bacalbasa [5] and Camelia Cristina Diaconu [6,7,*]

1. Department of Gastroenterology, "Carol Davila" University of Medicine and Pharmacy, 050474 Bucharest, Romania; gheorghe_gina2000@yahoo.com (G.G.); drmadalina@gmail.com (M.I.)
2. Department of Gastroenterology, Clinical Emergency Hospital of Bucharest, 105402 Bucharest, Romania
3. Department of Pharmacy, Faculty of Medicine and Pharmacy, University of Oradea, 410028 Oradea, Romania; simonabungau@gmail.com
4. Department of Diabetes, Nutrition and Metabolic Diseases, "Carol Davila" University of Medicine and Pharmacy, 020475 Bucharest, Romania; ancastoian@yahoo.com
5. Department of Visceral Surgery, Center of Excellence in Translational Medicine, Fundeni Clinical Institute, 022328 Bucharest, Romania; nicolae_bacalbasa@yahoo.ro
6. Department of Internal Medicine, "Carol Davila" University of Medicine and Pharmacy, 050474 Bucharest, Romania
7. Department of Internal Medicine, Clinical Emergency Hospital of Bucharest, 105402 Bucharest, Romania
* Correspondence: drcameliadiaconu@gmail.com; Tel.: +40-0726-377-300
† This author has equal contribution to the paper as the first author.

Abstract: Nowadays, humanity faces one of the most serious health crises, the severe acute respiratory syndrome coronavirus 2 (SARS-CoV-2) pandemic. The severity of coronavirus disease 2019 (COVID-19) pandemic is related to the high rate of interhuman transmission of the virus, variability of clinical presentation, and the absence of specific therapeutic methods. COVID-19 can manifest with non-specific symptoms and signs, especially among the elderly. In some cases, the clinical manifestations of hyponatremia may be the first to appear. The pathophysiological mechanisms of hyponatremia among patients with COVID-19 are diverse, including syndrome of inappropriate antidiuretic hormone secretion (SIADH), digestive loss of sodium ions, reduced sodium ion intake or use of diuretic therapy. Hyponatremia may also be considered a negative prognostic factor in patients diagnosed with COVID-19. We need further studies to evaluate the etiology and therapeutic management of hyponatremia in patients with COVID-19.

Keywords: SARS-CoV-2; COVID-19; SIADH; dyselectrolytemia; hyponatremia

1. Introduction

The severe acute respiratory syndrome coronavirus 2 (SARS-CoV-2) is part of the betacoronavirus family and causes coronavirus disease 2019 (COVID-19) [1,2]. In March 2020, the World Health Organization (WHO) declared COVID-19 a pandemic, one of the most severe pandemics that humanity has faced over time [1,2]. Worldwide, there have been 45,921,698 cases of SARS-CoV-2 infection and 1,193,909 deaths, these numbers increasing alarmingly with each passing day [3].

In most cases, this viral infection manifests with pneumonia, characterized by fever, dyspnea, cough, and bilateral interstitial infiltrates on chest X-ray examination [4]. According to one study from the USA, among the most frequent symptoms encountered in patients with COVID-19 are cough, fever, myalgia, headache, dyspnea, sore throat, diarrhea, nausea/vomiting, loss of smell or taste, abdominal pain, and rhinorrhea [5]. These patients can also present thrombotic manifestations, conjunctivitis, dermatological findings like maculopapular urticaria, vesicular eruptions, or transient livedo reticularis [6,7]. Some patients may even develop severe clinical forms, with acute respiratory distress syndrome (ARDS), respiratory failure and multiple organ dysfunction and death [8]. In contrast, an important part of the COVID-19 patients can remain asymptomatic, which makes the diagnosis more difficult [4].

2. COVID-19 and Hyponatremia

The clinical evolution of patients with COVID-19 can be unpredictable, as these patients can develop a series of complications, as it is summarized in Table 1) [4,9].

Table 1. Complications of patients with COVID 19 [2,5]

Complications	Syndromes, Diseases, Manifestations
Respiratory	Acute respiratory distress syndrome (ARDS) Pulmonary embolism
Cardiac	Arrhythmias Acute cardiac injury Cardiomyopathy Shock
Neurological	Acute disseminated encephalomyelitis (ADEM) Acute hemorrhagic necrotizing encephalopathy Encephalopathy Generalized myoclonus Gullain-Barré syndrome (acute polyradiculoneuritis) Meningoencephalitis Posterior reversible encephalopathy syndrome (PRES)
Inflammatory	Auto-antibody mediated manifestations Exuberant inflammatory response Kawasaki disease Toxic shock syndrome
Secondary infections	Bacterial/fungal coinfections

3. Incidence of Hyponatremia in Patients with COVID-19

Sometimes, patients with COVID-19 can present dyselectrolytemia, like hyponatremia, which is defined by serum sodium levels less than 135 mmol/L. In many cases, this electrolytic disorder is caused by a variety of factors [10,11]. Hyponatremia is the most common electrolyte disorder seen in clinical practice and is associated with increased risk of death [12]. This electrolytic disequilibrium is classified in hypovolemic, euvolemic, and hypervolemic hyponatremia, each category's therapeutic approach being different [2].

The most recognizable cause of hyponatremia is the syndrome of inappropriate antidiuretic hormone secretion (SIADH), found in about 40–50% of patients with this electrolyte disorder [13]. These percentages may be higher in some conditions, such as traumatic brain injury, subarachnoid haemorrhage or pneumonia [14]. SIADH can occur in the evolution of inflammatory diseases of infectious or non-infectious causes, malignant diseases, cardiovascular or hepatic diseases, but also in the evolution of acute respiratory distress syndrome (ARDS) [14,15]. Ho and colleagues reported the first case of COVID-19 associated with SIADH manifested by new-onset seizures [16]. Yousaf et al. published a series of cases of patients diagnosed with COVID-19 who also associated SIADH [17]. All patients included in this study had severe acute hyponatremia. After excluding other possible etiologies, these authors established that this hydro electrolytic disorder is secondary to SIADH [17].

4. Pathophysiology of Hyponatremia in Patients with COVID-19

In infectious diseases (i.e. COVID-19), haemodynamic disorders or an inadequate immune response may cause kidney damage [18]. It is also possible that kidney cells are directly affected by the infection, according to some studies that have demonstrated the presence of viral particles in the proximal tubules and podocytes [18]. Renal cells express receptors and enzymes used by viruses as gateways, such as angiotensin-converting enzyme 2 (ACE2) [9,18]. This enzyme is also found in the lungs, heart and intestines, which explains the damage of these organs in COVID-19 [18]. Another pathophysiological mechanism that may explain the renal impairment in COVID-19 is inflammatory cytokine-induced impairment. It is known that the cytokine cascade can cause a number of renal pathological changes, as well, such as acute kidney injury (AKI), tubular necrosis, dysfunction of the kidney proximal tubule, glomerulopathy and electrolyte abnormalities [9,18–20].

Hyponatremia was identified in approximately 35% of patients with pneumonia [2]. The presence of hyponatremia in patients with pneumonia has been associated with a higher mortality rate, indicating the need for an early diagnosis and proper therapeutic management, to improve the prognosis of these patients [2]. The literature also reports that approximately 60% of patients with COVID-19 and watery diarrhea have moderate hyponatremia. In this situation, hyponatremia is possibly secondary to viral replication in the intestinal epithelial cells [21]. Ata et al. report the case of a young patient, known with diabetes mellitus, who presented with diarrhea and abdominal pain. Laboratory investigations identified hyponatremia (120 mmol/L), and the patient subsequently tested positive for SARS-CoV-2 infection. In this case, the cause of hyponatremia was not clear, but the authors suspected the association between SIADH and stool sodium loss to be the culprit [22].

In order to establish the diagnosis and etiology of hyponatremia, a careful history and physical examination are required; investigations such as serum sodium level, urine sodium level, serum osmolality, urine osmolality, thyroid function tests and serum cortisol may be needed (Figure 1) [23].

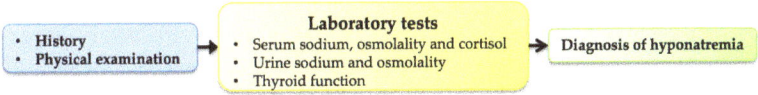

Figure 1. Diagnostic algorithm in hyponatremia.

In the pathogenesis of hyponatremia, interleukin-6 (IL-6) released by monocytes and macrophages plays an important role; it induces the non-osmotic release of vasopressin and secondary electrolyte disturbances [14]. IL-6 has also been shown to be involved in the pathophysiology of COVID-19 [13,17,24]. This explains the use and efficacy of tocilizumab, a humanized monoclonal antibody against the IL-6 receptor, in the treatment of patients with COVID-19 [25]. Other cause that may lead to increased ADH secretion among patients with SARS-CoV-2 infection is volume depletion through digestive loss (diarrhea or vomiting) or secondary to reduced oral fluid intake [26]. All these lead to water retention and the secondary increase of ADH secretion. Numerous SARS-CoV-2-induced comorbidities, such as pneumonia, respiratory failure, stroke etc., can also contribute to the development of SIADH [26]. The most common cause of death in patients with COVID-19 is ARDS; secondary, the inflammatory syndrome characterized by the massive release of cytokines and multiple organ failure may also contribute to the fatal evolution of these patients [13].

A retrospective study in Italy looked at the clinical impact of hyponatremia and the correlation with IL-6 levels in a group of patients diagnosed with COVID-19 [13]. Out of 29 patients, 15 had low serum sodium levels upon admission. There was an inversely proportional relationship between serum sodium level and IL-6 level and a directly proportional relationship between serum sodium level and PaO_2/FiO_2 ratio [14]. The relationship between serum IL-6 and sodium was also suggested by a significant increase in serum sodium 48 h after initiation of tocilizumab treatment [13]. Patients with hyponatremia and COVID-19 have a worse prognosis compared with patients without electrolyte disturbances [13].

A study that included 1099 patients hospitalized for COVID-19 in China showed an average serum sodium value of 138 mmol/L (range 135–141 mmol/L) in these patients [27]. Another study conducted in New York, that involved 5700 hospitalized patients with

COVID-19, including 55 solid organ transplant patients, showed an average serum sodium level of 136 mmol/L (133–138 mmol/L) [28].

An article presents the case of a 55-year-old woman with kidney transplant, diagnosed with COVID-19, who associated hyponatremia since hospitalization (serum sodium concentration upon admission <120mmol/L) [29]. This woman reported close contact with a confirmed patient with SARS-CoV-2 infection; she had also suggestive symptoms, respectively low-grade fever at home (temperature 37.4 °C), cough, dyspnea, headache, decreased appetite, nausea, and fatigue [29]. Under these conditions, there has been a suspicion of SARS-CoV-2 infection from the beginning. Another article presents the case of a 57-year-old man with a history of hypertension and type 2 diabetes who presented for dizziness, physical asthenia, headache, and nausea. This patient did not report close contact with a confirmed case; the electrocardiogram and chest X-ray were normal. On admission, however, laboratory tests showed severe hyponatremia (serum sodium level upon admission 112 mmol/L) and the RT-PCR test for SARS-CoV-2 proved to be positive [30]. In all cases of COVID-19 and hyponatremia reported until now, the patients presented with fever and radiological findings consistent with pneumonia [17].

Another study conducted in Hubei, China, evaluated the particularities of patients diagnosed with COVID-19 and disorders of sodium balance [31]. Thus, 1254 patients diagnosed with COVID-19 were enrolled. Of these, 9.9% (124 patients) associated hyponatremia (serum sodium below 135 mmol/L) and 2.4% associated hypernatremia (sodium over 145 mmol/L) [31]. The presence of hyponatremia among these patients was associated with old age, the existence of several comorbidities and diagnosis of severe pneumonia on chest X-ray. Regarding the etiology of hyponatremia, digestive sodium losses, by diarrhea or vomiting, could explain this hydro-electrolytic disorder only in a small number of patients (8.7% diarrhea, 3.3% vomiting) [31]. However, another reason that contributed largely to the development of hyponatremia in patients included in this study was renal failure, with elevated blood urea nitrogen and creatinine levels. A possible explanation could be the advanced age of patients with COVID-19 and hyponatremia and implicitly multiple comorbidities, with impaired renal function. On the other hand, liver function and serum albumin levels were normal in these patients, which significantly reduced the likelihood of hypervolemic hyponatremia of nephrotic or hepatic etiology. Another hypothesis is hyponatremia secondary to cardiac dysfunction. The pathophysiological mechanism incriminated in this situation is the expression by myocytes of angiotensin-converting enzyme 2 (ACE2), which acts as a viral receptor for SARS-CoV-2 and, implicitly, cardiac disease [31]. This study also provides additional evidence for the association of hyponatremia in COVID-19 patients with SIADH. The possible causes of SIADH in this situation include both the positive pressure ventilation (with non-osmotic stimulation of ADH secretion) and the usage of antibiotics and corticosteroids [31]. Regarding symptomatology, hyponatremia in SARS-CoV-2 positive patients was associated with a greater predisposition to fever and nausea, and in terms of biological changes, with increased leukocytes, neutrophils and high sensitivity C-reactive protein (HS-CRP). Hypernatremia was rarer in patients with COVID-19 compared with hyponatremia (2.4% vs. 9.9%) [31]. The only differences between patients with hypernatremia and those with normo-natremia were the clinical complications and biological anomalies [25]. In terms of treatment, patients with hypernatremia were treated more frequently with traditional Chinese medicine, as opposed to those with hyponatremia, who required intensive oxygen supply, high doses of antibiotics and corticosteroids [31]. Related to the duration of hospitalization, no significant differences were identified between patients with hypernatremia and those with normo-natremia, in contrast to patients with hyponatremia, who generally had more severe forms of the disease and required longer hospitalization [31].

In a study on 323 patients with COVID-19, Carvalho et al. concluded that hyponatremia may be a factor pointing towards a bad prognosis. The authors showed that patients with COVID-19 and hyponatremia had higher rates of admission to hospital, intensive care unit transfer, use of artificial ventilation and death, comparatively to patients with COVID-19 and normo-natremia (34% vs. 14%) [32].

Table 2 summarizes the existing studies offering information about the incidence of hyponatremia in COVID-19 patients.

Table 2. Original studies regarding the incidence of hyponatremia in COVID-19 patients.

Authors	Reference	Number of Patients	Incidence of Hyponatremia %
Berni, A.; et al.	[13]	29	51.72
Choi, K.W.; et al.	[21]	267	60
Hu, W.; et al.	[31]	1254	9.9
De Carvalho, H.; et al.	[32]	323	31

Until now, there are no studies published to show if there is a correlation between the incidence of hyponatremia and the severity of COVID-19, there are only data from case reports. This is an issue that should be clarified by future studies.

5. Hyponatremia Management in COVID-19 Patients

There are currently no clinical guidelines for the management of hyponatremia in patients diagnosed with COVID-19. The therapeutic approach of this hydro-electrolytic disorder depends, on one hand, on the etiology, and on the other hand on the volume status and comorbidities of the patient. As specified above, the hyponatremia etiology in patients with COVID-19 is multifactorial. According to existing data, the causes of hyponatremia include SIADH and digestive losses of sodium through diarrhea or vomiting [2]. The pathophysiological judgment is very important, because there are two therapeutic strategies, fluid restriction therapy and electrolytic substitution therapy. Thus, in the case of hypovolemic hyponatremia secondary to gastrointestinal fluid losses, reduced fluid intake or the use of diuretic therapy, guidelines impose initiation of electrolyte replacement therapy [2]. In the case of hyponatremia secondary to SIADH, fluid restriction is needed, that may associate hypertonic saline administration, depending on the level of neurological impairment. This therapeutic approach is relevant to avoid iatrogenic complications, such as pulmonary edema and lung damage exacerbation secondary to SARS-COV-2 infection [2].

6. Conclusions

Hyponatremia is frequent among patients with COVID-19, who sometimes may present only with symptoms and clinical signs secondary to this electrolytic imbalance. The diagnosis of hyponatremia upon admission of a patient, in the context of COVID-19 pandemic, should nowadays rise the suspicion of a possible SARS-CoV-2 infection. The causes of hyponatremia in these patients are diverse. It is very important to establish the exact etiology of this electrolytic disorder, because therapeutic management differs depending on its pathophysiological mechanism. Noteworthy, hyponatremia may be considered an unfavorable prognostic factor among patients with COVID-19. Future studies are needed to evaluate the exact incidence, pathogenesis, and therapeutic management of hyponatremia in patients with SARS-CoV-2 infection.

Author Contributions: Conceptualization, G.G. and C.C.D.; Methodology, C.C.D., and M.I.; Software, G.G.; N.B.; Validation, C.C.D. and S.B.; Formal Analysis, G.G.; M.I.; Investigation, G.G.; A.M.P.S.; Resources, N.B.; Data Curation, M.I.; A.M.P.S.; Writing—Original Draft Preparation, G.G.; Writing—Review & Editing, G.G., S.B. and C.C.D.; Visualization, C.C.D.; Supervision, C.C.D. and S.B.; Project Administration, C.C.D. All authors have read and agreed to the published version of the manuscript.

Funding: This research received no external funding.

Institutional Review Board Statement: Not applicable.

Informed Consent Statement: Not applicable.

Data Availability Statement: Not applicable.

Conflicts of Interest: The authors declare no conflict of interests.

References

1. Kabir, T.; Uddin, S.; Hossain, F.; Abdulhakim, J.A.; Alam, A.; Ashraf, G.; Bungau, S.G.; Bin-Jumah, M.N.; Abdel-Daim, M.M.; Aleya, L. nCOVID-19 pandemic from molecular pathogenesis to potential investigational therapeutics. *Front. Cell Dev. Biol.* **2020**, *8*. [CrossRef] [PubMed]
2. Carlos de la Flor Merino, J.; Amado, F.V.; Rodil, B.B.; Marschall, A.; Rodeles del Pozo, M. Hyponatremia in COVID-19 infection: Possible causal factors and management. *J. Allergy Infect Dis.* **2020**, *1*, 53–56. [CrossRef]
3. Worldometers. Available online: https://www.worldometers.info/coronavirus/ (accessed on 15 October 2020).
4. McIntosh, K. Coronavirus Disease 2019 (COVID-19): Clinical Features. UpToDate2020. Available online: https://www.uptodate.com/contents/coronavirus-disease-2019-covid-19-clinical-features? (accessed on 15 October 2020).
5. Stokes, E.K.; Zambrano, L.D.; Anderson, K.N.; Marder, E.P.; Raz, K.M.; Felix, S.E.B.; Tie, Y.; Fullerton, K.E. Coronavirus Disease 2019 Case Surveillance—United States, 22 January–30 May 2020. *MMWR Morb. Mortal. Wkly. Rep.* **2020**, *69*, 759–765. [CrossRef] [PubMed]
6. Colavita, F.; Lapa, D.; Carletti, F.; Lalle, E.; Bordi, L.; Marsella, P.; Nicastri, E.; Bevilacqua, N.; Giancola, M.L.; Corpolongo, A.; et al. SARS-CoV-2 isolation from ocular secretions of a patient with COVID-19 in Italy with prolonged viral RNA detection. *Ann. Intern. Med.* **2020**, *173*, 242–243. [CrossRef] [PubMed]
7. Wang, D.; Hu, B.; Hu, C.; Zhu, F.; Liu, X.; Zhang, J.; Wang, B.; Xiang, H.; Cheng, Z.; Xiong, Y.; et al. Clinical characteristics of 138 hospitalized patients with 2019 novel coronavirus–infected pneumonia in Wuhan, China. *JAMA* **2020**, *323*, 1061–1069. [CrossRef]
8. Huang, C.; Wang, Y.; Li, X.; Ren, L.; Zhao, J.; Hu, Y.; Zhang, L.; Fan, G.; Xu, J.; Gu, X.; et al. Clinical features of patients infected with 2019 novel coronavirus in Wuhan, China. *Lancet* **2020**, *395*, 497–506. [CrossRef]
9. Behl, T.; Kaur, I.; Bungau, S.; Kumar, A.; Uddin, S.; Kumar, C.; Pal, G.; Sahil; Shrivastava, K.; Zengin, G.; et al. The dual impact of ACE2 in COVID-19 and ironical actions in geriatrics and pediatrics with possible therapeutic solutions. *Life Sci.* **2020**, *257*, 118075. [CrossRef]
10. Elkind, M.S.V.; Cucchiara, B.L.; Koralnik, I.J. Coronavirus Disease 2019 (COVID-19): Neurologic Complications and Management of Neurologic Conditions. UpToDate2020. Available online: https://www.uptodate.com/contents/coronavirus-disease-2019-covid-19-neurologic-complications-and-management-of-neurologic-conditions? (accessed on 15 October 2019).
11. Sterns, R.H. Diagnostic Evaluation of Adults with Hyponatremia. Uptodate. 2020. Available online: https://www.uptodate.com/contents/diagnostic-evaluation-of-adults-with-hyponatremia? (accessed on 15 October 2020).
12. Corona, G.; Giuliani, C.; Parenti, G.; Norello, D.; Verbalis, J.G.; Forti, G.; Maggi, M.; Peri, A. Moderate hyponatremia is associated with increased risk of mortality: Evidence from a meta-analysis. *PLoS ONE* **2013**, *8*, e80451. [CrossRef]
13. Berni, A.; Malandrino, D.; Parenti, G.; Maggi, M.; Poggesi, L.; Peri, A. Hyponatremia, IL-6, and SARS-CoV-2 (COVID-19) infection: May all fit together? *J. Endocrinol. Investig.* **2020**, *43*, 1137–1139. [CrossRef]
14. Cuesta, M.; Thompson, C.J. The syndrome of inappropriate antidiuresis (SIAD). *Best Pract. Res. Clin. Endocrinol. Metab.* **2016**, *30*, 175–187. [CrossRef]
15. Ellison, D.H.; Berl, T. Clinical practice. The syndrome of inappropriate antidiuresis. *N. Engl. J. Med.* **2007**, *356*, 2064–2072. [CrossRef] [PubMed]
16. Ho, K.S.; Narasimhan, B.; Kumar, A.; Flynn, E.; Salonia, J.; El-Hachem, K.; Mathew, J.P. Syndrome of inappropriate antidiuretic hormone as the initial presentation of COVID-19: A novel case report. *Nefrologia* **2020**. [CrossRef] [PubMed]
17. Yousaf, Z.; Al-Shokri, S.D.; Al-Soub, H.; Mohamed, M.F.H. COVID-19 associated SIADH: A clue in the times of pandemic! *Am. J. Physiol. Endocrinol. Metab.* **2020**, *318*, E882–E885. [CrossRef] [PubMed]
18. Carlos De La Flor Merino, J.; Marschall, A.; Rodil, B.B.; Rodeles del Pozo, M. Hyponatremia in COVID-19 infection—Should only think about SIADH? *J. Clin. Nephrol. Renal Care* **2020**. [CrossRef]
19. Sanz, A.B.; Sanchez-Niño, M.D.; Ortiz, A. TWEAK, a multifunctional cytokine in kidney injury. *Kidney Int.* **2011**, *80*, 708–718. [CrossRef] [PubMed]
20. Werion, A.; Belkhir, L.; Perrot, M.; Schmit, G.; Aydin, S.; Chen, Z.; Penaloza, A.; De Greef, J.; Yildiz, H.; Pothen, L.; et al. SARS-CoV-2 causes a specific dysfunction of the kidney proximal tubule. *Kidney Int.* **2020**, *98*, 1296–1307. [CrossRef]
21. Choi, K.W.; Chau, T.N.; Tsang, O.; Tso, E.; Chiu, M.C.; Tong, W.L.; Lee, P.O.; Ng, T.K.; Ng, W.F.; Lee, K.C.; et al. Outcomes and prognostic factors in 267 patients with severe acute respiratory syndrome in Hong Kong. *Ann. Intern. Med.* **2003**, *139*, 715–723. [CrossRef]
22. Ata, F.; Almasri, H.; Sajid, J.; Yousaf, Z. COVID-19 presenting with diarrhoea and hyponatraemia. *BMJ Case Rep. CP* **2020**, *13*, e235456. [CrossRef]
23. Decaux, G.; Much, W. Clinical laboratory evaluation of the syndrome of inappropriate secretion of antidiuretic hormone. *Clin. J. Am. Soc. Nephrol.* **2008**, *3*, 1175–1184. [CrossRef]
24. Diaconu, C. COVID-19 and hyponatremia. *Arch. Balk. Med. Union* **2020**, *55*, 373–374. [CrossRef]

25. Luo, P.; Liu, Y.; Qiu, L.; Liu, X.; Liu, D.; Li, J. Tocilizumab treatment in COVID-19: A single center experience. *J. Med. Virol.* **2020**, *92*, 814–818. [CrossRef] [PubMed]
26. Using Osmolality to Diagnose and Treat Hyponatremia in COVID-19 Patients. Available online: https://www.aicompanies.com/wp-content/uploads/2020/05/Using_Osmolality_Diagnosis_and_Treat_Hyponatremia_in_COVID_19_patients_PCN01369.pdf (accessed on 15 October 2020).
27. Guan, W.J.; Ni, Z.Y.; Hu, Y.; Liang, W.H.; Ou, C.Q.; He, J.X.; Liu, L.; Shan, H.; Lei, C.I.; Hui, D.; et al. Clinical characteristics of coronavirus disease 2019 in China. *N. Engl. J. Med.* **2020**, *382*, 1708–1720. [CrossRef] [PubMed]
28. Richardson, S.; Hirsch, J.S.; Narasimhan, M.; Crawford, J.M.; McGinn, T.; Davidson, K.W. Northwell COVID-19 Research Consortium. Presenting characteristics, comorbidities, and outcomes among 5700 patients hospitalized with COVID-19 in the New York City Area. *JAMA* **2020**, *323*, 2052–2059. [CrossRef]
29. Tantisattamo, E.; Reddy, U.G.; Duong, D.K.; Ferrey, A.J.; Ichii, H.; Dafoe, D.C.; Kalantar-Zadeh, K. Hyponatremia: A possible immuno-neuroendocrine interface with COVID-19 in a kidney transplant recipient. *Transpl. Infect. Dis.* **2020**, e13355. [CrossRef] [PubMed]
30. Habib, M.B.; Sardar, S.; Sajid, J. Acute symptomatic hyponatremia in setting of SIADH as an isolated presentation of COVID-19. *ID Cases* **2020**, *21*, e00859. [CrossRef] [PubMed]
31. Hu, W.; Lv, X.; Li, C.; Xu, Y.; Qi, Y.; Zhang, Z.; Li, M.; Cai, F.; Liu, D.; Yue, J.; et al. Disorders of sodium balance and its clinical implications in COVID-19 patients: A multicenter retrospective study. *Intern. Emerg. Med.* **2020**, 1–10. [CrossRef]
32. De Carvalho, H.; Letellier, T.; Karakachoff, M.; Desvaux, G.; Caillon, H.; Papuchon, E.; Bentoumi-Loaec, M.; Benaouicha, N.; Canet, E.; Chapelet, G.; et al. Hyponatremia is associated with poor outcome in COVID-19. *Res. Sq.* **2020**. [CrossRef]

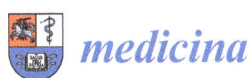

Review

Caudal Duplication Syndrome Systematic Review—A Need for Better Multidisciplinary Surgical Approach and Follow-Up

Spătaru Radu-Iulian [1,2], Avino Adelaida [3,4,*], Iozsa Dan-Alexandru [1,2], Ivanov Monica [2], Serban Dragos [5,6], Tomescu Luminița Florentina [7] and Cirstoveanu Cătălin [8,9]

1. Discipline of Pediatric Surgery, Faculty of Medicine, "Carol Davila" University of Medicine and Pharmacy, 020021 Bucharest, Romania; radu_spataru@yahoo.com (S.R.-I.); dan.iozsa@yahoo.com (I.D.-A.)
2. Department of Pediatric Surgery, Emergency Clinic Hospital for Children "Maria S. Curie", 41451 Bucharest, Romania; mqmivanov@yahoo.com
3. Department of Plastic and Reconstructive Surgery, Clinical Emergency Hospital "Prof. Dr. Agrippa Ionescu", 011356 Bucharest, Romania
4. Discipline of Plastic and Reconstructive Surgery, Faculty of Medicine, Doctoral School, "Carol Davila" University of Medicine and Pharmacy, 020021 Bucharest, Romania
5. Discipline of General Surgery, Faculty of Medicine, "Carol Davila" University of Medicine and Pharmacy, 020021 Bucharest, Romania; dragos.serban@umfcd.ro
6. Department of General Surgery, Emergency University Hospital, 050098 Bucharest, Romania
7. Department of Interventional Radiology, Clinical Emergency Hospital "Prof. Dr. Agrippa Ionescu", 011356 Bucharest, Romania; slumi2001@gmail.com
8. Discipline of Pediatrics, Faculty of Medicine, "Carol Davila" University of Medicine and Pharmacy, 020021 Bucharest, Romania; cirstoveanu@yahoo.com
9. Neonatal Intensive Care Unit, Emergency Clinic Hospital for Children "Maria S. Curie", 41451 Bucharest, Romania
* Correspondence: adelaida.avino@gmail.com; Tel.: +40-771-545

Received: 8 November 2020; Accepted: 24 November 2020; Published: 27 November 2020

Abstract: *Background and Objectives:* Caudal duplication syndrome is a rare association of anatomical anomalies describing duplication of the hindgut, spine, and uro-genital structures, leading to varied clinical presentations. The current literature focuses on case reports which describe the embryological etiology and anatomical spectrum of the condition giving little attention to the surgical preparation, the need for a well-structured follow-up program, or the transition into adult healthcare of these complex patients. No reviews have been published regarding this complex pathology. *Materials and Methods*: A review of caudal duplication syndrome cases was done to assess the range of the clinical malformations, timing, and types of surgical interventions. Inconsistencies in multidisciplinary care, follow-up, and risk events were described. *Results:* Hindgut duplication always involved the anorectal region. Anorectal malformations were evenly distributed as unilateral and bilateral. Colon duplication extended from the anal region to the transverse colon or ascending colon in most of the cases and less to terminal. In females, genital duplication was present in all cases. The follow-up period varied between 3 months and 12 years. In all adult females, the motive of presentation was related to pregnancy (complications after successful delivery, fertility evaluation) or late complications (fecalith obstruction of the end-to-side colon anastomosis, repeated UTIs with renal scarring). *Conclusions*: Complex malformations affecting multiple caudal organs may have a strong impact in many aspects of the long-term quality of life; therefore, patients with caudal duplication syndrome need increased awareness and joined multidisciplinary treatment.

Keywords: caudal duplication syndrome; colorectal duplication; genitourinary duplication; congenital malformation; pediatric surgery

1. Introduction

Caudal duplication syndrome (CDS) is a very rare congenital cluster of anomalies. Dominguez et al. (1993) defined it as an association of hindgut duplication, duplication of the lower uro-genital tract, spinal cord, and vertebral anomalies at heterogeneous degrees of severity resulting from a fetal insult at different stages of embryogenesis [1,2].

Considering the very low incidence of this malformation and the variety of clinical presentations, the majority of published literature focus on description of the anatomical spectrum and the possible embryological etiology and less on the short- and long-term surgical planning, implementation of a structured follow-up plan, and the responsibility for transition of care into adult healthcare of these complex patients [3,4].

Each type of gastrointestinal, genitourinary, and/or distal spine duplication, either partial or complete cannot be discussed separately but together and its management must be adjusted to each individual case. The purpose of treatment is to preserve or improve fecal and urinary continence, maintain reproductive potential, allow a satisfactory sexual life with acceptable cosmetic appearance of the perineum, and manage other neurological disabilities. All these will impact the long-term morbidities and quality of life [5].

The impact of the malformations severity on the prognosis and risks of potential complications of the surgical treatment can be reduced by a comprehensive anatomical and functional preoperative evaluation, prospective multidisciplinary surgical planning, and active involvement of the patient and family to assure collaboration and adherence to the follow-up plan.

The objective of this review is to recognize possible surgical management patterns used to treat different clinical presentations of CDS, to examine the presence of gaps in patients' care, to assess risk events which can occur during life and might signal the need for planned intervention and identify groups of patients with CDS which require special attention.

2. Materials and Methods

A literature review with the search term "caudal duplication syndrome" was done using open access search engines PubMed, Science Direct, and Google Scholar by two independent reviewers. We excluded duplicate references, conference abstracts, articles not in English, and cases which did not describe the surgical management. Articles which described patients with duplicated digestive system, genitourinary tract, spinal column, and the neural tube but also included duplications of the lower limb were not included. A total of 279 articles were retrieved during the systematic search using the specified criteria. The full text articles were reviewed, and the selected articles were saved using reference management software. A total of 17 articles (3 case series and 14 case reports) with a total of 23 patients were selected for meeting the criteria. No literature or systematic review articles could be found.

3. Results

Hindgut duplication in CDS always included the anorectal region (Table 1).

Table 1. Spectrum of malformations in patients with caudal duplication syndrome (CDS).

Author Name	Patient ID	Age at Presentation (Gender)	Colorectal Duplication Extension (Proximal Level)	Type of Anal Duplication	Urinary Duplication	Genital Duplication	Spinal Malformation	Follow-up Period
Dominguez et al.	1	Newborn (M)	No duplication	No duplication	Complete	Diphallia, scrotum duplication	Meningo-myelocele, duplication of L5 and sacrum	7 years
	2	Newborn (F)	Transverse colon	Unilateral ARM	Complete	Complete	Myelomeningocele, Chiari-Arnold syndrome, scoliosis, dislocated hip, equinovarus leg	9 years
	3	Newborn (F)	Transverse colon	ARM (not specified)	Complete	Complete	T10 hemivertebra	2 years
	4	Newborn (M)	Double appendix, double proximal colon, sigmoid triplication	Triple ani (not specified)	Complete	No duplication, 4 testicles	Hemivertebrae, sacrum duplication	No Follow-up
Acer et al.	5	Newborn (F)	Appendix, cecum duplication	Bilateral ARM	Complete	Complete	Bifid L5, sacrum	3 months
Swaika et al.	6	Newborn (M)	Ascending colon	Bilateral ARM	Complete	2 Hemi-phalluses	Spinal lipoma, normal vertebral spine	1 year
Samuk et al.	7	Newborn (M)	Hepatic flexure	Bilateral ARM	Complete	No Duplication	Tethered cord, lipomyelo-meningocele, splitting bellow dorso-lumbar junction	No Follow-up
Bajpai et al.	8	Newborn (M)	Transverse colon	ARM (unspecified)	Complete	Diphallia	Lipomeningo-myelocele, tethered cord, bifid sacrum, pelvis diastasis	No Follow-up
Chaussy et al.	9	Newborn (F)	Terminal ileum	Unilateral ARM	Complete	Complete	Hemivertebrae	5 years
	10	Newborn (F)	Colon (not specified)	Bilateral ARM	No duplication	Complete	Myelocele, duplication of lumbar and sacrum	1.5 years
Kroes et al.	11	Newborn (F)	Terminal ileum	Bilateral ARM	Complete	Complete	Hemivertebrae, sacrum malformation	12 years

Table 1. *Cont.*

Author Name	Patient ID	Age at Presentation (Gender)	Colorectal Duplication Extension (Proximal Level)	Type of Anal Duplication	Urinary Duplication	Genital Duplication	Spinal Malformation	Follow-up Period
Wisenbaugh et al.	12	Newborn (F)	Colon (unspecified)	Bilateral ARM	Complete	Complete	Myelomeningocele tethered cord	7 years
de Oliveira et al.	13	9 months (M)	Colon (not specified)	ARM (unspecified)	Complete	Diphallia	Intramedullary L4 cyst, tethered cord, lipoma, sacrum duplication	No Follow-up
Bansal et al.	14	2 years 10 months (F)	Ascending colon	Unilateral ARM	Complete	Complete	Lipomyelo-meningocele, tethered cord, hydrosyrinx, scoliosis, butterfly vertebrae, hemi-sacrum	8 months
	15	6 months (F)	Distal colon (unspecified)	Bilateral ARM	Complete	Complete	No malformation	13 years
Abdelhalim et al.	16	4 years (F)	Colon (unspecified)	Parasagittal duplication with intra sphincteric location	Complete	Complete	Hemivertebrae, lumbar scoliosis	15 months
	17	6 years (F)	No duplication	No duplication	Complete	Complete	No duplication	1 year
Salman et al.	18	8 years (F)	Ascending colon	Bilateral ARM	Complete	Complete	Spina bifida, hemivertebrae	Not specified
Liu et al.	19	13 years (M)	Transverse colon	Unilateral ARM	Complete	Glans duplication One shaft	Hemivertebrae, sacrum subfissure	2 years
Becker et al.	20	22 years (F)	Colon (not specified)	Unilateral ARM	Unspecified	Complete	Segmentation defects, lumbar and sacrum fusion defects	Not specified
Hu et al.	21	28 years (F)	Colon (not specified)	Unilateral ARM	Complete	Complete	Lumbar and sacrum fusion defects	Not specified
Ragab et al.	22	31 years (F)	Colon (not specified)	ARM Not specified	Complete	Complete	N/A	No Follow-up
Mei et al.	23	39 years (F)	N/A	N/A	Complete	Complete	N/A	Not specified

F—female, M—male; ARM—anorectal malformation; Complete—duplication of bladder and urethra or utero-vaginal duplication.

At anal level, anorectal malformation (ARM) was present at least on one duplicated side in all cases with the exception of three patients without hindgut duplication and one patient with intra-sphincteric location of both anal openings. Unilateral anorectal malformation was present in 7/23 cases (30.43%), bilateral ARM in 7/23 cases (30.43%), and five cases were not described. The most common types of anorectal malformation are perineal fistula or recto vestibular fistula. Colon duplication extended from anal region to the transverse colon in 5/23 cases (21.73%), to ascending colon in 4/23 cases (17.39%), and to terminal ileum in 2/23 (8.69%). In eight patients, the level of duplication was not specified. In one patient, the appendix and proximal colon was duplicated while the sigmoid and anorectal region was triplicated. Bladder and urethral duplication were always in the sagittal plane and was present in all cases with the exception of two female patients (one with unspecified anatomy). In males, genital involvement with complete or partial shaft duplication (glans duplication and one shaft) was present in five out of seven patients. In females, genital duplication was present in all cases. Spinal cord malformations (myelomeningocele, tethered cord, cord lipoma, hydrosyrix) were reported in half of the cases. The vertebral spine, most commonly defects of fusion and hemivertebrae, was involved in 14/23 cases (60.86%). Associated anomalies outside of the caudal region included the abdominal wall (omphalocele), cardiac malformations (patent ductus arteriosus, ventricular septal defect, atrial septal defect), gastro-intestinal (Meckel diverticulum, malrotation, duodenal atresia, small bowel atresia, esophageal duplication cyst), or limb malformations (unilateral lower leg hypoplasia), without being consistent in prevalence. Prenatal ultrasound evaluation was done in only 2 patients without a prenatal diagnosis of CDS and no further Magnetic resonance imaging (MRI) evaluation. In 19/23 cases (82.60%), the child was evaluated in the first year of life due to the evident malformations of the perineum. In cases with non-obstructive symptoms due to less severe malformations or inconsistent follow-up, evaluation was delayed until complications occurred. The most common surgical interventions in the first month of life were colostomy for anorectal malformation with obstructive symptoms, acute abdomen (entero-vesical fistula) or omphalocele repair. After this age, the motive of presentation was related to complications: severe dermatitis because continuous dribbling urine, fecal incontinence, long term constipation or for cosmetic correction of the perineal region in asymptomatic female patients. Functional evaluation of the bladder is inconsistently reported and was done in cases of urinary incontinence. The most common associated urologic pathology was unilateral or bilateral vesico-ureteral reflux. In male patients, penectomy or penile reconstruction was done in 3/5 cases or was planned for future reconstruction in the rest of the cases. Only one author opted for vaginoplasty with resection of the common wall for cosmetic reasons in two patients and in one other case one side of the duplication was removed. All adult cases (age between 22 and 39 years) were females and the motive of presentation was related to pregnancy (complications after successful delivery, fertility evaluation) or late complications (fecalith obstruction of the end-to-side colon anastomosis, repeated UTIs with renal scarring). All cases had limited surgical history (colorectal surgery in infancy) with no subsequent events. All four female patients were sexually active with one or bilateral side vaginal use retained the double vagina, all became pregnant and delivered by cesarean section. The main reasons for delayed presentation were non-obstructive colorectal malformation (stooling present with the help with suppository), no need for toilet training until school age (incases with urinary or fecal incontinence), or lack of caregiver awareness. The follow-up period varied between 3 months and 12 years and was longer in cases with fecal or urinary incontinence. Three of the adult females with history of colorectal surgery as infants had no reported follow-up until presentation for current problems as adults. The life events with the highest impact on occurrence of complications were the type of colorectal surgical procedure (end-to-side anastomosis with recurrent episodes of fecal impaction which required multiple hospital admissions and treatment), neglect or lack of awareness from caregivers (patients presented at 6 and 13 years old, respectively, with neurologic and continence problems) and pregnancy. A case of a 39-year-old female is presented with a history of three pregnancies, delivered with cesarean section and no prior medical history. After deliveries, the patient had one side hysterectomy for leiomyomas, two interventions for vaginal prolapse, one side ureteral reimplantation, three transurethral incisions of the bladder neck for inefficient bladder emptying, and one transurethral bulking agent injection in the bladder neck for stress incontinence.

4. Discussion

The very low incidence of caudal duplication syndrome makes it difficult to develop expertise and assemble a multidisciplinary team with participation in all the steps of care. Because of the evident clinical features of the perineum, these cases are first assessed at birth. Prenatal examination can diagnose clusters of severe anomalies which might not be recognized as CDS because of the low awareness of this syndrome [6,7].

- **Management of colorectal duplication**

If the baby has efficient bowel movements, is preferably breastfed, is gaining weight, and no other severe associated malformations require surgical intervention, we recommend delaying further treatment until a complete assessment of the types and extension of malformations is done and an individually tailored treatment plan can be made bringing the family together with the multidisciplinary team. The type of malformation determines the surgical strategy at birth: primary repair (not the best choice in these complex patients), temporary anal calibrations to ensure efficient bowel movements until definitive repair or colostomy creation. The purpose of surgical reconstruction is to have a single anal opening located within the complex muscle either by removal of the anal side opening outside of the sphincter [7,8] or joining of the two anorectal ends and positioning in the muscle sphincter [9]. Depending on the duplication length and anatomical variant, if the two duplicated colons are not fused and have a separate blood supply, one side should be removed if not, stripping of the mucosa on the non-dominant side [10] or stapling the common wall [9] (similar with stapling the common wall in Duhamel procedure [11]) to ensure efficient emptying, to avoid complications such as severe constipation [12] with fecal impaction, volvulus, or neoplastic changes. End-to-side anastomosis of the two colonic lumens should not be the first option because of the risk of stenosis at the anastomotic site in the long-term with fecal impaction and proximal colitis [3]. This can also make difficult efficient emptying of both lumens if antegrade continence will be required in patients with low the potential for fecal continence [9].

- **Management of bladder and urethral duplication**

Sagittal urethral duplication (side-by-side) is associated with bladder duplication and is specific for CDS. The two bladders can be completely separate or have a sagittal septum (most commonly two asymmetric sides) each with a ureter from the ipsilateral kidney and its own urethra. Urologic management in the first year of life is almost always conservative. Anatomic evaluation should be complemented with bladder function assessment especially in symptomatic patients. The goal is to avoid recurrent urinary infections, to ensure there is efficient emptying of both bladders and urinary continence. In most female patients, unilateral removal of the urethra is not necessary if asymptomatic. In males, the urethra will be excised when the decision for cosmetical penectomy is made [13], and it can be postponed until adolescence to let the patient decide, to assess penile growth and erectile function.

Assessment of continence potential is important in the development of any anorectal and urinary reconstruction plan. The type and severity of spinal cord and sacrum malformation have a direct role in predicting the fecal and urinary continence [14,15]. This can be assessed very early on and will influence the choice of surgical procedures as for example the decision to remove the bladder septum creating a bigger capacity bladder with bladder neck ligation and ipsilateral urethral removal or to keep the one or two appendices for antegrade continent enema (ACE)and/or appendicovesicostomy [16].

- **Management of genital duplication**

Gender distribution shows a predilection of CDS in females with a complete but well-developed duplicated external and internal genital organ and preserved ovarian function. Almost always, corrective genital surgery in females is not necessary unless one side is hypoplastic and might cause menstrual flow obstruction or for cosmetic concerns, in which case, it can be removed [10]. If congenital uterine anomalies such as septate or subseptate uteri have a risk for reduced conception rate, increased risk of first trimester miscarriage (especially with septal implantation), preterm birth, and fetal malpresentation, patients with didelphys uterus do not appear to have reduced fertility and have less pregnancy complications, but might be at increased risk for preterm labor [17]. All our adult female patients carried pregnancies to term and in three out the four cases [3,18–20] presented for pregnancy related issues (genetic counseling, symptomatic ureteral compression or vaginal prolapse, and voiding dysfunction after multiple pregnancies). Cesarean section was performed in all cases. In cases with a history of multiple abdominal surgeries and depending on the complexity of procedures, the cesarean surgery should be assisted by a colorectal surgeon and/or urologist. Male patients present with complete or partial penile duplication and are more likely to be corrected for cosmetic reasons with removal of one of the abnormal shafts [13] or penoplasty [12]. There are no reports assessing fertility and sexual function into adult age in CDS male patients.

- **Support groups and quality of life**

The importance of active involvement of family members and the patient itself is well recognized, but not always available. Parents must cope with the difficulty of accepting and adjusting to their child's condition, coordinate appointments with different healthcare providers, find information about their child's malformations, manage the financial demands of long-term medical care, and locate appropriate care centers [21,22]. Factors such as low income, socially disadvantaged groups, and inaccessible educational materials due to rarity of the malformations, limited access to information or lack of support groups can negatively influence adherence to the treatment plan. Quality of life in patients with CDS is unreported but it is known the long-term impact of incontinence and sexual dysfunction in patients with anorectal malformations. Spinal malformations such as myelomeningocele can lead to lower limb paralysis. The goal of management plan is to reduce disability early on by implementing bowel management programs in cases with low continence potential and the need for robust transitional care arrangements to enable continued management in adulthood [19,23]. The process of transition should start in early adolescence and the adult care provider who will assume care of the patient should be identified early in the process, when possible [3].

Our literature review has numerous limitations which influence the value and objectivity in making recommendations. We are aware of the difficulty of extracting consistent data and providing statistically significant results. There is a high heterogeneity in data reporting in case reports or case series articles, with ambiguous nomenclature used to describe the anatomy or details regarding surgical procedures and incomplete information about the extent of multi-organ malformations. The term "caudal duplication syndrome" was introduced in 1993, but there still are inconsistent ways of naming it (e.g., cloacal duplication).

5. Conclusions

Caudal duplication syndrome should receive more attention from the pediatric surgical community regarding team approach and data collection. It is not sufficient to report the anatomical particularities of a case. Similar to other rare and complex malformations which affect the caudal region and have an impact on the quality of life (for example, bladder exstrophy or cloacal exstrophy), patients with caudal duplication syndrome deserve a better integrated care to improve outcomes.

Author Contributions: Conceptualization, S.R.-I. and C.C.; methodology, I.D.-A. and S.D.; software, T.L.F.; validation, S.D. and I.M.; formal analysis, I.M.; investigation, I.D.-A. and S.D.; resources, S.R.-I.; data curation, C.C. and I.M.; writing—original draft preparation, I.D.-A. and C.C.; writing—review and editing, A.A.; visualization, A.A.; supervision, T.L.F.; project administration, S.R.-I. All authors have read and agreed to the published version of the manuscript.

Funding: This research received no external funding.

Conflicts of Interest: The authors declare no conflict of interest.

References

1. Acer, T.; Ötgün, İ.; SağnakAkıllı, M.; Gürbüz, E.E.; Güney, L.H.; Hiçsönmez, A. A newborn with caudal duplication and duplex imperforate anus. *J. Pediatr. Surg.* **2013**, *48*, E37–E43. [CrossRef] [PubMed]
2. Dominguez, R.; Rott, J.; Castillo, M.; Pittaluga, R.R.; Corriere, J.N., Jr. Caudal duplicationsyndrome. *Am. J. Dis. Child.* **1993**, *147*, 1048–1052. [PubMed]
3. Hu, T.; Browning, T.; Bishop, K. Caudal duplication syndrome: Imaging evaluation of a rareentity in an adult patient. *Radiol. Case Rep.* **2016**, *11*, 11–15. [CrossRef] [PubMed]
4. Cairo, S.B.; Gasior, A.; Rollins, M.D.; Rothstein, D.H. Challenges in Transition of Care for Patients with Anorectal Malformations: A Systematic Review andRecommendations for Comprehensive Care. *Dis. Colon Rectum* **2018**, *61*, 390–399. [CrossRef]
5. Kyrklund, K.; Pakarinen, M.P.; Rintala, R.J. Long-term bowel function, quality of life andsexual function in patients with anorectal malformations treated during the PSARP era. *Semin. Pediatr. Surg.* **2017**, *26*, 336–342. [CrossRef]
6. De Oliveira, A.; Nascimento, C.; Ramos, D.; Matushita, H. Surgical management of caudalduplication syndrome: A rare entity with a centered approach on quality of life. *Surg. Neurol. Int.* **2019**, *10*, 181, Published 20 September 2019. [CrossRef]
7. Chaussy, Y.; Mottet, N.; Aubert, D.; Auber, F. Caudal duplication syndrome. *J. Pediatr.* **2015**, *166*, 772-2.e1. [CrossRef]
8. Salman, A.B. Cloacal duplication. *J. Pediatr. Surg.* **1996**, *31*, 1587–1588. [CrossRef]
9. Samuk, I.; Levitt, M.; Dlugy, E.; Kravarusic, D.; Ben-Meir, D.; Rajz, G.; Konen, O.; Freud, E. Caudal Duplication Syndrome: The Vital Role of a Multidisciplinary Approach and Staged Correction. *Eur. J. Pediatr. Surg. Rep.* **2016**, *4*, 1. [CrossRef]
10. Bansal, G.; Ghosh, D.; George, U.; Bhatti, W. Unusual coexistence ofcaudal duplication and caudal regression syndromes. *J. Pediatr. Surg.* **2011**, *46*, 256–258. [CrossRef]
11. Spataru, R. The use of mechanical suture in the treatment of Hirschsprung's disease: Experience of 17 cases. *Chirurgia* **2014**, *109*, 208–212. [PubMed]
12. Liu, H.; Che, X.; Wang, S.; Chen, G. Multiple-stage correction of caudal duplication syndrome: A case report. *J. Pediatr. Surg.* **2009**, *44*, 2410–2413. [CrossRef] [PubMed]
13. Bajpai, M.; Das, K.; Gupta, A.K. Caudal duplication syndrome: More evidence for theory ofcaudal twinning. *J. Pediatr. Surg.* **2004**, *39*, 223–225. [CrossRef] [PubMed]
14. Kroes, H.Y.; Takahashi, M.; Zijlstra, R.J.; Baert, J.A.L.L.; Kooi, K.A.; Hofstra, R.M.W.; van Essenet, A.J. Two cases of the caudal duplication anomalyincluding a discordant monozygotic twin. *Am. J. Med. Genet.* **2002**, *112*, 390–393. [CrossRef] [PubMed]
15. Abdelhalim, A.; Arab, H.; Helmy, T.E.; Dawaba, M.E.; Abou-El-Ghar, M.E.; Hafez, A.T. Cloacalduplication: Single-center Experience in the Management of a Rare Anomaly. *Urology* **2017**, *108*, 171–174. [CrossRef]
16. Wisenbaugh, E.S.; Palmer, B.W.; Kropp, B.P. Successful management of a completelyduplicated lower urinary system. *J. Pediatr. Urol.* **2010**, *6*, 315–317. [CrossRef]
17. Chan, Y.Y.; Jayaprakasan, K.; Tan, A.; Thornton, J.G.; Coomarasamy, A.; Raine-Fenning, N.J. Reproductive outcomes in women with congenital uterine anomalies: A systematicreview. *Ultrasound Obstet. Gynecol.* **2011**, *38*, 371–382. [CrossRef]
18. Mei, J.Y.; Nguyen, M.T.; Raz, S. Female Caudal Duplication Syndrome: A Surgical CaseReportWith 10-Year Follow-up and Review of the Literature. *Female Pelvic Med. Reconstr. Surg.* **2018**, *24*, e16–e20. [CrossRef]
19. Becker, K.; Howard, K.; Klazinga, D.; Hall, C.M. Caudal duplication syndrome with unilateralhypoplasia of the pelvis and lower limb and ventriculoseptal heart defect in a mother andfeatures of VATER association in her child. *Clin. Dysmorphol.* **2009**, *18*, 139–141. [CrossRef]
20. Ragab, O.; Landay, M.; Shriki, J. Complete cloacal duplication imaged before and duringpregnancy. *J. Radiol. Case Rep.* **2009**, *3*, 24–28.
21. Mathiesen, A.M.; Frost, C.J.; Dent, K.M.; Feldkamp, M.L. Parental needs among children withbirth defects: Defining a parent-to-parent support network. *J. Genet. Couns.* **2012**, *21*, 862–872. [CrossRef] [PubMed]

22. Swaika, S.; Basu, S.; Bhadra, R.C.; Sarkar, R.; Maitra, S.K. Caudal duplication syndrome-reportof a case and review of literature. *Indian J. Surg.* **2013**, *75* (Suppl. S1), 484–487. [CrossRef] [PubMed]
23. Tarciuc, P.; Stănescu, A.M.A.; Diaconu, C.C.; Păduraru, L.; Duduciuc, A.; Diaconescu, S. Patterns and factors associated with self-medication among the pediatric population in Romania. *Medicina* **2020**, *56*, 312. [CrossRef] [PubMed]

Publisher's Note: MDPI stays neutral with regard to jurisdictional claims in published maps and institutional affiliations.

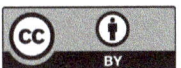

© 2020 by the authors. Licensee MDPI, Basel, Switzerland. This article is an open access article distributed under the terms and conditions of the Creative Commons Attribution (CC BY) license (http://creativecommons.org/licenses/by/4.0/).

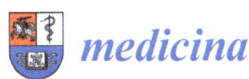

Case Report

Primary Pleural Hydatidosis—A Rare Occurrence: A Case Report and Literature Review

Cornel Savu [1,2], Alexandru Melinte [1], Vasile Grigorie [1], Laura Iliescu [2,3], Camelia Diaconu [2,4], Mihai Dimitriu [2,5], Bogdan Socea [6], Ovidiu Stiru [2,7], Valentin Varlas [2,8], Carmen Savu [9], Irina Balescu [10] and Nicolae Bacalbasa [2,11,*]

1. Department of Thoracic Surgery, "Marius Nasta" National Institute of Pneumophtisiology, 050152 Bucharest, Romania; drsavu25@yahoo.com (C.S.); alexandru.melinte@gmail.ro (A.M.); vasile.grigorie@gmail.ro (V.G.)
2. Internal Medicine Department, "Carol Davila" University of Medicine and Pharmacy, 020021 Bucharest, Romania; laura.iliescu@gmail.ro (L.I.); drcameliadiaconu@gmail.com (C.D.); mihai.dimitriu@gmail.ro (M.D.); ovidiu.stiru@gmail.ro (O.S.); valentine.varlas@gmail.ro (V.V.)
3. Department of Internal Medicine, "Fundeni" Clinical Institute, 022328 Bucharest, Romania
4. Department of Internal Medicine, Clinical Emergency Hospital of Bucharest, 105402 Bucharest, Romania
5. Department of Obstetrics and Gynecology, "Sf. Pantelimon" Emergency Clinical Hospital, 021661 Bucharest, Romania
6. Department of Surgery, "Sf. Pantelimon" Clinical Hospital, 021661 Bucharest, Romania; bogdan.socea@gmail.ro
7. Department of Cardiovascular Surgery, "Prof. Dr. C.C. Iliescu" Emergency Institute for Cardiovascular Diseases, 022322 Bucharest, Romania
8. Department of Obstetrics and Gynecology, "Filantropia" Hospital, 011171 Bucharest, Romania
9. Department of Anesthesiology, "Fundeni" Clinical Institute, 022328 Bucharest, Romania; carmen.savu@gmail.ro
10. Department of Visceral Surgery, "Ponderas" Academic Hospital, Bucharest, 021188 Bucharest, Romania; irina.balescu@ponderas-ah.ro
11. Center of Excellence in Translational Medicine, Department of Visceral Surgery, "Fundeni" Clinical Institute, 022328 Bucharest, Romania
* Correspondence: nicolae_bacalbasa@yahoo.ro; Tel.: +40-723-540-426

Received: 15 July 2020; Accepted: 20 October 2020; Published: 27 October 2020

Abstract: *Introduction*: The larvae of Echinococcus, a parasitic tapeworm, cause hydatid disease. The most commonly involved organ after the liver is the lung but there are cases of hydatid cysts in all systems and organs, such as brain, muscle tissue, adrenal glands, mediastinum and pleural cavity. Extra-pulmonary intrathoracic hydatidosis can be a diagnostic challenge and a plain chest x-ray can be misleading. It can also lead to severe complications such as anaphylactic shock or tension pneumothorax. The purpose of this paper is to present a severe case of primary pleural hydatidosis, as well as discussing the difficulties that come with it during diagnosis and treatment. *Case Report*: We present the case of a 43-year-old male, working as a shepherd, presenting with moderate dyspnea, chest pain and weight loss. Chest x-ray revealed an uncharacteristic massive right pleural effusion and thoracic computed tomography (CT) confirmed it, as well as revealing multiple cystic formations of various sizes and liquid density within the pleural fluid. Blood work confirmed our suspicion of pleural hydatidosis with an elevated eosinophil count, typical in parasite diseases. Surgery was performed by right lateral thoracotomy and consisted of removal of the hydatid fluid and cysts found in the pleura. Patient was discharged 13 days postoperative with Albendazole treatment. *Conclusion*: Cases of primary pleural hydatidosis are very rare but must be taken into consideration in patients from endemic regions with jobs that may have exposure to this parasite. Proper treatment, both surgical and antiparasitic medication, can lead to a full recovery and a low chance of recurrent disease.

Keywords: primary; pleural; hydatidosis; Albendazole; echinoccocus

1. Introduction

Hydatidosis is a parasitic disease caused by the Echinococcus larvae. There are four species of worms responsible for the presence of this disease in humans; however, the most frequent ones that cause cystic echinococcosis are granulosus, 95% of cases, and multilocularis. Echinococcus is a zoonotic disease requiring two mammals, one intermediate host (sheep or cattle) and the definitive host in dogs, wolves or foxes [1].

Batsch first described the form of Echinoccocus granulosus in 1786 and the first case described in the literature of a hydatid cyst is attributed to Bremser in 1821 [2]. In 1908, Rudolphi published a parasitology treaty where the term of hydatid cyst was first used [3]. In most cases, the primary localization of hydatid cysts is in the liver (60–80% of cases) with the lung being the second most common location (10–30%). In the remaining 10–15% of cases, either by haematogenous or lymphatic dissemination or through the veno-venous anastomosis of the Retzius space, the parasite can be found in any organ, tissue or cavity [4]. Primary pleural hydatid cyst is a very rare occurrence and is most often solitary [5].

Human contamination occurs by ingestion of parasite eggs by contaminated food, water or direct contact with the host. Even if hydatid cysts can develop anywhere in the body, liver and lung development are the most common. Pleural hydatidosis is a very rare disease, most cases being secondary to peripheral lung cysts that rupture or herniate in the pleural cavity.

Primary pleural hydatid cysts fall under the category of extra-pulmonary intrathoracic cysts, alongside those found in the parietal pleura, mediastinum, pericardium, diaphragm, fissures and chest wall, by either lymphatic or hematogenous dissemination.

2. Case Presentation

A 43-year-old male came into our department complaining of chest pain, dyspnea, persistent cough and weight loss; symptoms appeared during the last three months. From the patient history, we found that he was a heavy smoker, occasional consumer of ethanol as well as working with livestock as a shepherd. A routine chest x-ray showed a massive pleural effusion in the right hemithorax, with multiple round-shaped opacities within it. Blood work revealed an elevated eosinophil level (10%) with no other modified parameters. To confirm our suspicion of hydatid disease, we performed a thoracic CT scan, which revealed a large pleural effusion with multiple cystic formations of varying sizes within it (Figure 1).

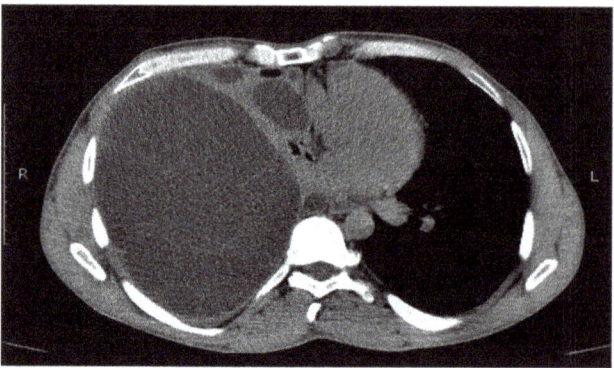

Figure 1. Computed tomography (CT) view of primary pleural hydatid disease.

After complete investigation of the patient, we started preoperative antiparasitic treatment with Albendazole 15 mg/kg/day for 6 days and then surgery was performed by using a lateral thoracotomy through the fifth intercostal space. After opening the pleural cavity, we introduced a hypertonic saline solution as well as oxygenated water 10% in order to inactivate the scolices. After draining approximately 4 L of ivory-colored fluid from the pleural cavity we discovered several hundred hydatid cysts with sizes ranging from 1–2 mm to 5–6 cm and the right lung was collapsed in the hilum. Cysts were round, well defined with a clear liquid content. Besides the intact cysts, we also found several ruptured ones, which evacuated and further contaminated the pleural cavity (Figure 2).

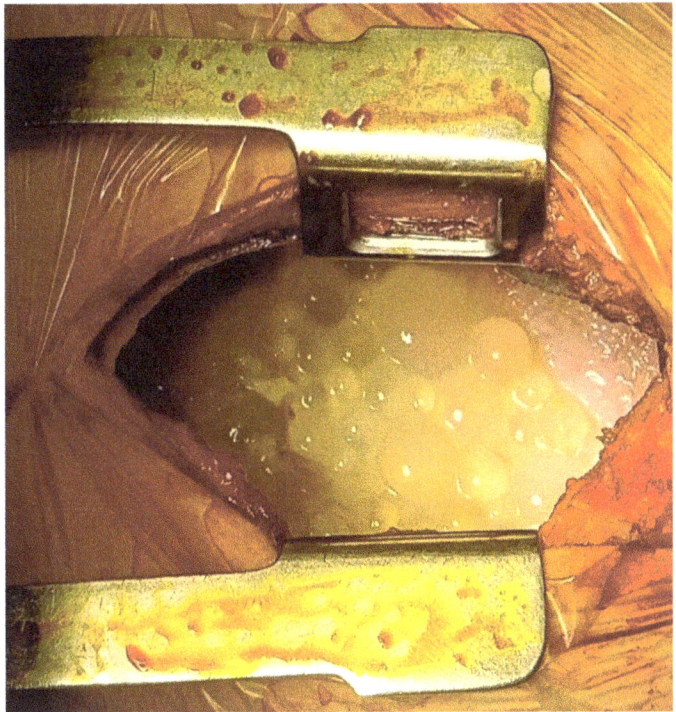

Figure 2. Intraoperative view of primary pleural hydatidosis.

After removing all the cysts from the pleural space, we performed several more pleural lavages using a hypertonic saline solution as well as an iodine solution. Further inspection revealed no other cysts in the lung, pleura, diaphragm, mediastinum or pericardium. In addition, there was no sign of rupture or migration of the cyst from any other thoracic organ, leading us to conclude that it was a primary pleural hydatidosis. Before closing, we inflated the lung and there was no air leakage and no other visible lesions on the parenchyma. We placed a single chest drain and the thoracotomy was closed in layers.

Parasitological tests performed on the pleural liquid as well as the parasitic material removed during surgery confirmed the presence of Echinoccocus. Additionally, IGG-specific ELISA tests performed from the pleural liquid confirmed the same.

Chest x-ray performed first day postoperative showed an almost fully expanded lung with no fluid or pneumothorax and a pleural drainage of approximatively 600 mL. The patient also received antiparasitic treatment with Albendazole 15 mg/kg/day. The patient spent 2 days in the intensive care unit (ICU) and was discharged on the 13th postoperative day with the indication of continuing Albendazole treatment for 1 year with 15 mg/kg/day due to the severity of the disease.

Follow-up showed no signs of recurrence with a normal chest x-ray and an improved lung volume function at one month, 6 months and 1 year.

3. Discussion

Larvae of the Echinoccocus parasite cause hydatid disease and humans are an accidental host either from consuming contaminated meat or from unwashed fruits and vegetables [1].

Dévé published the first significant study on secondary pleural hydatid disease in 1937 and his conclusions were that all pleural presentations of hydatidosis were secondary to either a lung or liver dome cyst that ruptured into the pleural space, stating that primary pleural hydatidosis does not exist [6]. However, future case reports, such as that of Rakower published in 1964, point to the existence of this pathology [7].

Although most hydatic cysts form in the liver or the lung, due to the possibility of haematogenous dissemination, lesions can develop anywhere in the body. Most common cause of pleural hydatidosis is by either trans-diaphragmatic contamination from cysts located in the right upper hepatic lobe or from the rupture of a peripheral lung cyst [8].

Primary pleural hydatid cysts fall under the category of extra-pulmonary intrathoracic cysts, alongside those found in the parietal pleura, mediastinum, pericardium, diaphragm, fissures and chest wall. Primary pleural hydatidosis manifests as the presence of either a solitary pleural hydatid cyst or as a parasitic pleural effusion [5]. Massive pleural effusions are usually of malignant origin (58% of cases), parapneumonic (23%), tuberculosis (10%), with the remaining cases having diverse origins [9]. Parasitic pleural effusion developed in the case of Echinoccocus is more frequently found as a complication of either a pulmonary hydatid cyst that ruptures in the pleura or as a liver hydatid cyst with intrathoracic development. Parasitic pleural effusion is extremely rare and unusual in medical practice [10].

Primary pleural hydatidosis is found in less than 1% of hydatidosis cases [11]. In our case, we could not find any lesions of the pulmonary parenchyma or any other thoracic lesion. Due to this, we concluded that in our case the diagnosis was that of primary pleural hydatidosis. Although not frequent, primary pleural hydatidosis has been presented as an exceptional situation for hepatic hydatidosis [12,13]. Primary development of a hydatid cyst within the parietal pleural structures is possible and can later lead to hydatid pleural effusion. The histological structure of the cystic membranes allows the passage of calcium, magnesium, water, urea as well as other nutritional substances that may pass through by diffusion and favor the development of the cyst [14].

The symptoms presented depend on the localization of the cyst and the degree of compression of the local organs [15]. There have also been reports of primary hydatid cysts in various organs such as the heart [16], soft tissue [17], adrenal gland [18] and brain [19].

Symptoms of pleural hydatidosis are similar to those found in pleural effusions such as dyspnea, mediastinal shift and reduction in lung volume. Even so, up to 15% of cases can be asymptomatic [20]. However, these can also be present alongside chest pain and other signs of cardiac or vascular involvement or compression [21]. Hydatid disease is also a rare cause of recurrent acute pulmonary embolism. This complication may develop after invasion of the cardiovascular system or direct invasion of the inferior vena cava [22].

In diagnosing hydatid disease, the most important part is played by imaging studies. Standard chest radiography alongside computed tomography, not only helps in diagnosing the disease but it also plays a role in the planning of surgery. Some radiological signs are pathognomonic for hydatid disease such as the presence of daughter cysts, water-lily sign (for ruptured cysts), and serpent sign (ruptured and completely evacuated cysts) [23]. Other tests such as skin tests, complement fixation, blood eosinophil count and indirect hemagglutination tests can be used, but must be interpreted carefully as they have a tendency towards false-positive results [24]. In addition, even if an ultrasound would be very useful in diagnosing liver cysts, it is rarely used for cysts in the thorax, with the exception of a chest wall hydatid cyst [25,26].

However, information provided by performing an ultrasound in such cases might bring significant information, complementary to those reported by other imagistic studies such as computed tomography; moreover, it can be safely performed in pregnant patients in whom such lesions are suspected [27,28]. Therefore, in pleural hydatidosis ultrasound might reveal suggestive aspects such as complex cystic lesions presenting double line sign whenever collapsed membranes exist [27]. In this respect, ultrasound has been successfully added as part of the examination tools in cases in which intrathoracic extrapulmonary hydatidosis is suspected, Gursoy et al. reporting the successful use of this method in a case series of 14 patients [14].

Although fine needle aspiration is recommended in the diagnosing of primary liver hydatid cysts, due to the high risk of complications such as pneumothorax, haemoptysis, cyst rupture, anaphylaxis and dissemination, performing this procedure on cysts located in the lung is not advised [29]. If we were to ignore the risks associated with this procedure and perform it, the most likely result is the discovery of hydatid material in the aspirated liquid.

However, in particular cases, puncture might orientate the diagnostic; therefore, in pregnant patients in whom the imagistic methods of evaluation are restricted due to the risk of fetal irradiation, performing an ultrasound examination and an ultrasound guided puncture might serve as an important diagnostic tool; therefore, in the case presented by a French study group and published in 2011 the authors reported the case of a 23-year-old patient who was investigated during the 22nd week of pregnancy for chest pain and dyspnea in association with pneumothorax; after performing puncture and establishing the diagnostic, the patient was further submitted to surgery, the cystic mass being removed; meanwhile, two bronchial fistulas were identified which were successfully sutured while the remaining cavity was capitonnaged [28].

The most common preoperative complications that may occur in pleural or lung hydatid disease include empyema and pneumothorax [30], but there are rare cases where, due to the rupture of the cysts, the patient can suffer from anaphylactic shock. There have even been cases of patients presenting with tension pneumothorax caused by the rupture of a lung cyst [31]. Several representative studies with patients with pulmonary hydatid cysts concluded that the rupture of the cyst in the pleural cavity is the most severe complication of the disease, alongside anaphylactic shock [32].

The main treatment in hydatid disease consists of surgery followed by medical treatment with antiparasitic medication. For pulmonary hydatid disease, the most common surgical approach is by thoracotomy and resection of the cysts. However, when the disease is present bilateral a median sternotomy is preferable [24]. The main goal of surgery is complete removal of the germinative membrane after inactivation using a hypertonic saline solution [33]. Standard surgical procedure consists of cystectomy and capitonnage; however, there are cases when an extended resection is necessary when the surrounding tissue is diffusely involved or there is presence of local infection or giant cysts. In all cases, local contamination during surgery must be avoided using a hypertonic saline solution to inactivate the cysts. If this is not performed thoroughly the chances of a recurrent disease increase significantly [34]. There are however several authors that consider that capitonnage is not necessary after cystectomy and that only the bronchial openings should be sutured and the cavity should be left open, arguing that capitonnage causes lung disfigurement, prolongs the operating time and increasing morbidity [35,36]. For primary pleural hydatidosis, the same surgical principles apply when it comes to approach and case management. Removal of the cysts and pleural fluid after inactivation with hypertonic saline solution is mandatory, followed by chest drainage paired with Albendazole treatment [14].

Antiparasitic treatment plays a key role in the management of any form of hydatidosis. Most authors recommend treatment with one of two benzimidazole carbamates, Albendazole or Mebendazole, which are the only drugs that interrupt larval growth of Echinoccocus species. Some authors consider that preoperative antiparasitic treatment is very useful, especially in severe forms of illness, and that it would reduce the recurrence by up to three and a half times [37]. In our opinion, preoperative antiparasitic treatment is extremely useful, especially in severe cases with a high risk of recurrence and intraoperative dissemination, such as the case we have presented.

The most used treatment is with Albendazole, while Mebendazole is only used as an alternative due to its adverse effects. However, antiparasitic treatment is recommended as anti-infection therapy, while the main course of treatment remains surgical [38].

As it can be observed, primary pleural hydatidosis is a rare entity, only rare cases being reported so far; experience gathered at this moment is rather related to case reports or case series presenting cases of patients diagnosed with intrathoracic extrapulmonary hydatidosis in general. Data published so far regarding this pathological entity are summarized into Table 1.

Table 1. Cases reported so far diagnosed with primary pleural hydatidosis.

Name, Year	Period of the Study	No. of Cases	Location of the Lesion	Surgical Treatment	Associated Resections (no. of Cases)	Medical Treatment	Postoperative Complications
Gursoy et al., 2009 [14]	2003–2007	14	Diaphragm Chest wall Mediastinum Pleura Pericardial cavity	Cystectomy Decortication Resection and repair of the adjacent organs	Costal resection-3 pericardial resection-1	Albendazole 10 mg/kg during the next 3 months postoperatively	None
Marghli et al., 2011 [28]	2011	1	Pleural hydatid cyst in a 23-year-old pregnant woman	Removal of the cyst, suture on the bronchial fistula, capitonnage	None	Not reported	Uneventful
Mardani et al., 2017 [13]	2017	1	Pleural hydatidosis in a 33-year-old woman	Removal of the cyst, complete lung expansion	None	Not reported	Uneventful
Tewari et al., 2009 [12]	2009	1	Pleural hydatidosis in a 28-year-old woman	Removal of the cyst	None	Albendazole	Uneventful
Rakower et al., 1964 [7]	1954–1964	3	Mediastinum Chest wall Pleura	Removal of the cysts	Pleural resection	Not reported	One patient died due to septic shock

4. Conclusions

There are very few cases of primary pleural hydatidosis reported in the literature. In our case, it was a diagnosis of exclusion for hydatid cysts within the pleural cavity, but with no obvious primary lesion that would explain the local contamination.

Cases of primary pleural hydatidosis are very rare but must be taken into consideration in patients from endemic regions with jobs that may have exposure to this parasite. Proper treatment, both surgical and antiparasitic medication, can lead to a full recovery and a low chance of recurrent disease.

Antiparasitic treatment plays a key role in the management of any form of hydatidosis; however, the main course of treatment is surgical.

Author Contributions: C.S. (Cornel Savu), V.G., A.M. —performed surgical procedures; I.B., M.D., B.S.—prepared the manuscript; I.B., C.D., C.S. (Carmen Savu), O.S. and V.V.—performed data analysis; L.I., N.B.—advised about the surgical oncology procedure, revised the final draft of the manuscript. All the authors agreed with the final version of the manuscript. All authors have read and agreed to the published version of the manuscript.

Funding: This research received no external funding.

Conflicts of Interest: The authors declare no conflict of interest.

References

1. Romig, T.; Deplazes, P.; Jenkins, D.; Giraudoux, P.; Massolo, A.; Craig, P.S.; Wassermann, M.; Takahashi, K.; De La Rue, M. Ecology and Life Cycle Patterns of Echinococcus Species. *Adv. Parasitol.* **2017**, *95*, 213–314. [PubMed]
2. Romero-Torres, R.; Campbell, J.R. An Interpretive Review of the Surgical Treatment of Hydatid Disease. *Surg. Gynecol. Obstet.* **1965**, *121*, 851–864. [PubMed]
3. Aletras, H.; Symbas, P.N. Hydatid disease of the lung. In *General Thoracic Surgery*; Shields, T.W., Ed.; Lippincott Williams & Wilkins: Philadelphia, PA, USA, 2000; Volume 1, pp. 1113–1122.
4. Barrett, N.R. The Anatomy and the Pathology of Multiple Hydatid Cysts in the Thorax. *Ann. R. Coll. Surg. Engl.* **1960**, *26*, 362–379. [PubMed]
5. Hormati, A.; Alemi, F.; Eshraghi, M.; Ghoddoosi, M.; Mohaddes, M.; Momeni, S. Trans-Diaphragmatic Rupture of Liver Hydatid Cyst in to the Pleural Cavity: A Case Report. *Arch. Clin. Infect. Dis.* **2020**, in press. [CrossRef]
6. Dévé, F. L'echinococcose secondaire de la plevre. *J. Chir.* **1937**, *4*, 497.
7. Rakower, J.; Milwidsky, H. Hydatid Pleural Disease. *Am. Rev. Respir. Dis.* **1964**, *90*, 623–631. [PubMed]
8. Pedrosa, I.; Saiz, A.; Arrazola, J.; Ferreiros, J.; Pedrosa, C.S. Hydatid Disease: Radiologic and Pathologic Features and Complications. *Radiographics* **2000**, *20*, 795–817. [CrossRef] [PubMed]
9. Porcel, J.M.; Vives, M. Etiology and Pleural Fluid Characteristics of Large and Massive Effusions. *Chest* **2003**, *124*, 978–983. [CrossRef] [PubMed]
10. Bajpai, J.; Jain, A.; Kar, A.; Kant, S.; Bajaj, D.K. "Necklace in the Lung:" Multilocularis Hydatid Cyst Mimicking Left-Sided Massive Pleural Effusion. *Lung India* **2019**, *36*, 550–552. [PubMed]
11. Erkoc, M.F.; Oztoprak, B.; Alkan, S.; Okur, A. A Rare Cause of Pleural Effusion: Ruptured Primary Pleural Hydatid Cyst. *BMJ Case. Rep.* **2014**, *2014*, bcr2013202959. [CrossRef] [PubMed]
12. Tewari, M.; Kumar, V.; Shukla, H.S. Primary Pleural Hydatid Cyst. *Indian J. Surg.* **2009**, *71*, 106. [CrossRef] [PubMed]
13. Mardani, P.; Karami, M.Y.; Jamshidi, K.; Zadebagheri, N.; Niakan, H. A Primary Pleural Hydatid Cyst in an Unusual Location. *Tanaffos* **2017**, *16*, 166–169. [PubMed]
14. Gursoy, S.; Ucvet, A.; Tozum, H.; Erbaycu, A.E.; Kul, C.; Basok, O. Primary Intrathoracic Extrapulmonary Hydatid Cysts: Analysis of 14 Patients with a Rare Clinical Entity. *Tex. Heart Inst. J.* **2009**, *36*, 230–233. [PubMed]
15. Elhassani, N.B.; Taha, A.Y. Management of Pulmonary Hydatid Disease: Review of 66 Cases from Iraq. *Case Rep. Clin. Med.* **2015**, *4*, 77–84. [CrossRef]
16. Debi, U.; Singh, L.; Maralakunte, M.; Karthik, R.; Singhal, M. Papillary Muscle Hydatid of Heart: A Rare Case of Disseminated Hydatidosis in A Young Female with Multisystemic Involvement. *Arch Clin. Med. Case Rep.* **2020**, *4*, 409–415. [CrossRef]
17. Alam, M.; Hasan, S.A.; Hashmi, S.F. Unusual Presentation of Hydatidosis—Neck Lump Causing Costo-Vertebral Erosion. *Iran J. Otorhinolaryngol.* **2016**, *28*, 363–367.
18. Zouari, S.; Marouene, C.; Bibani, H.; Saadi, A.; Sellami, A.; Haj, K.L.; Blel, A.; Bouzouita, A.; Derouiche, A.; Ben Slama, R.; et al. Primary Hydatid Cyst of the Adrenal Gland: A Case Report and a Review of the Literature. *Int. J. Surg. Case. Rep.* **2020**, *70*, 154–158. [CrossRef]
19. Alok, R.; Mahmoud, J. Successful Surgical Treatment of a Brain Stem Hydatid Cyst in a Child. *Case. Rep. Surg.* **2020**, *2020*, 5645812. [CrossRef]
20. Judson, M.A.; Sahn, S.A. Pulmonary physiologic abnormalities caused by pleural disease. In *Seminars in Respiratory and Critical Care Medicine*; Thieme Medical Publishers, Inc.: New York, NY, USA, 1995; Volume 16, pp. 346–353.
21. Horvat, T.; Savu, C.; Motaș, C.; Țețu, M. Pneumopericardium—Complication of an unknown tuberculosis in a HIV positive patient. *Eur. J. Cardio Thorac. Surg.* **2004**, *26*, 1043. [CrossRef]
22. Hirzalla, M.O.; Samara, N.; Ateyat, B.; Tarawneh, M.; Swaiss, A.; el Hussieni, T.; Ammari, B. Recurrent Hydatid Pulmonary Emboli. *Am. Rev. Respir. Dis.* **1989**, *140*, 1082–1085. [CrossRef]
23. Kervancioglu, R.; Bayram, M.; Elbeyli, L. CT Findings in Pulmonary Hydatid Disease. *Acta Radiol.* **1999**, *40*, 510–514. [CrossRef] [PubMed]

24. Ulku, R.; Eren, N.; Cakir, O.; Balci, A.; Onat, S. Extrapulmonary Intrathoracic Hydatid Cysts. *Can. J. Surg.* **2004**, *47*, 95–98. [PubMed]
25. Pendse, H.A.; Nawale, A.J.; Deshpande, S.S.; Merchant, S.A. Radiologic features of hydatid disease: The importance of sonography. *J. Ultrasound Med.* **2015**, *34*, 895–905. [CrossRef] [PubMed]
26. Dediu, M.; Horvat, T.; Tarlea, A.; Anghel, R.; Cordos, I.; Miron, G.; Iorga, P.; Alexandru, A.; Nistor, C.; Grozavu, C. Adjuvant chemotherapy for radically resected non-small cell lung cancer: A retrospective analysis of 311 consecutively treated patients. *Lung Cancer* **2005**, *47*, 93–101. [CrossRef] [PubMed]
27. Von Sinner, W.N. Ultrasound, CT and MRI of Ruptured and Disseminated Hydatid Cysts. *Eur. J. Radiol.* **1990**, *11*, 31–37. [CrossRef]
28. Marghli, A.; Ayadi-Kaddour, A.; Ouerghi, S.; Boudaya, M.S.; Zairi, S.; Smati, B.; Mestiri, T.; Kilani, T. Primary Heterotopic Pleural Hydatid Cyst Presenting As a Pneumothorax. *Rev. Mal. Respir.* **2011**, *28*, 344–347. [CrossRef]
29. Marla, N.J.; Marla, J.; Kamath, M.; Tantri, G.; Jayaprakash, C. Primary Hydatid Cyst of the Lung: A Review of the Literature. *J. Clin. Diagn. Res.* **2012**, *6*, 1313–1315.
30. Yousaf, A.; Badshah, A.; Khan, M.M.; Ahmad, M.; Ahmad, N. Hydatidosis; experience with surgical management of concomitant liver and lung disease. *KJMS* **2019**, *12*, 227–231.
31. Acharya, A.B.; Bhatta, N.; Mishra, D.R.; Verma, A.; Shahi, R. Rare Cause of Tension Pneumothorax: Hydatid Disease of Lung: A Case Report. *JNMA. J. Nepal. Med. Assoc.* **2020**, *58*, 265–268.
32. Issoufou, I.; Harmouchi, H.; Rabiou, S.; Belliraj, L.; Ammor, F.Z.; Diarra, A.S.; Lakranbi, M.; Sani, R.; Ouadnouni, Y.; Smahi, M. The Surgery of Diaphragmatic Hydatidosis and Their Complications. *Rev. Pneumol. Clin.* **2017**, *73*, 253–257. [CrossRef]
33. Tiwari, S.; Pate, R. Hydatid Cyst Presenting with Massive Unilateral Pleural Effusion. *Ann. Clin. Case Rep.* **2019**, *4*, 1768.
34. Tor, M.; Atasalihi, A.; Altuntas, N.; Sulu, E.; Senol, T.; Kir, A.; Baran, R. Review of Cases with Cystic Hydatid Lung Disease in a Tertiary Referral Hospital Located in an Endemic Region: A 10 Years' Experience. *Respiration* **2000**, *67*, 539–542. [CrossRef] [PubMed]
35. Taha, A.Y. To close or not to close: An enduring controversy. *Arch. Int. Surg.* **2013**, *3*, 254–255. [CrossRef]
36. Savu, C.; Melinte, A.; Posea, R.; Galie, N.; Balescu, I.; Diaconu, C.; Cretoiu, D.; Dima, S.; Filipescu, A.; Balalau, C. Pleural Solitary Fibrous Tumors—A Retrospective Study on 45 Patients. *Medicina* **2020**, *56*, 185. [CrossRef] [PubMed]
37. El On, J. Benzimidazole Treatment of Cystic Echinococcosis. *Acta Trop.* **2003**, *85*, 243–252. [CrossRef]
38. Wen, H.; Vuitton, L.; Tuxun, T.; Li, J.; Vuitton, D.A.; Zhang, W.; McManus, D.P. Echinococcosis: Advances in the 21st Century. *Clin. Microbiol. Rev.* **2019**, *32*, e00075-18. [CrossRef]

Publisher's Note: MDPI stays neutral with regard to jurisdictional claims in published maps and institutional affiliations.

© 2020 by the authors. Licensee MDPI, Basel, Switzerland. This article is an open access article distributed under the terms and conditions of the Creative Commons Attribution (CC BY) license (http://creativecommons.org/licenses/by/4.0/).

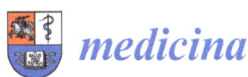

Article

Real-World Data Analysis of Pregnancy-Associated Breast Cancer at a Tertiary-Level Hospital in Romania

Anca A. Simionescu [1,*], Alexandra Horobeț [2], Lucian Belașcu [3] and Dragoș Mircea Median [4,*]

1. Department of Obstetrics and Gynecology, Carol Davila University of Medicine and Pharmacy, Filantropia Clinical Hospital, 011171 Bucharest, Romania
2. Department of International Business and Economics, The Bucharest University of Economic Studies, 010374 Bucharest, Romania; alexandra.horobet@rei.ase.ro
3. Department of Management, Marketing and Business Administration, Lucian Blaga University of Sibiu, 550024 Sibiu, Romania; lucian.belascu@ulbsibiu.ro
4. Gynecologic Oncology Department, Filantropia Clinical Hospital Bucharest, 011171 Bucharest, Romania
* Correspondence: anca.simionescu@umfcd.ro (A.A.S.); dragos.median@gmail.com (D.M.M.); Tel.: +40-021-3188937 (A.A.S. & D.M.M.)

Received: 27 August 2020; Accepted: 1 October 2020; Published: 6 October 2020

Abstract: *Background and objectives:* Breast cancer is among the most common cancer types encountered during pregnancy. Here, we aimed to describe the characteristics, management, and outcomes of women with pregnancy-associated breast cancer at a tertiary-level hospital in Romania. *Material and Methods:* We retrospectively and prospectively collected demographic, oncological, and obstetrical data for women diagnosed with cancer during pregnancy, and who elected to continue their pregnancy, between June 2012 and June 2020. Complete data were obtained regarding family and personal medical history and risks factors, cancer diagnosis and staging, clinical and pathological features (including histology and immunohistochemistry), multimodal cancer treatment, pregnancy management (fetal ultrasounds, childbirth, and postpartum data), and infant development and clinical evolution up to 2020. Cancer therapy was administered following national guidelines and institutional protocols and regimens developed for non-pregnant patients, including surgery and chemotherapy, while avoiding radiotherapy during pregnancy. *Results:* At diagnosis, 16.67% of patients were in an advanced/metastatic stage, while 75% were in early operable stages. However, the latter patients underwent neoadjuvant chemotherapy rather than up-front surgery due to aggressive tumor biology (triple negative, multifocal, or HER2+). No patient achieved complete pathological remission, but only one patient relapsed. No recurrence was recorded within 12 months among early-stage patients. *Conclusions:* In this contemporary assessment of real-world treatment patterns and outcomes among patients with pregnancy-associated breast cancer, our findings were generally consistent with globally observed treatment outcomes, underscoring the need for a multidisciplinary team and reference centers.

Keywords: breast cancer; pregnancy-associated breast cancer; Romania

1. Introduction

Breast cancer (BC) is the most frequent female cancer worldwide, and the leading cause of cancer-related death among women [1]. It is also one of the most common types of cancer encountered during pregnancy [2,3]. Data regarding the global burden of disease between 1990–2017 among Romanian women of fertile age (15–49 years) reveal that although the number of BC-related deaths has decreased, the importance of BC as a cause of mortality has increased by 38.51%. The estimated probability of pregnancy-associated breast cancer (PABC) is 1.29/100,000 among women aged 15–49 years, mainly due to pregnancy at an older age. We expect 59 new cases of PABC per year in Romania (Appendix A).

PABC guidelines were first introduced in 1999 [4]. Since then, substantial progress has been made regarding management and follow-up care. In 2017, Romania joined the International Network on Cancer, Infertility, and Pregnancy (INCIP). Globally, PABC accounts for 0.2–7% of BC cases [5–7]. PABC is not a single disease, but rather several diseases distinguished by the biological effects of pregnancy, variations in serum hormone levels [8], extracellular matrix modifications, and distinctive gene expression patterns in mammary epithelial cells [9]. Research over recent decades has focused on identifying potential PABC biomarkers [10]. Cancer screening can be performed in pregnant women by using a non-invasive prenatal screening test (NIPT) involving plasma cell-free DNA sequencing [11]. Higher maternal serum levels of cell-free DNA (cfDNA) are detected in cases of PABC with a euploid fetus, likely due to both harbored fragments of cell-free fetal DNA and cell-free tumoral DNA [12–14]. It has been hypothesized that hypertension during pregnancy or preeclampsia may decrease the risk of breast cancer development [15–17].

Traditionally, BC is considered PABC when the disease is diagnosed during pregnancy or in the first postpartum year [18,19]. Breast cancer diagnosed between 1 and 10 years after childbirth in women under 45 years of age seems to be a different entity, carrying increased risks of distant metastases and death, which can be explained at the molecular level by the phenomenon of breast involution [20,21].

In the recent past, the diagnosis of breast cancer during pregnancy has often been followed by induced abortion, as many doctors, patients, and patients' relatives have been concerned about the poor prognosis and high risk of maternal death or fetal adverse reaction following the disease or treatments. However, therapeutic abortion is no longer routinely recommended upon PABC diagnosis. With the application of a standard treatment, experts consider the prognosis of cancer during pregnancy to be similar to that in non-pregnant patients [22]. Studies have shown that BC diagnosis during pregnancy may be delayed due to the fact that this pathology is not specific to pregnancy, and because of the physiological increase of mammary gland size [23]. Staging and treatment regimens for PABC are similar in non-pregnant patients. Surgery and sentinel lymph nodes biopsy (SNB) are allowed during pregnancy, despite controversial findings regarding the safety and accuracy of the results [24,25]. SNB in pregnant breast cancer patients appears to be safe and accurate using either methylene blue dye or technetium 99 m (99 mTc) sulfur colloid and gamma probe according to a retrospective study [25]. However, recommendations from the American Society of Clinical Oncology (ASCO) still state that pregnant patients should not undergo sentinel lymph node biopsy (SLNB), based on cohort studies and informal consensus [26]. In contrast with ASCO, The National Comprehensive Cancer Network NCCN concluded that insufficient data exist on which to base recommendations regarding the use of SLNB in pregnant women and SLNB should not be offered to pregnant women under 30 weeks of gestation [27].

During surgery, pregnant women are considered at increased risk of hypoxemia, desaturation, and thrombosis. The more advanced the term, the more difficult it is to intubate, especially obese pregnant patients. The patient should be positioned as far as possible in the left lateral position to avoid aortocaval compression and hypotension that decreases uterine vascularization. Intraoperative cardiotocography for fetal heart rate monitoring may indicate a reduced fetal heart rate variability during general anesthesia. Administration of intravenous tocolytic drugs, e.g., betamimetics or atosiban may be used for the inhibition of uterine contractility [28,29].

In the second or third trimester, adjuvant or neoadjuvant chemotherapy (CMT) regimens include anthracycline-based treatment, followed by taxanes (paclitaxel and docetaxel) [30–33], and the main known fetal risks include intrauterine growth restriction and a small-for-gestational age newborn. During the postpartum period, the recommended treatment includes anti-HER-2 targeted therapy for HER-2+ tumors, and endocrine therapy for oestrogen-receptor (ER)-positive tumors. Radiotherapy is considered relatively safe during the first and second trimesters of pregnancy, although this is based on theoretical assumptions and few experiences [34,35]. In utero radiation exposure of >10 mGy has been associated with microcephaly, childhood cancers, and mental retardation [36–40]. Radiotherapy during pregnancy remains controversial. Some guidelines suggest that it can be safely used in the first or second trimester of pregnancy [19], while Romanian guidelines contraindicate radiotherapy for BC during pregnancy [41].

Upon diagnosis of cancer during pregnancy, selection of the optimal treatment approach requires a multidisciplinary team of healthcare professionals—including an obstetrician, a specialist in maternal–fetal medicine, a medical oncologist, an oncology surgeon, a pediatrician, a geneticist, a psycho-oncologist, and a radiotherapist. A multidisciplinary team can advise the patient and her family about the available treatment regimens, the potential risks for both the mother and the fetus, the prognosis, and the necessity of a long-term follow-up.

In the present study, we aimed to describe the characteristics, management, and follow-up care of women with PABC at a tertiary-level hospital in Romania.

2. Materials and Methods

We performed retrospective and prospective collection of data regarding women who were diagnosed with cancer during pregnancy and who elected to continue their pregnancy, between June 2012 and June 2020. All subjects gave their informed consent for inclusion before they participated in the study. The study was conducted in accordance with the Declaration of Helsinki, and the protocol was approved by the Hospital Ethics Committee (3299/20 March 2020). The "Filantropia" Clinical Hospital in Bucharest has departments specialized in gynecological oncology—including medical oncology, pathology, radiology, obstetrics, and maternal and fetal medicine—as well as a tertiary-level maternity ward equipped to provide neonatal resuscitation, and a counselling psychologist. Since 2015, a weekly multidisciplinary team (including gynecologic surgeons, radiotherapists, oncologists, and geneticists) meets to provide protocols for diagnoses and treatment plans (Figure 1) for any cancer patient.

Figure 1. Treatment algorithm. * For triple negative breast cancer (TNBC), HER2+ breast cancer (BC), and some Luminal B cases. ** For a gestational age of ≥28 weeks. Trim = trimester.

Data were retrieved from the hospital registries and patient files. We obtained complete data regarding family and personal medical history and risks factors; cancer diagnosis and staging; clinical and pathological features, including histology and immunohistochemistry (IHC); and multimodal cancer treatment. We also retrieved data about pregnancy management, including fetal ultrasound evaluations, childbirth, and the postpartum period. Finally, we collected data regarding infant development and clinical evolution after birth, up to 2020. In Romania, the National Insurance House does not reimburse genetic testing for a tumor genome, for cancer risk or NIPT in pregnancy. Thus, cancer genetic tests were available for few patients. Diagnoses were mostly suspected based on patient self-examination, rather than a scheduled medical exam. Staging was generally established by ultrasound assessment—with mammography or other imaging studies recommended only for postpartum patients. Breast cancer was staged according to the American Joint Committee on Cancer

(AJCC) Tumor-Node-Metastasis (TNM)-staging system [42,43]. Immunohistochemistry assessment was used to categorize breast cancer into the following subtypes: Luminal A, Luminal B HER2−, Luminal B HER2+, HER2+ (non-luminal), and triple-negative [44]. Data were analyzed descriptively.

Surgery was performed regardless of the gestational age of the pregnancy. For all cases, axillary staging was performed by axillary lymph node dissection (ALND). For tumors greater than 2 cm (determined by ultrasound), we offered neoadjuvant chemotherapy (NACT) starting in the second trimester of pregnancy. Systemic therapy was performed using the same regimens and schedules as in non-pregnant patients, including anthracyclines (epirubicin or doxorubicin/cyclophosphamide) and taxane-based chemotherapy (paclitaxel, docetaxel). No dose-dense regimen was used. Chemotherapy was stopped no later than 35 weeks of gestation, according to available international guidelines [19], to avoid the delivery occurring during the time-frame of maternal pancytopenia, which could lead to fetal complications (hematologic toxicities or infection) [19]. Due to the different gestational ages at the start of systemic treatment, taxanes were usually given postpartum. Patients with HER2+ disease received anti-HER2 targeted therapy (i.v. or s.c. trastuzumab, pertuzumab, or trastuzumab emtansine) after delivery, according to the drugs' label. The delayed administration of anti-HER2 therapy, for a few weeks, after delivery, is unlikely to impact the outcome negatively. The four-year follow-up of the HERA study suggested that patients who received delayed treatment with Herceptin at a median of 2 years following chemotherapy had a lower risk of relapse compared to patients who remained in the observational, non-treated group [45]. For patients with luminal disease, postpartum endocrine therapy disease was recommended. When indicated, radiotherapy was administered after delivery.

These high-risk pregnancy management options included fetal ultrasound assessment for structural abnormalities and fetal growth, including Doppler evaluation (umbilical artery Doppler assessment, *ductus venosus* (DV), middle cerebral artery, cerebroplacental ratio, uterine arteries) and amniotic fluid level measurements after systemic chemotherapy, according to our local protocols. Maternal and fetal echocardiography monitoring of the serial left ventricular ejection fraction was performed before and after anthracycline-based chemotherapy administration. Corticosteroid treatment for lung maturation was offered at between 28 and 32 gestational weeks. Birth induction was rare and was mostly performed for obstetric indications (breech presentation, intrauterine growth restriction with abnormal DV blood flow, placenta previa, first twin in non-cephalic presentation), or if the maternal condition had deteriorated. Vaginal birth was preferred and recommended after 37 weeks. Breastfeeding was contraindicated while a mother was undergoing systemic treatment or radiation therapy. Lactation was suppressed when continued cancer treatment was needed. Newborns were clinically evaluated, subjected to echocardiography, and, if the mother agreed, monitored every six months for physical and neurologic development and age-appropriate scores on echocardiography evaluation.

3. Results

During the studied time period, 13 cases of PABC were managed at our hospital, with an average of 1.62 new cases per year. Of these 13 cases, 12 are included in our analysis. One was excluded because, while the patient underwent surgery, oncological treatment was postponed due to severe acute respiratory syndrome coronavirus 2 (SARS-CoV-2) infection. The 12 analyzed patients with PABC gave birth to 13 babies (one pair of twins). During the investigation period, 30,355 children were born in the Department of Obstetrics, and 295 new cases of breast cancer in women of childbearing age (16–49 years) were treated in our Medical Oncology Department. Among age-matched women, the incidence rate of PABC was 4.4%.

Table 1 presents the patients' characteristics. The mean age at diagnosis was 35 years (range, 24–38 years), with 91.67% of patients being over 30 years old. Two-thirds of the cases were among patients 36–40 years of age. BC was diagnosed during the second trimester in 41.67% of cases, and during the third trimester in 33.33% of cases. Two patients were multigravida, five (41.67%) primigravida, and five secundigravida. In all cases of multigravidity, <5 years had passed since the previous pregnancy. The lump was more frequently found in the right breast. Four patients had a positive family history of cancer. None of the patients smoked or drank alcohol.

Table 1. Characteristics of the studied population.

Characteristics		Number (N)	%
Age at diagnosis			
	16–25 yrs.	0	0
	26–30 yrs.	1	8.33
	31–35 yrs.	3	25.00
	36–40 yrs.	8	66.67
	>40 yrs.	0	0
Gestational age at diagnosis			
	1st Trim	1	8.33
	2nd Trim	5	41.67
	3rd Trim	4	33.33
	Post-partum	2	16.67
Reproductive factors			
	Menarche < 12 yrs	1	8.33
	Menarche > 12 yrs	11	91.67
	Spontaneous pregnancy	11	91.67
	FIV	1	8.33
	Primigravida	5	41.67
	Secundigravida	5	41.67
	Multigravida	2	16.67
	Time since last birth < 5 yrs.	7	58.33
	Time since last birth > 5 yrs.	5	41.67
Maternal BMI (kg/m^2)			
	< 18.5	1	8.33
	18.5–24.9	6	50
	25.0–29.9	5	41.67
	>30	0	0
Tobacco use			
	Yes	0	0
	No	12	100
Alcohol use			
	Yes	0	0
	No	12	100
Family history of cancer			
	Yes	4	33.33
	No	8	66.67

Table 2 presents the cancer characteristics, management, and issues. Disease-free survival (DFS) was defined as the interval (in months) from the date of primary surgery to the first locoregional recurrence or distant metastasis, as of 1 August 2020. Overall survival (OS) was the interval (in months) from the date of diagnosis to breast cancer-related death. The majority of cases (75%) were diagnosed in early stages. However, due to aggressive tumor biology, treatment was started with NACT in 8 of 12 patients. Among the analyzed cases, two were triple negative breast cancer (TNBC), five were HER2+ disease, one was multifocal multicentric disease, and two patients presented in the metastatic stage. Among the 12 patients, 5 underwent treatment during pregnancy, which included anthracycline-based chemotherapy, followed by treatment with taxanes. Taxanes were most commonly administered in the postpartum period. Conventional adverse events were recorded, including nausea (grade 1); hematologic toxicities, such as anemia and leukopenia (grade 1); alopecia (grade 1); and sensitive neuropathy (grade 2). No experienced adverse events required that treatment be stopped or postponed.

Table 2. Cancer characteristics and management.

Case No.	Stage T	Stage N	M	Grade	Molecular Subtype	Gene Mut Status	Chemo during preg	NACT	Response	Surgery	Adj Chemo	Adj RT	Adj HT	HER2 Treat	DFS (mo)	OS (mo)	Comments
1	2	1	0	3	TNBC	UNK	No	N/A	N/A	R	A,T	Yes	No	No	101	101	
2	4b	0	0	2	Luminal B	UNK	Yes	A,T	PR	R	No	Yes	Yes	No	66	98	A
3	2	1	0	x	HER2+	UNK	No	A	UNK	R	No	No	No	No	N/A	3	B
4	2	1	0	2	Luminal A	UNK	Yes	A,T	PR	R	No	No	Yes	No	77	85	
5	3	0	1	2	HER2+	UNK	No	N/A	N/A	N/A	T (M1 setting)	N/A	No	Yes (H adj)	N/A	9	C
6	4b	3	1	3	Luminal B	UNK	No	N/A	N/A	N/A	N/A	N/A	N/A	N/A	N/A	N/A	D
7	2	0	0	3	Luminal B	Neg	Yes	A,T	PR	R (+PCM)	No	No	Yes	No	28	36	
8	m2	0	0	2	HER2+	VUS (CDH1)	Yes	A,T	PR	R (+PCM)	No	No	Yes	Yes (H adj)	22	36	
9	2	1	0	3	TNBC	BRCA1 mut	No	A,T	N/A	R (+PCM)	Xel	No	No	No	24	32	
10	1	0	0	1	Luminal A	VUS (Rad50)	No	N/A	N/A	R	No	N/A	Yes	No	21	22	
11	3	0	0	2	HER2+	UNK	No	A,T	PR	R (+PCM)	No	No	Yes	Yes (H, P neoadj)	5	10	
12	2	1	0	3	HER2+	UNK	Yes	A,T	PR	R	No	Yes	No	Yes (H, P neoadj; TDM1 adj)	1	10	E

Chemo=chemotherapy; preg=pregnancy; mo=months; mut = mutational; NACT = neoadjuvant chemotherapy; adj = adjuvant; FIV = fertilization in vitro; DFS = disease-free survival; OS = overall survival; RT = radiotherapy; HT = hormonal therapy; TNBC = triple negative breast cancer; UNK = unknown; VUS = variant of unknown significance; N/A = not applicable; A = anthracyclines; T = taxanes; PR = partial response; R = radical; PMC = prophylactic contralateral mastectomy; H = trastuzumab (Herceptine); P = pertuzumab (Perjeta); TDM1 = trastuzumab emtansine (Kadcyla); BRA = brain; HEP = liver; OSS = bone; PUL = lung; BC = breast cancer; FU = follow-up. A: M1 BRA, HEP, OSS, PUL, controlat BC. B: Perioperative death. C: Lost to FU. D: Postpartum maternal death M1 SK BRA HEP PUL. E: Treatment ongoing.

Patient No. 9 had TNBC and exhibited non-pathologic complete response (non-pCR), and received capecitabine in the adjuvant setting. No patient achieved pCR with NACT. The same regimens were used in the adjuvant setting for the patients with upfront surgery if chemotherapy was considered.

For the patients with HER2+ disease, trastuzumab was offered in one case, and trastuzumab plus pertuzumab in two cases. One patient with non-pCR was offered trastuzumab emtansine in the adjuvant setting. For the other patients, treatment was followed with trastuzumab alone. Only one patient (No. 3) did not receive anti-HER2 treatment. After four cycles of AC, she opted for surgery. On postoperative day 5, the patient·s general status worsened. She was diagnosed with metabolic encephalopathy and brain edema and died six days after the surgical intervention. The family refused the necropsy, so we do not have a conclusion for this case.

One patient (No. 5) received taxanes (docetaxel) and trastuzumab in the metastatic setting (lung, liver, and bone). She achieved a partial response, but she left the country. After disease progression, her treatment was switched to capecitabine, trastuzumab, and pertuzumab. However, after a few months, we were unable to contact her anymore. She was the only patient lost to follow-up.

The most eventful follow-up was for patient No. 2, who was diagnosed at 32 years old during her second pregnancy. She received NACT and underwent radical mastectomy. After four years of adjuvant endocrine therapy (tamoxifen and goserelin), the patient developed bone metastasis. Treatment was changed to fulvestrant and the bone-modifying agent zoledronic acid. Two years later, liver metastasis occurred, and the patient resumed chemotherapy with capecitabine, gemcitabine, and PLD. Meanwhile, several brain metastases were diagnosed and radiotherapy performed. In May 2020, the patient was diagnosed with contralateral BC, and a simple mastectomy was performed. The pathology report showed a triple-negative disease in contrast with the initial luminal B tumor.

Except for two patients (No.5 and No.10) who were in the metastatic stage, all patients underwent surgery, including radical modified mastectomy and ALND. A prophylactic contralateral mastectomy was also performed in four cases: in one patient with BRCA1 mutation, one with Rad50 mutation (variant of unknown significance (VUS), and two with no or unknown gene mutation. Five patients (including the four with prophylactic contralateral mastectomy) underwent breast reconstruction—four immediately after surgery, one delayed.

Patient No. 6 died immediately postpartum. This patient was a 37-year-old multiparous woman with invasive ductal carcinoma G3, ER+, PgR+, HER2−, T4bN3M1 with skin metastases. She had presented with a lump since her previous pregnancy and had been hospitalized due to general condition degradation [46].

After birth, two patients (No. 11 and No. 12) received anti-HER2-targeted therapy with trastuzumab and pertuzumab, in a neoadjuvant setting, but no pCR was achieved. They went on with an anti-HER2 treatment in an adjuvant setting, but the short follow-up did not allow any DFS consideration.

Adjuvant radiotherapy was offered to three patients. Hormonal therapy was offered to all six patients with ER+ or PgR+ disease.

No patients were diagnosed with obstetrical complications of pregnancy, structural malformation, or restrictive intrauterine growth. No cases involved premature rupture of membranes after NACT. All patients gave birth by cesarean section, 50% due to obstetrical indications, and 50% due to maternal request. All infants were in the 10th to 90th percentile for weight, with Apgar scores of ≥8 at 1, 5, and 10 min. For the two patients with a deteriorated general condition, induction of labor or cesarean section was indicated at 33 weeks, and these patients died in the postpartum period. Their babies were admitted in NICU due to prematurity.

None of the patients in this series wanted an additional pregnancy after completing the treatment. Two-thirds of the patients are currently free of disease with a follow-up of 5–101 months. All infants have exhibited healthy development.

4. Discussion

In this study, we performed a contemporary analysis of real-world treatment patterns and outcomes among cases of PABC in a tertiary-level hospital in Romania. This hospital treated an average of two PABC cases per year. Although this may seem small, it suggests that approximately 1568 women of fertile age may suffer PABC throughout the European Union each year (Appendix A). We found that PABC incidence was increased in association with increasing maternal age, with a mean age at diagnosis of 35 years, and 91.67% of patients over 30. We also found that PABC was associated with multiparity and shorter time (≤5 years) between pregnancies. BC is commonly associated with genetic, environmental, reproductive, and lifestyle factors. First childbirth at a young age (under 25 years) [47] reduces the risk of luminal subtype tumors [48,49] and might provide a lesser degree of protection against TP53 mutant premalignant lesions. TP53 has long been recognized as a potential mediator of pregnancy-induced resistance to mammary carcinogenesis [47]. Later age at first pregnancy, and pregnancy by in vitro fertilization in premenopausal or menopausal aged women are associated with an increased possibility of PABC. PABC is considered rare, but its incidence shows an increasing trend in parallel to increasing age at childbirth [6,35].

Our analysis confirmed that PABC was associated with prognosis factors, similar to those reported among BC patients over 35 years of age. PABC is considered to have a worse outcome than BC in non-pregnant women, partly due to its intrinsic biological aggressivity (TNBC, HER2+). When diagnosed during pregnancy, BC exhibits aggressive behavior, more frequently occurring as triple-negative or HER2+ positive disease. Apart from the hormonal influences on mammary glands during pregnancy, we do not fully understand the interaction between pregnancy and breast cancer carcinogenesis. Studies have demonstrated that young age (under 35 years) is a negative prognostic factor for breast cancer. Compared to older patients, younger patients with breast cancer more commonly exhibit factors associated with local recurrence and worse survival—including non-luminal types, grade 3 tumors, lymphatic vessel invasion, necrosis, and lack of ER expression [50]. However, among total breast cancer deaths, 6.7% occur among women less than 45 years of age [51]. A multicentric analysis published in 2013 suggests that DFS and OS in BC patients under the age of 45 did not significantly differ between patients diagnosed and treated during pregnancy compared with non-pregnant patients when controlled for stage, and with a median follow-up of 61 months [22].

Additionally, PABC diagnosis can be delayed because it is a rare pathology that is not obvious for clinicians, and because diagnosis can be complicated due to physiological mammary modifications and limited investigation possibilities in pregnant women [52]. In our study, 58.33% (7/12) of cases were HER2+ and/or triple-negative. Of the 12 cases, 2 were diagnosed in the metastatic stage, and another 7 cases were locally advanced (T3–T4 and/or N1).

Since 2012, all PABC cases at our hospital have received a standard regimen of chemotherapy in the second and third trimester of pregnancy, resulting in incomplete remission. In cases of TNBC and HER2+ disease, pathologic complete response is correlated with DFS and OS [53]. However, although none of our patients achieved pCR, only one case exhibited recurrence (at five years). One possible explanation for the lack of pCR is that no dose-dense regimen was used in order to avoid the use of granulocyte colony-stimulating factor (G-CSF); although this is allowed by current guidelines [54]. For TNBC cases, NACT regimens did not include platinum-based therapy due to the limited data available at that time; however, guidelines now consider this approach acceptable [55].

Our present analysis could be biased by the different lengths of the follow-up periods (very short for recent patients), and by the differences in the therapeutic approach, which reflect updates of oncology guidelines. In one case (No. 9), we used an adjuvant treatment with capecitabine, which is reportedly associated with improved OS in non-pCR patients with TNBC after NACT [56]. In two cases (Nos. 11 and 12), we used a neoadjuvant treatment with trastuzumab and pertuzumab, instead of trastuzumab alone (the previous standard), to increase the pCR rate [57]; however, this regimen was not used for case No. 8 (not reimbursed at that time). Additionally, for one HER2+ patient (No. 12) with residual disease after NACT, we administered adjuvant treatment with trastuzumab emtansine

(TDM1), which is associated with a decreased risk of recurrence and improved DFS [58]. This treatment was not available for the other HER2+ patients.

Guidelines recommend genetic testing for BRCA mutations in all breast cancer patients of <50 years. This test was only performed in 33% of patients in our series. The increased frequency of genetic mutation (VUS and BRCA1 mutations) in young BC patients may explain the different pathogenesis. Genetic testing of all patients can allow treatment personalization and improved outcomes [59].

Although cases of PABC are considered high-risk pregnancies with known potential complications (premature rupture of membranes and intrauterine growth restriction), our present series exhibited no obstetrical events or infant-related complications.

The two cases of maternal death can be explained by the very long delay of diagnosis and treatment, such that both cases showed advanced metastases at diagnosis and exhibited rapid general clinical deterioration. In the case lost to follow-up in February 2017, the patient was diagnosed during the postpartum period with invasive ductal carcinoma cT3N0 (ER−, PgR−, and HER2+) with liver, lung, and bone metastases. We obtained a partial response with first-line chemotherapy (docetaxel q3w and trastuzumab q3w). Grade 2 sensitive neuropathy occurred after 10 cycles of chemotherapy and taxane treatment; therefore, taxanes and anti-HER2 therapy were switched to capecitabine, trastuzumab, and pertuzumab. Targeting HER2, e.g., with transtuzumab and lapatinib, is a major step towards improvement of new cancer therapies, and is similar to targeting the estrogen receptor through hormone therapy.

Our present results are in accordance with prior studies, confirming that pregnancy itself does not seem to influence breast cancer outcome, with the therapeutic approach being similar between PABC and BC in non-pregnant patients, according to the disease type and stage [60]. All infants exhibited healthy development, and no cardiac side effects from chemotherapy were reported for either the mothers or infants.

Our study has several limitations. Our analysis includes only a small number of patients due to the rarity of PABC. INCIP register (including 37 centers from 16 countries) includes 462 cases of PABC reported between 2005 and 2020, representing an average of 28 cases per year, and 12 cases per center, over 16 years [35]. Additionally, a recent study including 11,846,300 deliveries between 1999 and 2012 reports an PABC incidence of 6.5 cases/100,000 pregnancies [61]. Our study only included patients who underwent chemotherapy at our hospital. Since the patients had their diagnoses established by the attending physician, we do not know the number of abortions performed upon request due to PABC. Moreover, this study was non-analytical; there were no control patients for cases, and the treatment protocols differed across the time period.

5. Conclusions

In conclusion, our present findings indicate that it is important for pregnant women to undergo clinical examination of the breasts, to promote timely detection of the rare pathology of PABC, especially in patients over 30 years of age. Pregnancy itself seems to be an independent factor affecting prognosis. Case management and prognosis in PABC are similar in non-pregnant BC patients, determined according to clinical stage, timely treatment, and patient age. Chemotherapy during pregnancy is allowed after a gestational age of 16 weeks. No intrauterine growth restriction or small-for-gestational age newborns were observed in our study. Due to the rarity of PABC, strengthening the means for a global partnership may improve PABC survival.

Author Contributions: Conceptualization, A.A.S. and D.M.M.; methodology, A.A.S., and D.M.M.; software, A.A.S., A.H., L.B., and D.M.M.; validation, A.A.S. and D.M.M.; formal analysis, A.A.S., D.M.M., A.H., and L.B.; investigation, A.A.S., D.M.M., A.H., and L.B.; data curation, A.A.S. and D.M.M.; writing—original draft preparation, A.A.S., D.M.M., A.H., and L.B.; writing—review and editing, A.A.S., D.M.M., A.H., and L.B.; visualization, A.A.S., D.M.M., A.H., and L.B.; supervision, A.A.S. and D.M.M. Appendix A: A.H. and L.B. All authors have read and agreed to the published version of the manuscript.

Funding: This research received no external funding.

Conflicts of Interest: The authors declare no conflict of interest.

Appendix A

In 2017, 28% of pregnant women between the age of 30 and 34 years, 9.92% between 35 and 39 years, 0.09% aged 40–49, and three women older than 50 years were diagnosed with breast cancer in Romania. Breast cancer (BC) remains a significant cause of death among Romanian women of fertile age (15–49 years), with a share of 8.8% in all causes of death in 2017. While the number of deaths caused by breast cancer declined by 19.42% between 1990 and 2017, the importance of the disease as cause of death increased by 38.51%. The incidence of BC in women of fertile age has increased by 39.44% between 1990 and 2017 with an average annual growth rate of approximately 1.24%. A substantial increase of BC was noted between 1990 and 1999 (26.70%), and between 2010 and 2017 (16.22%), although the number of deaths decreased by 4.95% between 2000 and 2009. BC prevalence also increased between 1990 and 2017, by 76.20%, or by 2.12% on average annually. Romanian women's age at first birth has increased between 1990 and 2019—from 22.3 to 27.4 years. Maternal age at birth has surged from 25 years in 1990 to 28.8 years in 2019, but the decade with the steepest increase was 1990–1999 (12%), followed by the 2000–2009 decade (7%) and the 2010–2019 decade (4.34%) with a similar trend in the incidence of BC.

Table A1. Estimated probability of PABC

No.	Indicator	Romania	EU
(1)	Number of women of reproductive age (15–49 years)	4,585,074	113,108,086
(2)	Number of pregnancies 15–49 years	120,344.00	2,467,790.00
(3)	% incidence of pregnancies = (2): (1)	2.625%	2.182%
(4)	Prevalence of BC 15–49 years	2260	71,890
(5)	% incidence of BC = (4): (1)	0.049%	0.064%
(6)	% incidence of PABC = (5) × (3)	0.001%	0.001%
(7)	Number of PABC cases/100,000 women = (6) × 100,000	1.29	1.39
(8)	Number of PABC cases 15–49 years = (7) × (1): 100,000	254	7091

EU—European Union, PABC—Pregnancy-associated breast cancer.

The estimated probability of pregnancy-associated breast cancer (PABC) is 1.29/100,000 among women aged 15–49 years in Romania, mainly due to pregnancy at an older age. We expect 59 new cases of PABC per year in Romania. Throughout the EU, we expect that 1568 women of fertile age may suffer from BC each year.

Data sets used for modeling the estimated probability of pregnancy-associated breast cancer (PABC) in Romania and throughout the EU were the following:

- National Institute of Statistics, Romania—Tempo Database. Available online: http://statistici.insse.ro:8077/tempo-online/ [62];
- Eurostat Database of the European Commission—https://ec.europa.eu/eurostat/data/database [63];
- Romania Global Cancer Observatory 2020—https://gco.iarc.fr [64];
- Global Burden of Disease Collaborative Network. Global Burden of Disease Study 2017 (GBD 2017) Reference Life Table. Seattle, United States: Institute for Health Metrics and Evaluation (IHME), 2018. Available online: http://ghdx.healthdata.org/gbd-2017 [65].

References

1. Fitzmaurice, C.; Allen, C.; Barber, R.M.; Barregard, L.; Bhutta, Z.A.; Brenner, H. Global Burden of Disease Cancer Collaboration, Global, Regional, and National Cancer Incidence, Mortality, Years of Life Lost, Years Lived With Disability, and Disability-Adjusted Life-years for 32 Cancer Groups, 1990 to 2015: A Systematic Analysis for the Global Burden of Disease Study. *JAMA Oncol.* **2017**, *3*, 524–548. [PubMed]
2. Eibye, S.; Kjær, S.K.; Mellemkjær, L. Incidence of pregnancy-associated cancer in Denmark, 1977–2006. *Obstet. Gynecol.* **2013**, *122*, 608–617. [CrossRef] [PubMed]
3. Cottreau, C.M.; Dashevsky, I.; Andrade, S.E.; Li, D.-K.; Nekhlyudov, L.; Raebel, M.A.; Ritzwoller, D.P.; Partridge, A.H.; Pawloski, P.A.; Toh, S. Pregnancy-Associated Cancer: A U.S. Population-Based Study. *J. Womens Health* **2019**, *28*, 250–257. [CrossRef]
4. Berry, D.L. Management of breast cancer during pregnancy using a standardized protocol. *J. Clin. Oncol.* **1999**, *17*, 855–861. [CrossRef] [PubMed]
5. Rojas, K.E.; Bilbro, N.; Manasseh, D.-M.; Borgen, P.I. A Review of Pregnancy-Associated Breast Cancer: Diagnosis, Local and Systemic Treatment, and Prognosis. *J. Womens Health* **2019**, *28*, 778–784. [CrossRef]
6. Andersson, T.M.-L.; Johansson, A.L.V.; Hsieh, C.-C.; Cnattingius, S.; Lambe, M. Increasing Incidence of Pregnancy-Associated Breast Cancer in Sweden. *Obstet. Gynecol.* **2009**, *114*, 568–572. [CrossRef]
7. Stensheim, H.; Møller, B.; Van Dijk, T.; Fosså, S.D. Cause-Specific Survival for Women Diagnosed With Cancer During Pregnancy or Lactation: A Registry-Based Cohort Study. *J. Clin. Oncol.* **2009**, *27*, 45–51. [CrossRef]
8. Iqbal, J.; Kahane, A.; Park, A.L.; Huang, T.; Meschino, W.S.; Ray, J.G. Hormone Levels in Pregnancy and Subsequent Risk of Maternal Breast and Ovarian Cancer: A Systematic Review. *J. Obstet. Gynaecol. Can.* **2019**, *41*, 217–222. [CrossRef]
9. Perou, C.M.; Jeffrey, S.S.; Van De Rijn, M.; Rees, C.A.; Eisen, M.B.; Ross, D.T.; Pergamenschikov, A.; Williams, C.F.; Zhu, S.X.; Lee, J.C.F.; et al. Distinctive gene expression patterns in human mammary epithelial cells and breast cancers. *Proc. Natl. Acad. Sci. USA* **1999**, *96*, 9212–9217. [CrossRef]
10. Thanmalagan, R.R.; Naorem, L.D.; Venkatesan, A. Expression Data Analysis for the Identification of Potential Biomarker of Pregnancy Associated Breast Cancer. *Pathol. Oncol. Res.* **2017**, *23*, 537–544. [CrossRef]
11. Amant, F.; Verheecke, M.; Wlodarska, I.; Dehaspe, L.; Brady, P.; Brison, N.; Bogaert, K.V.D.; Dierickx, D.; Vandecaveye, V.; Tousseyn, T.; et al. Presymptomatic Identification of Cancers in Pregnant Women During Noninvasive Prenatal Testing. *JAMA Oncol.* **2015**, *1*, 814–819. [CrossRef] [PubMed]
12. Bianchi, D.W.; Chudova, D.; Sehnert, A.J.; Bhatt, S.; Murray, K.; Prosen, T.L.; Garber, J.E.; Wilkins-Haug, L.; Vora, N.L.; Warsof, S.; et al. Noninvasive Prenatal Testing and Incidental Detection of Occult Maternal Malignancies. *JAMA* **2015**, *314*, 162–169. [CrossRef] [PubMed]
13. Karin-Kujundzic, V.; Sola, I.M.; Predavec, N.; Potkonjak, A.; Somen, E.; Mioc, P.; Serman, A.; Vranic, S.; Serman, L. Novel Epigenetic Biomarkers in Pregnancy-Related Disorders and Cancers. *Cells* **2019**, *8*, 1459. [CrossRef] [PubMed]
14. A Leon, S.; Shapiro, B.; Sklaroff, D.M.; Yaros, M.J. Free DNA in the serum of cancer patients and the effect of therapy. *Cancer Res.* **1977**, *37*, 646–650.
15. Opdahl, S.; Romundstad, P.R.; Alsaker, M.D.K.; Vatten, L.J. Hypertensive diseases in pregnancy and breast cancer risk. *Br. J. Cancer* **2012**, *107*, 176–182. [CrossRef]
16. Vatten, L.J.; Romundstad, P.R.; Trichopoulos, D.; Skjærven, R. Pre-eclampsia in pregnancy and subsequent risk for breast cancer. *Br. J. Cancer* **2002**, *87*, 971–973. [CrossRef]
17. Nechuta, S.; Paneth, N.; Velie, E.M. Pregnancy characteristics and maternal breast cancer risk: A review of the epidemiologic literature. *Cancer Causes Control.* **2010**, *21*, 967–989. [CrossRef]
18. A Petrek, J.; Dukoff, R.; Rogatko, A. Prognosis of pregnancy-associated breast cancer. *Cancer* **1991**, *67*, 869–872. [CrossRef]
19. Amant, F.; Deckers, S.; Van Calsteren, K.; Loibl, S.; Halaska, M.; Brepoels, L.; Beijnen, J.; Cardoso, F.; Gentilini, O.D.; Lagae, L.; et al. Breast cancer in pregnancy: Recommendations of an international consensus meeting. *Eur. J. Cancer* **2010**, *46*, 3158–3168. [CrossRef]
20. Goddard, E.T.; Bassale, S.; Schedin, T.; Jindal, S.; Johnston, J.; Cabral, E.; Latour, E.; Lyons, T.R.; Mori, M.; Schedin, P.J.; et al. Association Between Postpartum Breast Cancer Diagnosis and Metastasis and the Clinical Features Underlying Risk. *JAMA Netw. Open* **2019**, *2*, e186997. [CrossRef]

21. Goddard, E.T.; Hill, R.C.; Nemkov, T.; D'Alessandro, A.; Hansen, K.C.; Maller, O.; Mongoue-Tchokote, S.; Mori, M.; Partridge, A.H.; Borges, V.F.; et al. The rodent liver undergoes weaning-induced involution and supports breast cancer metastasis. *Cancer Discov.* **2017**, *7*, 177–187. [CrossRef] [PubMed]
22. Amant, F.; von Minckwitz, G.; Han, S.N.; Bontenbal, M.; Ring, A.E.; Giermek, J.; Wildiers, H.; Fehm, T.; Linn, S.C.; Schlehe, B.; et al. Prognosis of women with primary breast cancer diagnosed during pregnancy: Results from an international collaborative study. *J. Clin. Oncol.* **2013**, *31*, 2532–2539. [CrossRef] [PubMed]
23. Azim, H.A.; Santoro, L.; Russell-Edu, W.; Pentheroudakis, G.; Pavlidis, N.; Peccatori, F. Prognosis of pregnancy-associated breast cancer: A meta-analysis of 30 studies. *Cancer Treat. Rev.* **2012**, *38*, 834–842. [CrossRef] [PubMed]
24. Veronesi, U.; Viale, G.; Paganelli, G.; Zurrida, S.; Luini, A.; Galimberti, V.; Veronesi, P.; Intra, M.; Maisonneuve, P.; Zucca, F.; et al. Sentinel Lymph Node Biopsy in Breast Cancer. *Ann. Surg.* **2010**, *251*, 595–600. [CrossRef]
25. Gropper, A.B.; Calvillo, K.Z.; Dominici, L.; Troyan, S.; Rhei, E.; Economy, K.E.; Tung, N.M.; Schapira, L.; Meisel, J.L.; Partridge, A.H.; et al. Sentinel Lymph Node Biopsy in Pregnant Women with Breast Cancer. *Ann. Surg. Oncol.* **2014**, *21*, 2506–2511. [CrossRef]
26. Lyman, G.H.; Temin, S.; Edge, S.B.; Newman, L.A.; Turner, R.R.; Weaver, D.L.; Benson, A.B.; Bosserman, L.D.; Burstein, H.J.; Cody, H.; et al. Sentinel Lymph Node Biopsy for Patients With Early-Stage Breast Cancer: American Society of Clinical Oncology Clinical Practice Guideline Update. *J. Clin. Oncol.* **2014**, *32*, 1365–1383. [CrossRef]
27. Recently updated NCCN Clinica Practice Guidelines in Oncology. Available online: https://www.nccn.org/professionals/physician_gls/pdf/breast.pdf (accessed on 22 September 2020).
28. Eskandari, A.; Alipour, S. Aspects of Anesthesia for Breast Surgery during Pregnancy. *Adv. Exp. Med. Biol.* **2020**, *1252*, 107–114. [CrossRef]
29. Non Obstetric Surgery during Pregnancy. ACOG Clinical Committee Opinion Number 775. Available online: https://www.acog.org/clinical/clinical-guidance/committee-opinion/articles/2019/04/nonobstetric-surgery-during-pregnancy (accessed on 21 September 2020).
30. Cardonick, E.; Iacobucci, A. Use of chemotherapy during human pregnancy. *Lancet Oncol.* **2004**, *5*, 283–291. [CrossRef]
31. Cardonick, E.; Gringlas, M.B.; Hunter, K.; Greenspan, J. Development of children born to mothers with cancer during pregnancy: Comparing in utero chemotherapy-exposed children with nonexposed controls. *Am. J. Obstet. Gynecol.* **2014**, *212*, 658.e1–658.e8. [CrossRef]
32. Amant, F.; Vandenbroucke, T.; Verheecke, M.; Fumagalli, M.; Halaska, M.; Boere, I.; Han, S.N.; Gziri, M.M.; Peccatori, F.; Rob, L.; et al. Pediatric Outcome after Maternal Cancer Diagnosed during Pregnancy. *N. Engl. J. Med.* **2015**, *373*, 1824–1834. [CrossRef]
33. Simionescu, A.A.; Median, D. Chemotherapy for breast cancer during pregnancy and postpartum:a retrospective descriptive study. *Farmacia* **2015**, *63*, 417–421.
34. Antypas, C.; Sandilos, P.; Kouvaris, J.; Balafouta, E.; Karinou, E.; Kollaros, N.; Vlahos, L. Fetal Dose Evaluation During Breast Cancer Radiotherapy. *Int. J. Radiat. Oncol. Biol. Phys.* **1998**, *40*, 995–999. [CrossRef]
35. De Haan, J.; Verheecke, M.; Van Calsteren, K.; Van Calster, B.; Shmakov, R.G.; Gziri, M.M.; Halaska, M.; Fruscio, R.; Lok, C.A.R.; A Boere, I.; et al. Oncological management and obstetric and neonatal outcomes for women diagnosed with cancer during pregnancy: A 20-year international cohort study of 1170 patients. *Lancet Oncol.* **2018**, *19*, 337–346. [CrossRef]
36. Stewart, A.; Kneale, G. Radiation Dose Effects In Relation To Obstetric X-Rays And childhood Cancers. *Lancet* **1970**, *1*, 1185–1188. [CrossRef]
37. Kneale, G.W.; Stewart, A.M. Mantel-Haenszel analysis of Oxford data. I.Independent effects of several birth factors including fetal irradiation. *J. Natl. Cancer Inst.* **1976**, *56*, 879. [CrossRef] [PubMed]
38. Kneale, G.W.; Stewart, A.M. Mantel-Haenszel Analysis of Oxford Data. II. Independent Effects of Fetal Irradiation Subfactors23. *J. Natl. Cancer Inst.* **1976**, *57*, 1009. [CrossRef] [PubMed]
39. Doll, R.; Wakeford, R. Risk of childhood cancer from fetal irradiation. *Br. J. Radiol.* **1997**, *70*, 130–139. [CrossRef] [PubMed]
40. Gardner, M.J. Leukemia in children and paternal radiation exposure at the Sellafield nuclear site. *J. Natl. Cancer Inst. Monogr.* **1992**, *12*, 133–135.

41. Sogr.ro/ghidurile-revizuite-2019. Available online: https://sogr.ro/wp-content/uploads/2019/03/cancerul-mamar-09.03.2019.pdf (accessed on 18 June 2020).
42. Hayes, D.F.; Allred, C.; Anderson, B.O.; Andreson, S.; Ashley, P.; Barlow, W.; Berry, D.; Carlson, R.W.; Gelman, R.; Hilsenbeck, S.; et al. Breast. In *AJCC Cancer Staging Manual*, 7th ed.; Edge, S., Byrd, D.R., Compton, C.C., Fritz, A.G., Greene, F., Trotti, A., Eds.; Springer: New York, NY, USA, 2010; pp. 345–376. ISBN 978-0-387-88440-0.
43. Hortobagyi, G.N.; Conolly, J.L.; D'Orsi, C.J.; Edge, S.B.; Mittendorf, E.A.; Rugo, H.S.; Solin, L.J.; Weaver, D.L.; Winchester, D.J.; Giuliano, A. Breast. In *AJCC Cancer Staging Manual*, 8th ed.; Amin, M.B., Edge, S.B., Greene, F.L., Byrd, D.R., Brookland, R.K., Washington, M.K., Gershenwald, J.E., Compton, C.C., Hess, K.R., Sullivan, D.C., et al., Eds.; Springer: New York, NY, USA, 2017; pp. 589–636. ISBN 978-3-319-40617-6.
44. Cardoso, F.; Kyriakides, S.; Ohno, S.; Penault-Llorca, F.; Poortmans, P.; Rubio, I.T.; Zackrisson, S.; Senkus, E. Early Breast Cancer: ESMO Clinical Practice Guidelines. *Ann. Oncol.* **2019**, *30*, 1194–1220. [CrossRef]
45. Gianni, L.; Dafni, U.; Gelber, R.D.; De Azambuja, E.; Muehlbauer, S.; Goldhirsch, A.; Untch, M.; Smith, I.; Baselga, J.; Jackisch, C.; et al. Treatment with trastuzumab for 1 year after adjuvant chemotherapy in patients with HER2-positive early breast cancer: A 4-year follow-up of a randomised controlled trial. *Lancet Oncol.* **2011**, *12*, 236–244. [CrossRef]
46. Simionescu, A.A.; Georgescu, C.V.; Ghiluși, M.C.; Stoica, S.I.; Median, M.D. Advanced metastatic breast cancer in pregnancy: The imperative of physical breast examination in pregnancy. *Rom. J. Morphol. Embryol.* **2017**, *58*, 645–650. [PubMed]
47. Nguyen, B.; Venet, D.; Lambertini, M.; Desmedt, C.; Salgado, R.; Horlings, H.M.; Rothé, F.; Sotiriou, C. Imprint of parity and age at first pregnancy on the genomic landscape of subsequent breast cancer. *Breast Cancer Res.* **2019**, *21*, 25. [CrossRef] [PubMed]
48. Ellingjord-Dale, M.; Vos, L.; Tretli, S.; Hofvind, S.S.H.; Dos-Santos-Silva, I.; Ursin, G. Parity, hormones and breast cancer subtypes—results from a large nested case-control study in a national screening program. *Breast Cancer Res.* **2017**, *19*, 10. [CrossRef] [PubMed]
49. Lambertini, M.; Santoro, L.; Del Mastro, L.; Nguyen, B.; Livraghi, L.; Ugolini, N.; Peccatori, F.; Azim, H.A., Jr. Reproductive behaviors and risk of developing breast cancer according to tumor subtype: A systematic review and meta-analysis of epidemiological studies. *Cancer Treat. Rev.* **2016**, *49*, 65–76. [CrossRef] [PubMed]
50. Nixon, A.J.; Neuberg, D.; Hayes, D.F.; Gelman, R.; Connolly, J.L.; Schnitt, S.; Abner, A.; Recht, A.; Vicini, F.; Harris, J.R. Relationship of patient age to pathologic features of the tumor and prognosis for patients with stage I or II breast cancer. *J. Clin. Oncol.* **1994**, *12*, 888–894. [CrossRef]
51. National Cancer Institute. Available online: Seer.cancer.gov (accessed on 5 June 2020).
52. Amant, F.; Loibl, S.; Neven, P.; van Calsteren, K. Breast cancer in pregnancy. *Lancet* **2012**, *379*, 570–579. [CrossRef]
53. Von Minckwitz, G.; Kaufmann, M.; Kuemmel, S.; Fasching, P.A.; Eiermann, W.; Blohmer, J.-U.; Costa, S.-D.; Hilfrich, J.; Jackisch, C.; Gerber, B.; et al. Correlation of various pathologic complete response (pCR) definitions with long-term outcome and the prognostic value of pCR in various breast cancer subtypes: Results from the German neoadjuvant meta-analysis. *J. Clin. Oncol.* **2011**, *29* (Suppl. S15), 1028–1028. [CrossRef]
54. Loibl, S.; Schmidt, A.P.; Gentilini, O.; Kaufman, B.; Kuhl, C.; Denkert, C.; Von Minckwitz, G.; Parokonnaya, A.; Stensheim, H.; Thomssen, C.; et al. Breast Cancer Diagnosed During Pregnancy. *JAMA Oncol.* **2015**, *1*, 1145–1153. [CrossRef]
55. Loibl, S.; Lederer, B. *Managing Cancer during Pregnancy*; Hatem, A.A., Jr., Ed.; Springer: Berlin, Germany, 2016. [CrossRef]
56. Masuda, N.; Lee, S.-J.; Ohtani, S.; Im, Y.-H.; Lee, E.-S.; Yokota, I.; Kuroi, K.; Im, S.-A.; Park, S.; Kim, S.-B.; et al. Adjuvant Capecitabine for Breast Cancer after Preoperative Chemotherapy. *N. Engl. J. Med.* **2017**, *376*, 2147–2159. [CrossRef]
57. Gianni, L.; Pienkowski, T.; Im, Y.-H.; Tseng, L.-M.; Liu, M.-C.; Lluch, A.; Starosławska, E.; De La Haba-Rodriguez, J.; Im, S.-A.; Pedrini, J.L.; et al. 5-year analysis of neoadjuvant pertuzumab and trastuzumab in patients with locally advanced, inflammatory, or early-stage HER2-positive breast cancer (NeoSphere): A multicentre, open-label, phase 2 randomised trial. *Lancet Oncol.* **2016**, *17*, 791–800. [CrossRef]
58. Von Minckwitz, G.; Huang, C.-S.; Mano, M.S.; Loibl, S.; Mamounas, E.P.; Untch, M.; Wolmark, N.; Rastogi, P.; Schneeweiss, A.; Redondo, A.; et al. Trastuzumab Emtansine for Residual Invasive HER2-Positive Breast Cancer. *N. Engl. J. Med.* **2019**, *380*, 617–628. [CrossRef] [PubMed]

59. Tung, N.M.; Boughey, J.C.; Pierce, L.J.; Robson, M.E.; Bedrosian, I.; Dietz, J.R.; Dragun, A.; Gelpi, J.B.; Hofstatter, E.W.; Isaacs, C.J.; et al. Management of Hereditary Breast Cancer: American Society of Clinical Oncology, American Society for Radiation Oncology, and Society of Surgical Oncology Guideline. *J. Clin. Oncol.* **2020**, *38*, 2080–2106. [CrossRef] [PubMed]
60. Paluch-Shimon, S.; Cardoso, F.; Partridge, A.; Abulkhair, O.; Azim, H.; Bianchi-Micheli, G.; Cardoso, M.-J.; Curigliano, G.; Gelmon, K.; Harbeck, N.; et al. ESO–ESMO 4th International Consensus Guidelines for Breast Cancer in Young Women (BCY4). *Ann. Oncol.* **2020**, *31*, 674–696. [CrossRef] [PubMed]
61. Maor, G.S.; Czuzoj-Shulman, N.; Spence, A.R.; Abenhaim, H.A. Neonatal outcomes of pregnancy-associated breast cancer: Population-based study on 11 million births. *Breast J.* **2019**, *25*, 86–90. [CrossRef] [PubMed]
62. National Institute of Statistics, Romania. Available online: https://insse.ro (accessed on 5 June 2020).
63. Database-Eurostat-European Commission. Available online: https://ec.europa.eu/eurostat/data/database (accessed on 5 June 2020).
64. Romania Global Cancer Observatory. Available online: https://gco.iarc.fr (accessed on 5 June 2020).
65. GBD data. Institute for Health Metrics and Evaluation. Available online: http://www.healthdata.org/gbd/data (accessed on 5 June 2020).

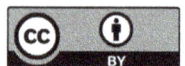

© 2020 by the authors. Licensee MDPI, Basel, Switzerland. This article is an open access article distributed under the terms and conditions of the Creative Commons Attribution (CC BY) license (http://creativecommons.org/licenses/by/4.0/).

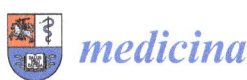

Case Report

A Very Rare Case of Colosalpingeal Fistula Secondary to Diverticulitis: An Overview of Development, Clinical Features and Management

Natalia Darii Plopa [1], Nicolae Gica [2,*], Marie Gerard [3], Marie-Cécile Nollevaux [4], Milenko Pavlovic [5] and Emil Anton [6]

1. Department of Gynecology, CHU de Charleroi, 6000 Charleroi, Belgium; plopa_nati@yahoo.com
2. Carol Davila University of Medicine and Pharmacy, 020021 Bucharest, Romania
3. Department of Radiology, CHU Dinant Godinne|UCL Namur, 5530 Yvoir, Belgium; marie.gerard@uclouvain.be
4. Department of Pathology, CHU Dinant Godinne|UCL Namur, 5530 Yvoir, Belgium; marie-cecile.nollevaux@uclouvain.be
5. Department of Gynecology, Faculty of Medicine, Pontificia Universidad Católica de Chile, 833-0073 Santiago, Chile; mpavlovicv@gmail.com
6. University of Medicine and Pharmacology Gr T Popa, 700115 Iasi, Romania; emil.anton@yahoo.com
* Correspondence: gica.nicolae@umfcd.ro; Tel.: +40-727-827-815

Received: 26 August 2020; Accepted: 15 September 2020; Published: 17 September 2020

Abstract: Background: Colosalpingeal fistula is a rare complication secondary to diverticular disease. The pathogenesis is still not clearly understood. We present the case of a colosalpingeal fistula and a review of the management of this pathology. Case report: A 69-year-old patient with uncomplicated diverticular disease was referred to our department for recurrent vaginal discharge. The clinical examination was unremarkable, hysteroscopy revealed the presence of air in the uterine cavity in the absence of a uterine fistula. A preliminary diagnosis of colosalpingeal fistula was made and was confirmed by computed tomography (CT) scan and hysterosalpingography. A one-stage surgery via laparotomy was successfully performed with remission of the symptoms. Conclusion: Colotubal fistula is a rare complication resulting from intestinal diverticular disease. The purpose of this paper was to emphasize the presence of a rare, but serious complication occurring in diverticular disease with atypical symptoms and one-stage surgery treatment.

Keywords: colosalpingeal fistula; enterotubal fistula; diverticular fistulation; diagnosis; hysteroscopy management

1. Introduction

The colotubal (or colosalpingeal or salpingo-intestinal) fistula occurs in 2% of the cases with fistulas secondary to diverticular disease [1]. The initial symptoms of this disease are not specific, but this complication must be suspected in patients with persistent or recurrent vaginal discharge and a history of diverticular disease. The specific diagnostic tests for this condition are computed tomography (CT) scan and hysterosalpingography. The management options depend on the patient's age and desire to preserve fertility. We report a case of a menopausal women with known diverticular disease and colosalpingeal fistula, managed in our gynecology department, with a review of the literature.

2. Case Report

A 69-year-old postmenopausal caucasic woman with previous two pregnancies and two deliveries was referred to our department for a vaginal recurrent leucorrhoea which lasted for over one year despite multiple vaginal local treatments. Her past medical and surgical histories revealed two episodes of diverticulitis managed with antibiotics, appendectomy, and breast cancer treated with breast-conserving surgery followed by radiotherapy and hormonotherapy with complete remission of the disease. Unlike other cases from the literature reports, our patient presented with gynecological problems and her only symptom was the vaginal discharge, the patient did not complain about abdominal pain, fever, or other symptoms. The clinical examination was unremarkable, and vaginal swab revealed the presence of *Escherichia coli* and *Streptococcus constellatus*. The transvaginal ultrasound examination showed a heterogeneous intrauterine collection. Hysteroscopy was performed as an additional exam. The presence of air in the uterine cavity in the absence of uterine fistula or neoplasic process made us suspect the tubo-intestinal fistula. The endometrial biopsy was compatible with endometritis secondary to *E. coli*. To confirm the diagnosis, CT scan and hysterosalpingography were performed and the communication between the tube and sigmoidal diverticulum was visualized (Figures 1 and 2).

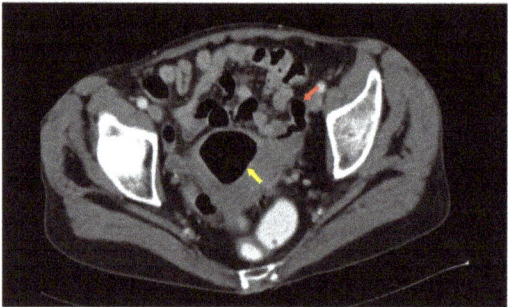 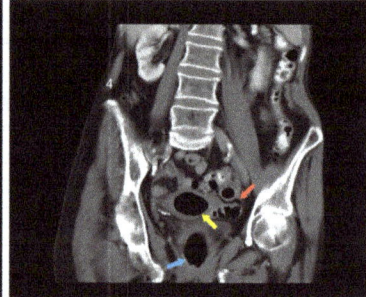

Figure 1. Computed tomography (CT) scan: **Left side**—axial contrast—enhanced CT scan of pelvis shows the presence of air in the uterine cavity (yellow arrow) and enlargement of left adnexa which contains gas (red arrow); **right side**—coronal contrast—enhanced CT pelvis image with rectal lumen (blue arrow), the air presence in the uterine cavity (yellow arrow), and the air in the tubal lumen (red arrow).

Based on the medical history, age, and symptoms, elective surgical treatment was performed by gastrointestinal surgeons. This was a one-stage surgery with sigmoidal and concomitant left salpingo-oophorectomy and primary anastomosis. Intraoperative, the affected area of the colon was densely adherent to the left fallopian tube. Inflammation was present in the proximal rectum, therefore dissection was extended more distally and a low anterior resection with primary anastomosis was performed. The colon and fallopian tubes were successfully separated using finger fracture technique. Pathological examination confirmed the diverticular disease associated with neutrophilic cryptitis and serosal inflammation. The 6.5 cm length fallopian tube was characterized by a dilated lumen. At the microscopic level, the fallopian tube showed evidence of chronic and subacute salpingitis whereas the peritubal environment revealed some stercoral debris mixed with extensive abscessation beaches (see Figure 3A,B). There were no intraoperative complications. The patient had a favorable evolution during hospitalization and was discharged home on day 7 post surgery. One month later, she remained asymptomatic.

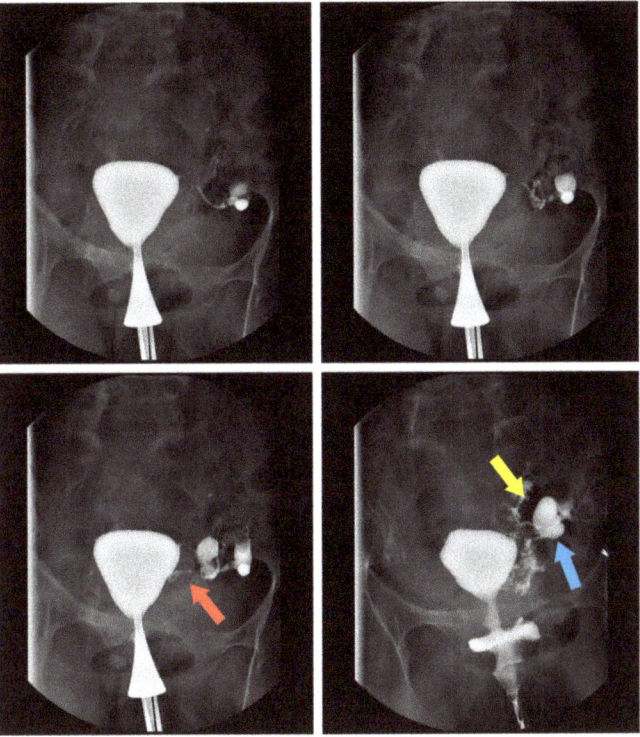

Figure 2. Hysterosalpingography: (red arrow)—tubal lumen; (blue arrow)—intestinal lumen; (yellow arrow)—tubal fistula.

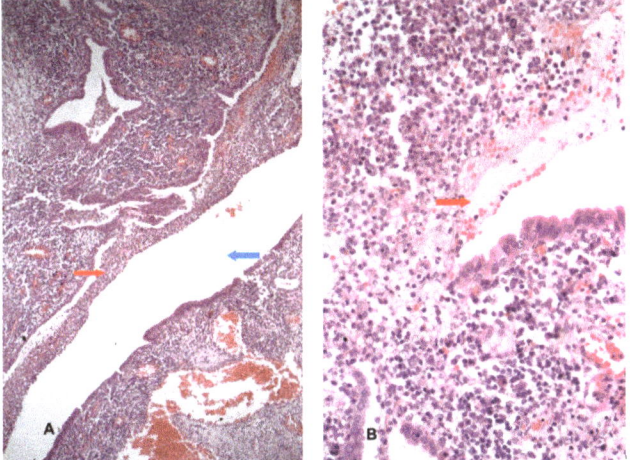

Figure 3. Microscopic examination: (**A**) H&E slide ×5 magnification. Chronic and subacute salpingitis (red arrow; tubal lumen—blue arrow). (**B**) H&E slide ×10 magnification. Stercoral debris mixed with extensive abscessation beaches (red arrow).

3. Discussion

Diverticular disease is becoming more common, affecting up to 71.4% of the population over 80 years [2]. Literature reports an increase from 49,000 cases of diverticular disease in 2000 to more than 70,000 in 2006, the complicated diseases almost doubled between 1990 and 2005 [3]. Many conditions of diverticular disease are described, from asymptomatic form to complicated aspects such as inflammation and fistulation to the surrounding burden organs. The incidence of enteric fistula in diverticular disease is about 2–4%, reaching up to 20% in patients with history of surgical treatment of diverticular disease [4]. Spontaneous colosalpingeal fistula secondary to diverticulosis is very rare (only 10 cases reported in the literature) and may appear even during pregnancy [5,6]. The first case of sigmoidotubal fistula was described in 1956 [7]. The prevalence of colotubal fistula is about 2% [1].

The colosalpingeal fistula is rare due to the tubal obstruction secondary to inflammatory process at the tubal level. Although the pathogenesis is not fully understood, some authors hypothesized that chronic inflammation is involved in the development of this pathology. The adhesions between intestinal wall and the fallopian tube may occur during an acute episode of diverticulitis, resulting in necrosis and fistula formation. This pathogenesis may explain the colosalpingeal fistula secondary to diverticulitis or Crohn's disease [8]. Fistula can occur also due to a diverticulum perforation with local abscess formation and weakening of adjacent structures [9]. Moreover, the neoplastic fistula is formed following the same mechanism of inflammation, epithelial necrosis, and destruction associated with ulceration [10].

Colosalpingeal fistula occurs in the left tube in 93% of the cases, with the right tube affected in only 7% of the cases, due to cecal diverticulosis [11]. Until now, only one case of bilateral salpingocolic fistula was reported in the literature [12].

Colotubal fistulas are uncommon and difficult to diagnose. Clinical manifestations may be nonspecific, and the symptoms appear later in the evolution of the disease. Although clinical manifestations may vary, the most frequent symptom is persistent or recurrent vaginal discharge with the presence of enterocolic germs at the vaginal swab. Gynecologic examination is mandatory to exclude vaginal fistula and verify vaginal integrity. Endovaginal ultrasonography examination may indicate the presence of an intrauterine collection and may rarely reveal a parauterine collection or fistulous trajectory. Uterine cavity exploration by hysteroscopy should be performed to exclude the presence of a uterine fistula or a fistulized endometrial neoplasia. The presence of air in the uterine cavity associated with the absence of uterine communication or cancerous process may suggest the presence of a colosalpingeal fistula. The endometrial biopsy may reveal the presence of granulation tissue and exclude a neoplasic process.

CT scan is the gold standard test for the diagnosis of abdominal and pelvic organs fistulas [13]. The sensitivity and specificity of the CT scan for the diagnosis of colorectal fistula is 88% and 100%, respectively [11]. The presence of adnexal gas, adnexal fluid, intraabdominal gas, or intraabdominal collections associated with enlarged inflammatory adnexa was described in the cases of the colosalpingeal fistula [14]. The sensitivity and the specificity of CT scan and hysteroscopy for the diagnosis of colosalpingeal fistula remains to be established due to the low incidence of this pathology.

The hysterosalpingography is the imaging method with the highest sensitivity for the diagnosis of colosalpingeal fistula [15]. Colonoscopy helps to identify bowel pathology that caused an enteral fistula in 8.5–55% of cases [16].

Colosalpingeal fistula can also occur as a consequence of other conditions, different from diverticular disease, such as tuberculosis [17,18], appendicitis, or pelvic inflammatory disease [19,20]; primary tubo-ovarian abscess; endometriosis; and neoplasic conditions.

The treatment is a surgical one, only one case has been shown to resolve spontaneously [21], and it depends on the age of the patient, the medical and surgical history, and especially the desire of fertility preservation. The recommended surgical treatment is the resection of the affected bowel segment with primary anastomosis and resection of the complete adjacent organ or only the affected part of it. The primary intestinal anastomosis is possible in the absence of sepsis or severe malnutrition [22]. Meticulous treatment of the fistula is required if a conservative surgical approach is needed. Radical surgical treatment, such as Hartmann´s opereation, should be reserved only for emergencies, and secondary anastomosis should be performed once the acute inflammation has resolved. In the presence of acute diverticulitis, a preoperative medical treatment is preferred to decrease the risk of postoperative complications [23].

The recommended surgical treatment for colosalpingeal fistula in postmenopausal women is total hysterectomy with bilateral salpingo-oophorectomy coupled with sigmoid resection. In premenopausal women who want to preserve fertility, an ipsilateral salpingo-oophorectomy or salpingectomy with sigmoid resection is the treatment of choice [21]. Laparoscopy has the advantage of shorter hospitalization, compared with the classical approach, has fewer complications, but requires a longer operating time [22]. This surgical option seems to be safe, but there is lack of randomised clinical trials in the literature [24].

The conservative, nonsurgical treatment (antibiotics, standard intravenous fluids, and artificial nutrition) is an ineffective therapy and it is associated with a higher recurrence risk [25]. This management option is only reserved for the patients with comorbidities and high anesthesia risk or those who decline surgical treatment.

The novelty of this case report is that, unlike the literature reports, our patient presented with gynecological problems and her only symptom was the vaginal discharge, managed in our gynecology department.

4. Conclusions

Colosalpingeal fistula is a rare complication of intestinal diverticulosis, and the diagnosis should be suspected by the gynecologist in a patient with abdominal pain and known diverticular disease, especially in the presence of persistent or recurrent vaginal discharge. The purpose of our paper is to bring attention to the recurrent vaginal discharge and to make the differential diagnosis with the colotubal fistula, especially in patients with diverticular or inflammatory disease.

Author Contributions: Conceptualization, N.G. and N.D.P.; methodology, N.D.P.; software, E.A.; validation, M.G., M.-C.N., and M.P.; formal analysis, N.D.P.; investigation, N.G., M.G. and E.A.; resources, N.D.P.; data curation, N.G., M.G.; writing—Original draft preparation, N.D.P., M.P. and N.G.; writing—Review and editing, M.-C.N. and E.A.; visualization, M.P.; supervision, M.-C.N.; project administration, N.G.; funding acquisition, N.G., N.D.P. All authors have read and agreed to the published version of the manuscript.

Funding: This research received no external funding.

Acknowledgments: All authors had equal contributions to this article. There were no additional sources of technical help, and no financial or material sources supported the work.

Conflicts of Interest: The authors declare no conflict of interest.

References

1. Vasilevsky, C.A.; Belliveau, P.; Trudel, J.L.; Stein, B.L.; Gordon, P.H. Fistulas complicating diverticulitis. *Int. J. Colorect. Dis.* **1998**, *13*, 57–60. [CrossRef] [PubMed]
2. Tursi, A.; Scarpignato, C.; Strate; Lanas, A.; Kruis, W.; Lahat, A.; Danese, S. Colonic diverticular disease. *Nat. Rev. Dis. Primers* **2020**, *6*, 20. [CrossRef] [PubMed]
3. Lanas, A.; Abad-Baroja, D.; Lanas-Gimeno, A. Progress and challenges in the management of diverticular disease: Which treatment? *Therap. Adv. Gastroenterol.* **2018**, *11*, 1756284818789055. [CrossRef] [PubMed]
4. Marcucci, T.; Giannessi, S.; Giudici, F.; Riccadonna, S.; Gori, A.; Tonelli, F. Management of colovesical and colovaginal diverticular fistulas Our experience and literature reviewed. *Ann. Itali. Chir.* **2017**, *88*, 55–61.
5. Raidh, B.H.S.; Khalil, B.M.; Mohamed, B.B.; Mounir, B.M.; Abdeljelil, Z. Sigmoïdite diverticulaire compliquée d'une fistule colo-tubaire survenant au cours d'une grossesse. *La Tunis Médicale* **2011**, *89*, 574–575.
6. Botezatu, R.; Marian, R.; Gica, N.; Iancu, G.; Peltecu, G.; Panaitescu, A.M. Axial torsion and infarction of Meckel's diverticulum in the 3rd trimester of pregnancy. *Chirurgia* **2018**, *113*, 266–269. [CrossRef]
7. Tancer, M.L.; Veridiano, N.P. Genital fistulas caused by diverticular disease of the sigmoid colon. *Am. J. Obstet. Gynecol.* **1996**, *174*, 1547–1550. [CrossRef]

8. Maun, D.; Vine, A.; Slater, G. Ileosalpingeal fistula: An unusual complication of Crohn's disease. *Mt. Sinai J. Med.* **2006**, *73*, 1115–1116.
9. Chaikof, E.L.; Cambria, R.P.; Warshaw, A.L. Colouterine fistula secondary to diverticulitis. *Dis. Colon Rectum* **1985**, *28*, 358–360. [CrossRef]
10. McDaid, J.; Reichl, C.; Hamzah, I.; Fitter, S.; Harbach, L.; Savage, A.P. Diverticular fistulation is associated with nicorandil usage. *Ann. R. Coll. Surg. Engl.* **2010**, *92*, 463–465. [CrossRef]
11. Panghaal, V.S.; Chernyak, V.; Patlas, M.; Rozenblit, A.M. CT features of adnexal involvement in patients with diverticulitis. *Am. J. Roentgenol.* **2009**, *192*, 963–966. [CrossRef] [PubMed]
12. Al Sinani, N.S. Bi-salpingocolonic fistula report of both fallopian tubes fistulizing with sigmoid diverticulum with literature review. *J. King Abdulaziz Univ. Med. Sci.* **2012**, *19*, 3.
13. Birnbaum, B.A.; Balthazar, E.J. CT of appendicitis and diverticulitis. *Radiol. Clin. N. Am.* **1994**, *32*, 885–898. [PubMed]
14. Ruiz-Tovar, J.; Gamallo, C. Pneumosalpynx caused by colosalpingeal fistula secondary to acute colonic diverticulitis. *Int. J. Colorectal. Dis.* **2011**, *26*, 1357–1358. [CrossRef]
15. Williams, S.M.; Nolan, D.J. Colosalpingeal fistula: A rare complication of colonic diverticular disease. *Eur. Radiol.* **1999**, *9*, 1432–1433. [CrossRef]
16. Golabek, T.; Szymanska, A.; Szopinski, T.; Bukowczan, J.; Furmanek, M.; Powroznik, J.; Chlosta, P. Enterovesical Fistulae: Aetiology, Imaging, and Management. *Gastroenterol. Res. Pract.* **2013**, *2013*, 617967. [CrossRef]
17. Kumar, A.; Bhargava, S.K.; Mehrotra, G.; Pushkarna, R. Enterotubal fistulae secondary to tuberculosis: Report of three cases and review of literature. *Clin. Radiol.* **2001**, *56*, 858–860. [CrossRef]
18. Clotteau, J.E.; Premont, M.; Belkaid, A.; Habib, E. Female genital tuberculosis. Apropos of a case of salpingo-sigmoidal fistula. *Chirurgie* **1983**, *109*, 374–377.
19. Hoffer, F.A.; Ablow, R.C.; Gryboski, J.D.; Seashore, J.H. Primary appendicitis with an appendoci-tuboovarian fistula. *AJR* **1982**, *138*, 742–743. [CrossRef]
20. Simstein, N.L. Colo-tubo-ovarian fistula as complication of pelvic inflammatory disease. *S. Med. J.* **1981**, *74*, 512–513. [CrossRef]
21. Hain, J.M.; Sherick, D.G. Salpingo colonic Fistula Secondary to Diverticulitis. *Am. Surg.* **1996**, *62*, 984–988. [PubMed]
22. Poulin, E.C.; Schlachta, C.M.; Mamazza, J.; Seshadri, P. Should enteric fistulas from Crohn's disease or diverticulitis be treated laparoscopically or by open surgery? *Dis. Colon Rectum* **2000**, *43*, 621–626. [CrossRef] [PubMed]
23. Zonca, P.; Jacobi, C.A.; Meyer, G.P. The current view of surgical treatment of diverticular disease. *Rozhl. Chir.* **2009**, *88*, 568–576. [PubMed]
24. Cirocchi, R.; Arezzo, A.; Renzi, C.; Cochetti, G.; D'Andrea, V.; Fingerhut, A.; Mearini, E.; Binda, G.A. Is laparoscopic surgery the best treatment in fistulas complicating diverticular disease of the sigmoid colon? A systematic review. *Int. J. Surg.* **2015**, *24*, 95–100. [CrossRef]
25. Garcea, G.; Majid, I.; Sutton, C.D.; Pattenden, C.J.; Thomas, W.M. Diagnosis and management of colovesical fistulae; six-year experience of 90 consecutive cases. *Colorectal Dis.* **2006**, *8*, 347–352. [CrossRef]

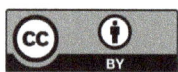

© 2020 by the authors. Licensee MDPI, Basel, Switzerland. This article is an open access article distributed under the terms and conditions of the Creative Commons Attribution (CC BY) license (http://creativecommons.org/licenses/by/4.0/).

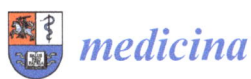

Article

Methotrexate and Adalimumab Decrease the Serum Levels of Cardiovascular Disease Biomarkers (VCAM-1 and E-Selectin) in Plaque Psoriasis

Natalia Zdanowska [1],*, Agnieszka Owczarczyk-Saczonek [1], Joanna Czerwińska [1], Jacek J. Nowakowski [2], Anna Kozera-Żywczyk [3], Witold Owczarek [3], Wojciech Zdanowski [4] and Waldemar Placek [1]

1. Department of Dermatology, Sexually Transmitted Diseases and Clinical Immunology, The University of Warmia and Mazury, 10-229 Olsztyn, Poland; aganek@wp.pl (A.O.-S.); joannaj061@gmail.com (J.C.); w.placek@wp.pl (W.P.)
2. Department of Ecology and Environmental Protection, The University of Warmia and Mazury, 10-727 Olsztyn, Poland; jacek.nowakowski@uwm.edu.pl
3. Department of Dermatology, Military Institute of the Health Services, 04-141 Warsaw, Poland; annakozera@o2.pl (A.K.-Ż.); witold.owczarek@dermedicus.pl (W.O.)
4. Department of Gynecology and Obstetrics, The University of Warmia and Mazury, 10-561 Olsztyn, Poland; wojciechzdanowskiw@gmail.com
* Correspondence: natalia.zdanowska@uwm.edu.pl; Tel.: +48-89-6786670

Received: 1 August 2020; Accepted: 14 September 2020; Published: 15 September 2020

Abstract: *Background and objectives:* The shared pathogenesis of psoriasis and atherosclerosis may be determined by assaying the levels of endothelial activation molecules. This study aimed at evaluating vascular cell adhesion molecule 1 (VCAM-1) and E-selectin serum concentrations, and atherosclerosis severity in patients with plaque psoriasis. It also aimed to determine the effects of methotrexate/adalimumab treatment for 12 weeks on the plasma levels of the aforementioned molecules. *Materials and Methods:* The study included 34 psoriasis patients (17 treated with methotrexate and 17 treated with adalimumab) and eight controls. The 10-year risk of a fatal cardiovascular disease, body mass index, Psoriasis Area and Severity Index, and body surface area were calculated for each subject. VCAM-1 and E-selectin levels were determined via an enzyme-linked immunosorbent assay at baseline and after 12 weeks. *Results:* Baseline E-selectin and VCAM-1 levels were higher in the adalimumab group than in the methotrexate and control groups. VCAM-1 levels decreased in the adalimumab ($p = 0.02$) and methotrexate groups ($p = 0.008$), while E-selectin levels decreased in the methotrexate group ($p = 0.004$). *Conclusions:* The results indicate a correlation between systemic psoriasis treatment and E-selectin and VCAM-1 plasma concentrations, which may be associated with the risk of cardiovascular disease development.

Keywords: VCAM-1; E-selectin; psoriasis; methotrexate; adalimumab

1. Introduction

Epidemiological data have provided evidence of an association between psoriasis and adverse cardiovascular outcomes [1]. This association may be determined by assessing their shared pathogenesis involving endothelial dysfunction [2,3]. Vascular cell adhesion molecule 1 (VCAM-1) is an inducible glycoprotein, and E-selectin is a soluble cell adhesion molecule. Both molecules are primarily expressed in the endothelium [4–7]. The serum levels of soluble VCAM-1 appear to be correlated with the degree of atherosclerosis and may be used for diagnosing the early stages of the condition [8]. Endothelial activation, resulting in E-selectin expansion, induces leukocyte rolling along the vascular wall and mediates inflammation in various diseases, including atherosclerosis [9]. A common feature of the inflammatory process in psoriasis and atherosclerosis is leukocyte migration, to which VCAM-1 and E-selectin significantly contribute. These adhesion molecules, being the indicators of endothelial activation, might be potential biomarkers of inflammatory activity and of the severity of atherosclerosis and cardiovascular disease coexisting with psoriasis [10].

In clinical practice, atherosclerosis and its severity are assessed by determining the 10-year risk of fatal cardiovascular disease, which is estimated using the European Risk Chart: Systematic Coronary Risk Evaluation (SCORE) [11,12]. Methotrexate (MTX) is used to treat psoriasis, and one of its main mechanisms of action is believed to be based on its effect of decreasing E-selectin expression [13,14]. Endothelial function, which is significantly altered in psoriasis patients, may also improve during treatment with tumor necrosis factor alpha (TNF-alpha) inhibitors [15].

This study aimed at determining VCAM-1 and E-selectin levels and evaluating their relationship with psoriasis severity compared to those in healthy controls. We also estimated atherosclerosis severity by evaluating cardiovascular risk in patients with plaque psoriasis who were assigned to receive a systemic treatment. The objective was also to assess the impact of 12-week MTX and adalimumab (ADA) treatments on the VCAM-1 and E-selectin concentrations in psoriasis patients. We believe our research will supplement information concerning cardiovascular and atherosclerosis risks in patients with plaque psoriasis, as well as the effects of MTX and ADA on endothelial activation markers in psoriasis. Understanding the impact of systemic psoriasis treatment on E-selectin and VCAM-1 serum levels will enable the selection of the appropriate therapy for both cardiovascular disease and skin lesions as coexisting conditions.

2. Materials and Methods

Study Group

This prospective cohort study was conducted in 34 patients (27 men and seven women) with plaque psoriasis (age: 30–73 years) and eight healthy volunteers (age: 30–57 years) as the control group. The study was approved by the Bioethics Commission at the University of Warmia and Mazury in Olsztyn, Poland (Resolution 16/2019). Each patient included in the study provided informed consent for participation. The inclusion criteria included being of an age higher than 18 years and a diagnosis of moderate-to-severe plaque psoriasis. The exclusion criteria were as follows: age below 18 years, mild plaque psoriasis, pregnancy, breastfeeding, and previous biological treatment (in the case of patients who qualified for MTX treatment). Due to the requirements of the treatment program for moderate-to-severe plaque psoriasis in Poland, patients starting ADA treatment confirmed the contraindications and/or side effects associated with the use of at least two classic methods of systemic psoriasis treatment or a history of ineffective systemic treatment. The systemic treatment is understood as the use of at least two of the following agents: MTX, cyclosporine, acitretin, and psoralen ultraviolet A (PUVA).

Of the patients, 17 were treated only with MTX and the remaining 17 were treated with ADA only. The patients received oral MTX at a dose of 7.5–20 mg per week and subcutaneous ADA at an initial dose of 80 mg followed by 40 mg every 2 weeks. The observation period lasted 12 weeks. The following parameters were evaluated for each subject: body mass index (BMI), the severity of psoriasis based on the Psoriasis Area and Severity Index (PASI), and body surface area (BSA). Depending on risk factors, such as age, sex, systolic blood pressure, smoking, and total cholesterol, the risk of fatal cardiovascular disease events over the next 10-year period was estimated using SCORE charts [16]. Laboratory tests to determine E-selectin and VCAM-1 serum levels were performed via an enzyme-linked immunosorbent assay (commercial ELISA kit, EIAab Science Co., Ltd., Wuhan, China) by using fasting blood samples obtained before and after 12 weeks of treatment.

Statistical analyses were performed using Statistica 13.1 (StatSoft Poland). Mean values and standard deviations (±SD) were used to describe the level of variables (PASI, BSA, VCAM-1, E-selectin) and demographic characteristics of the studied groups. The distributions of all studied explanatory metric variables in the groups were compared to the normal distribution using the Shapiro–Wilk test, and the homogeneity of variance was tested using the Bartlett test. The one-way ANOVA model was used when the important assumptions for the analysis of variance were met. In case of failure to meet the assumption with a distribution close to normal, the Kruskal–Wallis test was used. The Mann–Whitney test was used to test the differentiation of variable levels between two groups: MTX vs. control and ADA vs. control. Comparisons of variables over time (baseline (W0) vs. the end of the study (W12)) were made using the paired samples Student's T-test if a parametric analysis was possible. For other cases, the nonparametric Wilcoxon test was used. Correlations were analyzed using Spearman's correlation coefficient. The χ^2 test was used to compare the distribution of two demographic nominal characteristics (sex, smoking) between the experimental and control groups. The Kruskal–Wallis test was also used for the comparison of the level of VCAM-1 and E-selectin between four groups of patients classified as presenting different SCORE risk levels. Differences and correlations were considered statistically significant at $p < 0.05$.

3. Results

The demographic data of the patients included in the study are listed in Table 1. BMI was significantly higher in the psoriasis group than in the control group ($p = 0.001$). Likewise, the BMI in psoriasis patients was significantly and positively correlated with PASI and BSA (Spearman's correlation coefficients 0.5 and 0.56; $p = 0.0007$ and $p = 0.0001$, respectively). The healthy volunteers were nonsmokers. They were significantly younger ($p = 0.01$), and had significantly lower systolic blood pressure ($p = 0.04$) than the patients qualifying for MTX treatment. Therefore, the 10-year risk of fatal cardiovascular disease and atherosclerosis risk (estimated via the European Risk Chart SCORE) among the healthy volunteers were significantly lower than the corresponding risks among psoriasis patients assigned to receive MTX ($p = 0.001$).

Table 1. Demographic characteristics of the study groups at baseline (W0).

	MTX (n = 17)	ADA (n = 17)	Control (n = 8)	p
Age (years) (mean ± SD)	33–73 (52.9 ± 11.97)	24–72 (46.1 ± 13.55)	30–57 (34.6 ± 9.38)	0.005 [1] 0.25 * 0.01 ** 0.15 ***
Sex (M/F)	14/3	13/4	2/6	0.01 [2,4]
Height (cm) (mean ± SD)	158–190 (174.2 ± 8.49)	161–186 (174.6 ± 20.62)	160–192 (172.4 ± 11.59)	0.832 [3,6]
Weight (kg) (mean ± SD)	63–129 (88.3 ± 17.29)	60–115 (93.4 ± 25.40)	48–98 (68.6 ± 19.03)	0.014 [3] 0.58 * 0.18 ** 0.01 ***
BMI (kg/m^2) (mean ± SD)	23.1–39.8 (29 ± 5.24)	24–42.4 (30.7 ± 8.69)	19.1–33 (22.6 ± 5.14)	0.001 [1] 0.57 * 0.03 ** 0.005 ***
Cholesterol, total (mg/dL) (mean ± SD)	144–303 (212 ± 44.52)	144–276 (203 ± 43.28)	173–244 (210.5 ± 24.63)	0.805 [1,5]
Smoking: yes/no	10/7	5/12	0/8	0.01 [2,4]
Systolic blood pressure (mmHg) (mean ± SD)	125–177 (140.9 ± 16.4)	109–156 (134.4 ± 13.35)	110–135 (123.6 ± 9.4)	0.049 [3] 1.0 * 0.04 ** 0.2 ***
SCORE (%) (mean ± SD)	<1–10 (6.9 ± 7.36)	<1–8 (3.2 ± 2.23)	<1–1 (1 ± 0)	0.0012 [3] 0.31 * 0.001 ** 0.07 ***

Abbreviations: MTX: patients qualified for treatment with methotrexate; ADA: patients qualified for treatment with adalimumab; BMI: body mass index; SCORE: estimation of the risk of fatal cardiovascular disease events over the next 10-year period via Systematic Coronary Risk Evaluation charts. [1] One-way ANOVA model, [2] χ^2 test, [3] Kruskal–Wallis tests, [4] nonrandomized group structure, [5] no level of differentiation between the study groups, [6] no significant differentiation was found by testing the hypothesis with the Kruskal–Wallis test, and there are no post hoc results, * post hoc test: MTX vs. ADA, ** post hoc test: MTX vs. control, *** post hoc test: ADA vs. control.

Figures 1 and 2 show the levels of VCAM-1 and E-selectin in patients depending on the ten-year risk of fatal cardiovascular disease estimated via SCORE charts. At baseline, the serum levels of VCAM-1 and E-selectin were significantly higher in patients with an estimated SCORE risk >= 10% compared to patients with a risk of <1% ($p = 0.02$ and $p = 0.012$, respectively).

The evaluation of the severity of psoriasis is shown in Table 2. Patients who qualified for treatment with ADA presented more severe psoriatic lesions than those who qualified for MTX therapy. As shown in Table 3, baseline VCAM-1 and E-selectin levels were significantly correlated with disease activity (PASI and BSA) in psoriasis patients. Interestingly, when examining only the patients assigned for treatment with MTX or ADA, the correlation between these values was not significant. Table 4 shows the VCAM-1 and E-selectin levels at W0 and W12 in groups of patients treated with MTX and ADA. In the control group, only W0 values were noted, as the group included healthy volunteers who did not require treatment.

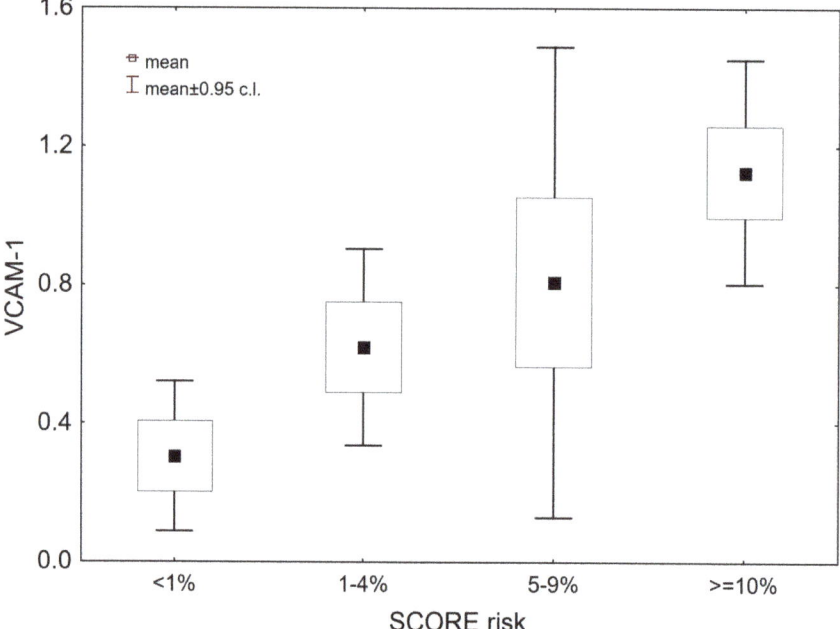

Figure 1. Vascular cell adhesion molecule 1 serum levels in patients with ten-year risk of fatal cardiovascular disease estimated via SCORE charts. Abbreviations—VCAM-1: vascular cell adhesion molecule 1, SCORE risk: ten-year risk of fatal cardiovascular disease estimated via SCORE (Systemic Coronary Risk Evaluation) charts.

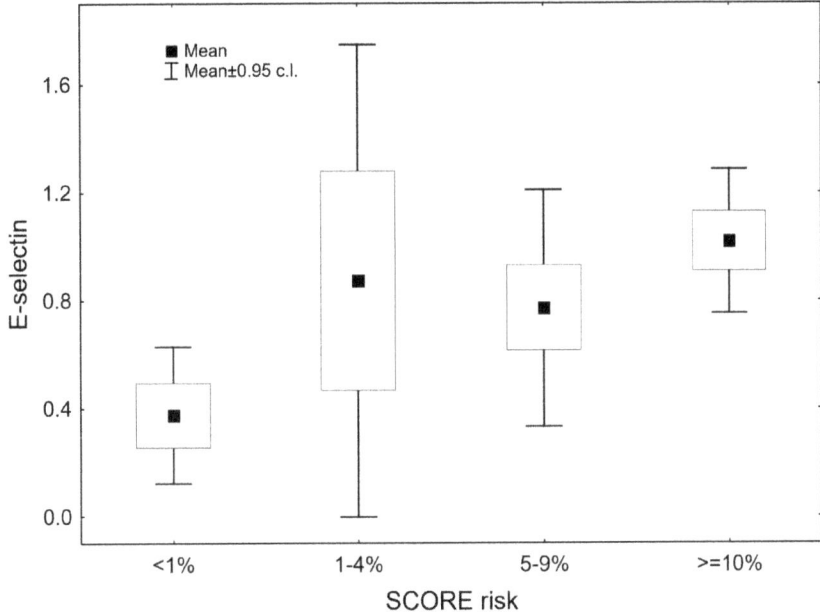

Figure 2. E-selectin serum levels in patients with ten-year risk of fatal cardiovascular disease estimated via SCORE charts. Abbreviations—SCORE risk: ten-year risk of fatal cardiovascular disease estimated via SCORE (Systemic Coronary Risk Evaluation) charts.

Table 2. Severity of psoriasis (Psoriasis Area and Severity Index (PASI) and Body Surface Area (BSA)) during the study period.

	MTX (n = 17)		ADA (n = 17)	
	W0	W12	W0	W12
PASI (mean ± SD)	6.5–26.2 (12 ± 5.0)	0–15 (4.5 ± 4.05)	12.1–33.2 (20.6 ± 5.41)	0–11.8 (3.6 ± 3.11)
	$p = 0.001$ [1]		$p = 0.0003$ [1]	
BSA (%) (mean ± SD)	10–46 (19.8 ± 9.43)	0–20 (6.9 ± 6.30)	12.5–77 (33.8 ± 17.57)	0–22.5 (8.9 ± 8.77)
	$p = 0.002$ [1]		$p = 0.0005$ [1]	

Abbreviations: PASI: Psoriasis Area and Severity Index; BSA: body surface area; W0: baseline; W12: end of the study; [1] Wilcoxon test.

Table 3. Correlation of VCAM-1 and E-selectin levels with PASI and BSA at W0.

Values at Baseline (W0)		Ps (n = 34)		MTX (n = 17)		ADA (n = 17)	
		Spearman's Correlation Coefficient	p	Spearman's Correlation Coefficient	p	Spearman's Correlation Coefficient	p
VCAM-1	PASI	−0.4	0.01	−0.21	0.4	−0.07	0.76
	BSA	−0.38	0.02	−0.15	0.54	−0.21	0.4
E-selectin	PASI	−0.4	0.01	−0.27	0.29	−0.06	0.81
	BSA	−0.35	0.03	−0.21	0.4	−0.1	0.7

Abbreviations: VCAM-1: vascular cell adhesion molecule 1; Ps: psoriasis patients; MTX: patients qualified for treatment with methotrexate; ADA: patients qualified for treatment with adalimumab; PASI: Psoriasis Area and Severity Index; BSA: body surface area.

Table 4. VCAM-1 and E-selectin serum levels at W0 and W12.

		Methotrexate		Adalimumab		Control	Comparisons between the Groups		
		Mean (ng/mL) ± SD	p (W0 vs. W12)	Mean (ng/mL) ± SD	p (W0 vs. W12)	Mean (ng/mL) ± SD	MTX vs. ADA (p)	MTX vs. C (p)	ADA vs. C (p)
VCAM-1	W0	0.45 ± 0.32	0.008 [1]	1.03 ± 0.46	0.02 [1]	0.04 ± 0.03	0.01 [2]	0.02 [2]	0.000002 [2]
	W12	0.2 ± 0.22		0.91 ± 0.33		N/A	0.000005 [3]	N/A	N/A
E-selectin	W0	0.46 ± 0.39	0.004 [1]	1.24 ± 1.26	0.16 [1]	0.04 ± 0.05	0.027 [2]	0.034 [2]	0.00001 [2]
	W12	0.16 ± 0.19		0.9 ± 0.33		N/A	0.000005 [3]	N/A	N/A

Abbreviations: VCAM-1: vascular cell adhesion molecule 1; W0: baseline; W12: end of the study; MTX: patients qualified for treatment with methotrexate; ADA: patients qualified for treatment with adalimumab; C: control group.
[1] Wilcoxon test, [2] Kruskal–Wallis test, and [3] Mann–Whitney test.

At W0, the highest levels of VCAM-1 and E-selectin were found in the subjects assigned to receive ADA, and the lowest levels were noted in the control group. Regarding the plasma levels of VCAM-1, a comparison between the groups showed significant differences among patients starting treatment with ADA versus MTX ($p = 0.01$) and versus the control group ($p = 0.000002$). Differences were also significant between patients starting treatment with MTX and the control group ($p = 0.02$). With regard to the levels of E-selectin, significant differences were found among patients starting treatment with ADA versus MTX ($p = 0.027$) and versus the control group ($p = 0.00001$). Furthermore, significant differences were observed in patients starting treatment with MTX versus the control group ($p = 0.034$). At W12, the difference between the MTX and ADA groups in terms of the levels of both E-selectin ($p = 0.000005$) and VCAM-1 ($p = 0.000005$) was also significant. A significant decrease was noted in the VCAM-1 serum levels (W0 vs. W12) in patients treated with ADA ($p = 0.02$) or MTX ($p = 0.008$). The reduction in E-selectin level was significant only in patients treated with MTX ($p = 0.004$).

4. Discussion

The results of our study highlight a relationship between the severity of psoriasis as described via PASI and BSA with BMI and the levels of VCAM-1 and E-selectin. They also prove the relationship between the level of studied particles and the ten-year risk of fatal cardiovascular events estimated via SCORE charts. A significant decrease in the serum levels of both studied adhesion molecules was observed in patients receiving MTX. However, only VCAM-1 levels decreased in patients treated with ADA.

The interaction of endothelial adhesion molecules (such as VCAM-1) with selectins (including E-selectin) mediates the migration of activated T cells and macrophages from blood vessels. It also initiates adherence between the vascular endothelium and neutrophils, monocytes, eosinophils, and T lymphocytes during the inflammatory process, resulting in plaque formation in both psoriasis and atherosclerosis [17–19]. Several studies showed higher levels of E-selectin and VCAM-1 in psoriasis [19–22]. The E-selectin serum level is correlated with the severity of psoriasis (as indicated by PASI), so it appears to be an indicator of disease activity [21]. Furthermore, Szepietowski et al. confirmed that the plasma levels of E-selectin significantly decreased after treatment in psoriasis patients [19].

The present study demonstrated the highest VCAM-1 and E-selectin levels in the group of patients assigned to receive ADA, lower values in patients beginning MTX treatment, and the lowest values in the control group. Baseline VCAM-1 and E-selectin levels were significantly and negatively correlated with PASI and BSA in psoriasis patients. Interestingly, the correlation between these levels was not significant after the patients were divided into MTX and ADA treatment groups. Similarly, BMI was significantly correlated with the severity and extent of skin lesions (as indicated by PASI and BSA) in psoriasis patients. No correlation of BMI with either VCAM-1 or E-selectin was found. A high BMI appears to be positively correlated with the severity of psoriasis and defines the clinical response to systemic treatment [23–25]. Long-term anti-TNF-alpha therapy was related to BMI elevation in psoriasis patients [26,27].

Few reports demonstrated the correlation of adhesion molecules with BMI. Most of them concerned E-selectin, whose level positively correlated with BMI [28–30]. However, Abd El-Kader et al. demonstrated that a reduction in BMI resulted in the modulation of VCAM-1 levels in obese patients with type 2 diabetes [31]. The essential mechanism of action of MTX in psoriasis might relate to a decrease in E-selectin expression during treatment. Torres-Alvares et al. showed that a reduced expression of E-selectin and VCAM-1 in the blood vessels of psoriasis patients after therapy [13,14]. Endothelial function, which is significantly altered in psoriasis patients, may also improve during treatment with TNF-alpha inhibitors. Furthermore, several studies provided evidence of a decrease in E-selectin levels in the sera of psoriasis patients during treatment with infliximab or ADA [2,10,15,32].

In our study, E-selectin and VCAM-1 levels significantly decreased during MTX treatment. Moreover, contrary to E-selectin levels, the decrease in VCAM-1 was significant in patients treated with ADA. The results suggest that endothelial function and the cardiovascular risk of patients with plaque psoriasis are influenced to a larger extent by MTX than ADA.

The most significant limitations of our study were the low number of patients (34 psoriasis patients and eight healthy volunteers), short observation time (12 weeks), and volunteer self-selection of the control group. Volunteer serum samples were not obtained for VCAM-1 and E-selectin determination at W12 because, as healthy individuals, they were not treated. The present results will be verified in a larger study group over an extended period to draw more general conclusions, including the impact of systemic therapy of psoriasis on cardiovascular risk.

5. Conclusions

The results of our study demonstrate a possible impact of psoriasis itself and its systemic treatment on serum E-selectin and VCAM-1 levels. Therefore, they indicate the risk of developing cardiovascular disease. VCAM-1 and E-selectin serum levels appear to be correlated with psoriasis severity as indicated by PASI and BSA. After 12 weeks of MTX administration, E-selectin and VCAM-1 levels significantly decreased. However, treatment with ADA resulted in a significant decrease only in VCAM-1 levels. Therefore, compared to ADA, MTX may have a greater impact on the levels of adhesion molecules, so it might help determine the risk of cardiovascular disease development in psoriasis patients.

Author Contributions: Conceptualization, N.Z. and A.O.-S.; data curation, N.Z., J.C., J.J.N., and W.Z.; investigation, N.Z. and J.C.; methodology, J.C.; resources, N.Z., A.K.-Ż., and W.O.; supervision, A.O.-S. and W.P.; writing—original draft, N.Z.; writing—review and editing, N.Z. and A.O.-S. All authors have read and agreed to the published version of the manuscript.

Funding: This study was supported by the Ministry of Science and Higher Education (Ministerstwo Nauki i Szkolnictwa Wyższego) of Poland, Grant No. 61.610. 001-300.

Acknowledgments: The authors would like to thank Abbvie for its help in purchasing research reagents.

Conflicts of Interest: The authors declare no conflict of interest.

References

1. Masson, W.; Lobo, M.; Molinero, G. Psoriasis and Cardiovascular Risk: A Comprehensive Review. *Adv. Ther.* **2020**, *37*, 2017–2033. [CrossRef] [PubMed]
2. Brezinski, E.A.; Follansbee, M.R.; Armstrong, E.J.; Armstrong, A.W. Endothelial dysfunction and the effects of TNF inhibitors on the endothelium in psoriasis and psoriatic arthritis: A systematic review. *Curr. Pharm. Des.* **2014**, *20*, 513–528. [CrossRef]
3. Haberka, M.; Bańska-Kisiel, K.; Bergler-Czop, B.; Biedroń, M.; Brzezińska-Wcisło, L.; Okopień, B.; Gąsior, Z. Mild to moderate psoriasis is associated with oxidative stress, subclinical atherosclerosis, and endothelial dysfunction. *Pol. Arch. Intern. Med.* **2018**, *128*, 434–439. [PubMed]

4. Kong, D.-H.; Kim, Y.K.; Kim, M.R.; Jang, J.H.; Lee, S. Emerging roles of vascular cell adhesion molecule-1 (VCAM-1) in immunological disorders and cancer. *Int. J. Mol. Sci.* **2018**, *19*, 1057. [CrossRef] [PubMed]
5. Milstone, D.S.; O'Donnell, P.E.; Stavrakis, G.; Mortensen, R.M.; Davis, V.M. E-selectin expression and stimulation by inflammatory mediators are developmentally regulated during embryogenesis. *Lab. Investig.* **2000**, *80*, 943–954. [CrossRef] [PubMed]
6. Rossi, B.; Constantin, G. Anti-selectin therapy for the treatment of inflammatory diseases. *Inflamm. Allergy Drug Targets* **2008**, *7*, 85–93. [CrossRef]
7. Dowlatshahi, E.A.; Van Der Voort, E.A.M.; Arends, L.R.; Nijsten, T. Markers of systemic inflammation in psoriasis: A systematic review and meta-analysis. *Br. J. Dermatol.* **2013**, *169*, 266–282. [CrossRef]
8. Peter, K.; Weirich, U.; Nordt, T.K.; Ruef, J.; Bode, C. Soluble vascular cell adhesion molecule-1 (VCAM-1) as potential marker of atherosclerosis. *Thromb. Haemost.* **1999**, *82* (Suppl. 1), 38–43.
9. Tsoref, O.; Tyomkin, D.; Amit, U.; Landa, N.; Cohen-Rosenboim, O.; Kain, D.; Golan, M.; Naftali-Shani, N.; David, A.; Leor, J. E-selectin-targeted copolymer reduces atherosclerotic lesions, adverse cardiac remodeling, and dysfunction. *J. Control. Release* **2018**, *288*, 136–147. [CrossRef]
10. Genre, F.; Armesto, S.; Corrales, A.; López-Mejías, R.; Remuzgo-Martínez, S.; Pina, T.; Ubilla, B.; Mijares, V.; Martín-Varillas, J.L.; Rueda-Gotor, J.; et al. Significant sE-Selectin levels reduction after 6 months of anti-TNF-α therapy in non-diabetic patients with moderate-to-severe psoriasis. *J. Dermatol. Treat.* **2017**, *28*, 726–730. [CrossRef]
11. Yalcin, M.; Kardesoglu, E.; Aparci, M.; Isilak, Z.; Uz, O.; Yiginer, O.; Ozmen, N.; Cingozbay, B.Y.; Uzun, M.; Cebeci, B.S. Cardiovascular risk scores for coronary atherosclerosis. *Acta Cardiol.* **2012**, *67*, 557–563. [CrossRef] [PubMed]
12. Versteylen, M.O.; Joosen, I.A.; Shaw, L.J.; Narula, J.; Hofstra, L. Comparison of Framingham, PROCAM, SCORE, and Diamond Forrester to predict coronary atherosclerosis and cardiovascular events. *J. Nucl. Cardiol.* **2011**, *18*, 904–911. [CrossRef] [PubMed]
13. Sigmundsdottir, H.; Johnston, A.; Gudjonsson, J.E.; Bjarnason, B.; Valdimarsson, H. Methotrexate markedly reduces the expression of vascular E-selectin, cutaneous lymphocyte-associated antigen and the numbers of mononuclear leucocytes in psoriatic skin. *Exp. Dermatol.* **2004**, *13*, 426–434. [CrossRef] [PubMed]
14. Torres-Alvarez, B.; Castanedo-Cazares, J.P.; Fuentes-Ahumada, C.; Moncada, B. The effect of methotrexate on the expression of cell adhesion molecules and activation molecule CD69 in psoriasis. *J. Eur. Acad. Dermatol. Venereol.* **2007**, *21*, 334–339. [CrossRef]
15. Gkalpakiotis, S.; Arenbergerova, M.; Gkalpakioti, P.; Potockova, J.; Arenberger, P.; Kraml, P. Impact of adalimumab treatment on cardiovascular risk biomarkers in psoriasis: Results of a pilot study. *J. Dermatol.* **2017**, *44*, 363–369. [CrossRef]
16. Piepoli, M.F.; Hoes, A.W.; Agewall, S.; Albus, C.; Brotons, C.; Catapano, A.L.; Cooney, M.T.; Corrà, U.; Cosyns, B.; Deaton, C.; et al. 2016 European Guidelines on cardiovascular disease prevention in clinical practice: The Sixth Joint Task Force of the European Society of Cardiology and Other Societies on Cardiovascular Disease Prevention in Clinical Practice (constituted by representatives of 10 societies and by invited experts) Developed with the special contribution of the European Association for Cardiovascular Prevention & Rehabilitation (EACPR). *Eur. Heart J.* **2016**, *37*, 2315–2381.
17. Conroy, R.M.; Pyörälä, K.; Fitzgerald, A.P.; Sans, S.; Menotti, A.; De Backer, G.; De Bacquer, D.; Ducimetière, P.; Jousilahti, P.; Keil, U.; et al. Estimation of ten-year risk of fatal cardiovascular disease in Europe: The SCORE project. *Eur. Heart J.* **2003**, *24*, 987–1003. [CrossRef]
18. Sigurdardottir, G.; Ekman, A.K.; Ståhle, M.; Bivik, C.; Enerbäck, C. Systemic treatment and narrowband ultraviolet B differentially affect cardiovascular risk markers in psoriasis. *J. Am. Acad. Dermatol.* **2014**, *70*, 1067–1075. [CrossRef]
19. Kim, J.; Tomalin, L.; Lee, J.; Fitz, L.J.; Berstein, G.; da Rosa, J.C.; Garcet, S.; Lowes, M.A.; Valdez, H.; Wolk, R.; et al. Reduction of inflammatory and cardiovascular proteins in the blood of patients with psoriasis: Differential responses between tofacitinib and etanercept after 4 weeks of treatment. *J. Investig. Dermatol.* **2018**, *138*, 273–281. [CrossRef]
20. Szepietowski, J.C.; Wasik, F.; Bielicka, E.; Nockowski, P.; Noworolska, A. Soluble E-selectin serum levels correlate with disease activity in psoriatic patients. *Clin. Exp. Dermatol.* **1999**, *24*, 33–36. [CrossRef]

21. Teixeira, G.G.; Mari, N.L.; de Paula, J.C.C.; de Alcantara, C.C.; Flauzino, T.; Lozovoy, M.A.B.; Martin, L.M.M.; Reiche, E.M.V.; Maes, M.; Dichi, I.; et al. Cell adhesion molecules, plasminogen activator inhibitor type 1, and metabolic syndrome in patients with psoriasis. *Clin. Exp. Med.* **2020**, *20*, 39–48. [CrossRef] [PubMed]
22. Bonifati, C.; Trento, E.; Carducci, M.; Sacerdoti, G.; Mussi, A.; Fazio, M.; Ameglio, F. Soluble E-selectin and soluble tumour necrosis factor receptor (60 kD) serum levels in patients with psoriasis. *Dermatology* **1995**, *190*, 128–131. [CrossRef] [PubMed]
23. Cordiali-Fei, P.; Trento, E.; D'Agosto, G.; Bordignon, V.; Mussi, A.; Ardigò, M.; Mastroianni, A.; Vento, A.; Solivetti, F.; Berardesca, E.; et al. Decreased levels of metalloproteinase-9 and angiogenic factors in skin lesions of patients with psoriatic arthritis after therapy with anti-TNF-alpha. *J. Autoimmune Disord.* **2006**, *3*, 5. [CrossRef] [PubMed]
24. Kacalak-Rzepka, A.; Kiedrowicz, M.; Maleszka, R. Analysis of the chosen parameters of metabolic status in patients with psoriasis. *Ann. Acad. Med. Stetin.* **2013**, *59*, 12–17.
25. Naldi, L.; Addis, A.; Chimenti, S.; Giannetti, A.; Picardo, M.; Tomino, C.; Maccarone, M.; Chatenoud, L.; Bertuccio, P.; Caggese, E.; et al. Impact of body mass index and obesity on clinical response to systemic treatment for psoriasis. Evidence from the Psocare project. *Dermatology* **2008**, *217*, 365–373. [CrossRef]
26. Hercogová, J.; Ricceri, F.; Tripo, L.; Lotti, T.; Prignano, F. Psoriasis and body mass index. *Dermatol. Ther.* **2010**, *23*, 152–154. [CrossRef]
27. Gisondi, P.; Cotena, C.; Tessari, G.; Girolomoni, G. Anti-tumour necrosis factor-α therapy increases body weight in patients with chronic plaque psoriasis: A retrospective cohort study. *J. Eur. Acad. Dermatol. Venereol.* **2008**, *22*, 341–344. [CrossRef]
28. Wu, M.Y.; Yu, C.L.; Yang, S.J.; Chi, C.C. Change in body weight and body mass index in psoriasis patients receiving biologics: A systematic review and network meta-analysis. *J. Am. Acad. Dermatol.* **2020**, *82*, 101–109. [CrossRef]
29. Lee, C.H.; Kuo, F.C.; Tang, W.H.; Lu, C.H.; Su, S.C.; Liu, J.S.; Hsieh, C.H.; Hung, Y.J.; Lin, F.H. Serum E-selectin concentration is associated with risk of metabolic syndrome in females. *PLoS ONE* **2019**, *14*, e0222815. [CrossRef]
30. Ponthieux, A.; Herbeth, B.; Droesch, S.; Haddy, N.; Lambert, D.; Visvikis, S. Biological determinants of serum ICAM-1, E-selectin, P-selectin and L-selectin levels in healthy subjects: The Stanislas study. *Atherosclerosis* **2004**, *172*, 299–308. [CrossRef]
31. El-Kader, S.M.A.; Al-Jiffri, O.H. Impact of weight reduction on insulin resistance, adhesive molecules and adipokines dysregulation among obese type 2 diabetic patients. *Afr. Health Sci.* **2018**, *18*, 873–883. [CrossRef] [PubMed]
32. Mastroianni, A.; Minutilli, E.; Mussi, A.; Bordignon, V.; Trento, E.; D'Agosto, G.; Cordiali-Fei, P.; Berardesca, E. Cytokine profiles during infliximab monotherapy in psoriatic arthritis. *Br. J. Dermatol.* **2005**, *153*, 531–536. [CrossRef] [PubMed]

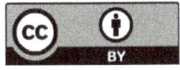

© 2020 by the authors. Licensee MDPI, Basel, Switzerland. This article is an open access article distributed under the terms and conditions of the Creative Commons Attribution (CC BY) license (http://creativecommons.org/licenses/by/4.0/).

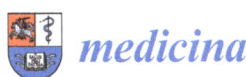

Case Report

Management of a Patient with Tuberous Sclerosis with Urological Clinical Manifestations

Vlad Padureanu [1,†], Octavian Dragoescu [2,†], Victor Emanuel Stoenescu [2,†], Rodica Padureanu [3,*], Ionica Pirici [4,*], Radu Cristian Cimpeanu [5], Dop Dalia [6], Alexandru Radu Mihailovici [7] and Paul Tomescu [2]

1. Department of Internal Medicine, University of Medicine and Pharmacy Craiova, 200349 Craiova, Romania; vldpadureanu@yahoo.com
2. Department of Urology, University of Medicine and Pharmacy Craiova, 200349 Craiova, Romania; pdragoescu@yahoo.com (O.D.); victorstoenescu@yahoo.com (V.E.S.); paul.tomescu@yahoo.com (P.T.)
3. Department of Biochemistry, University of Medicine and Pharmacy of Craiova, 200349 Craiova, Romania
4. Department of Anatomy, University of Medicine and Pharmacy of Craiova, 200349 Craiova, Romania
5. Student, University of Medicine and Pharmacy Craiova, 200349 Craiova, Romania; cimpeanu_r@yahoo.com
6. Department of Pediatrics, University of Medicine and Pharmacy of Craiova, 200349 Craiova, Romania; dalia_tastea@yahoo.com
7. Department of Cardiology, University of Medicine and Pharmacy of Craiova, 200349 Craiova, Romania; drmihailovici@yahoo.com
* Correspondence: zegheanurodica@yahoo.com (R.P.); danapirici@yahoo.com (I.P.)
† All these authors contributed equally to this work.

Received: 8 June 2020; Accepted: 19 July 2020; Published: 23 July 2020

Abstract: The tuberous sclerosis complex (TSC) is highly variable as far as its clinical presentation is concerned. For the implementation of appropriate medical surveillance and treatment, an accurate diagnosis is compulsory. TSC may affect the heart, skin, kidneys, central nervous system (epileptic seizures and nodular intracranial tumors—tubers), bones, eyes, lungs, blood vessels and the gastrointestinal tract. The aim of this paper is to report renal manifestations as first clinical signs suggestive of TSC diagnosis. A 20-year-old patient was initially investigated for hematuria, dysuria and colicky pain in the left lumbar region. The ultrasound examination of the kidney showed bilateral hyperechogenic kidney structures and pyelocalyceal dilatation, both suggestive of bilateral obstructive lithiasis, complicated by uretero-hydronephrosis. The computer tomography (CT) scan of the kidney showed irregular kidney margins layout, undifferentiated images between cortical and medullar structures, with non-homogenous round components, suggestive of kidney angiomyolipomas, bilateral renal cortical retention cysts, images of a calculous component in the right middle calyceal branches and a smaller one on the left side. The clinical manifestations and imaging findings (skull and abdominal and pelvis CT scans) sustained the diagnosis.

Keywords: tuberous sclerosis; angiomyolipomatosis; uretero-hydronephrosis; angiofibromas

1. Introduction

The tuberous sclerosis complex (TSC) is an extremely variable disease that can affect any organs, from the brain, eyes, kidneys, skin, heart, and lungs, to occasionally the bones, because of growing benign tumors [1]. Until the 1980s, TSC was underdiagnosed when individuals with less severe manifestations of the disease began to be recognized. Nowadays, it has been established that the genetic component of this disease is linked to TSC1 and TSC2 genes' alterations [2]. Pathogenic mutations in either the TSC2 gene at chromosome 16p13.3, or the TSC1 gene at chromosome 9q34, cause a multisystem disorder that greatly varies in extent and severity [3]. TSC has an autosomal dominant mode of inheritance, with almost complete penetrance, but variable expressivity [1]. Both genders and all ethnic groups could be affected by TSC [1]. More so, since 2010 the m-TOR inhibitor drugs are administrated as a medical treatment for the benign tumors, in combination with a possible surgical management [2].

2. Case Report

A 30-year-old Romanian patient, female, from urban background, with significant family history, came to the Emergency Department of our hospital for colicky pain in the left lumbar region, pollakiuria, hematuria, dysuria, nausea, unspecified vomiting, fever, chills and cough. All these symptoms had started 2 days prior to the presentation and had intensified in the last 3–4 h. The patient had a suggestive family history for neurological diseases (a grandfather with a kidney tumor, father with epilepsy, uncle (brother of father)—epilepsy and intellectual disability, aunt (sister of father)—intellectual disability, and a sister with epilepsy). At the admission the patient had a Glasgow Coma Scale score of 15, a respiratory rate of 16 rpm, 99% Oxygen Saturation, blood pressure of 135/95 mmHg, with a heart rate of 90 beats/minute, and body temperature of 37,7 °C.

The findings of the physical examination were: normal body build, pale skin and mucosae, facial angiofibromas on the nasal wings, cheek and chin (Figure 1), hypopigmented plaques on the lower limbs (Figure 2), confetti-like lesions on the legs (Figure 3), small shagreen spots on the posterior hemithorax (Figure 4), tachycardia, painful abdomen and highly sensitive left flank, left costovertebral angle tenderness, pollakiuria. Due to the presence of typical skin lesions TSC diagnosis was suspected.

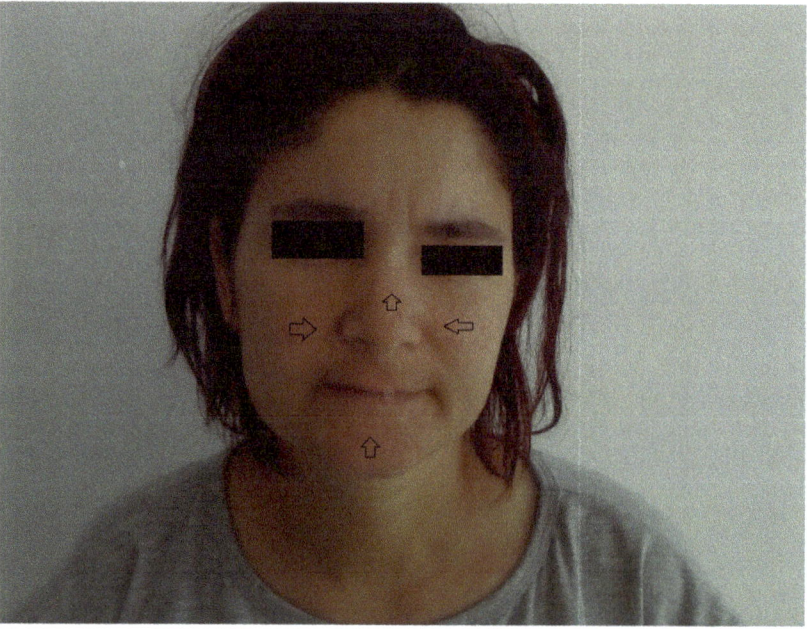

Figure 1. Facial angiofibromas on the nasal wings, cheek and chin.

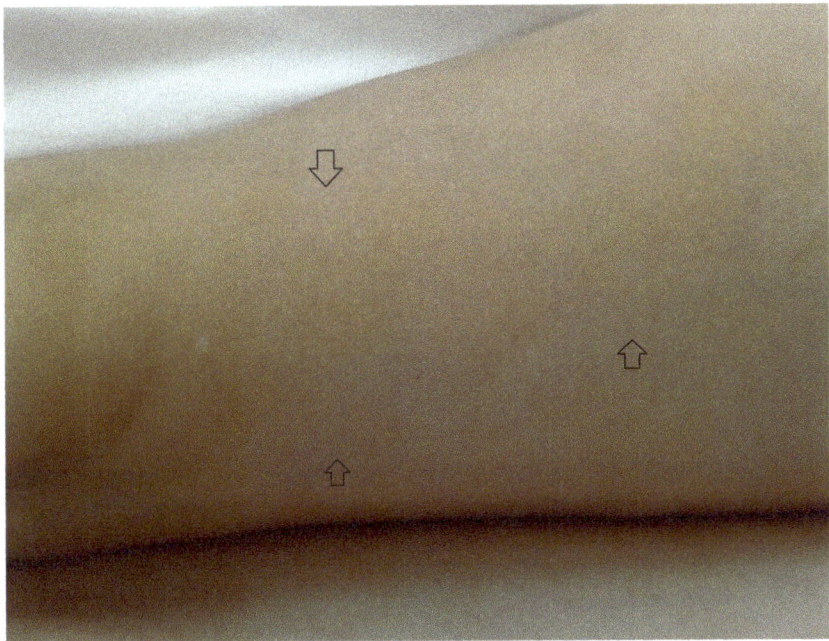

Figure 2. Hypopigmented plaques on the lower limbs.

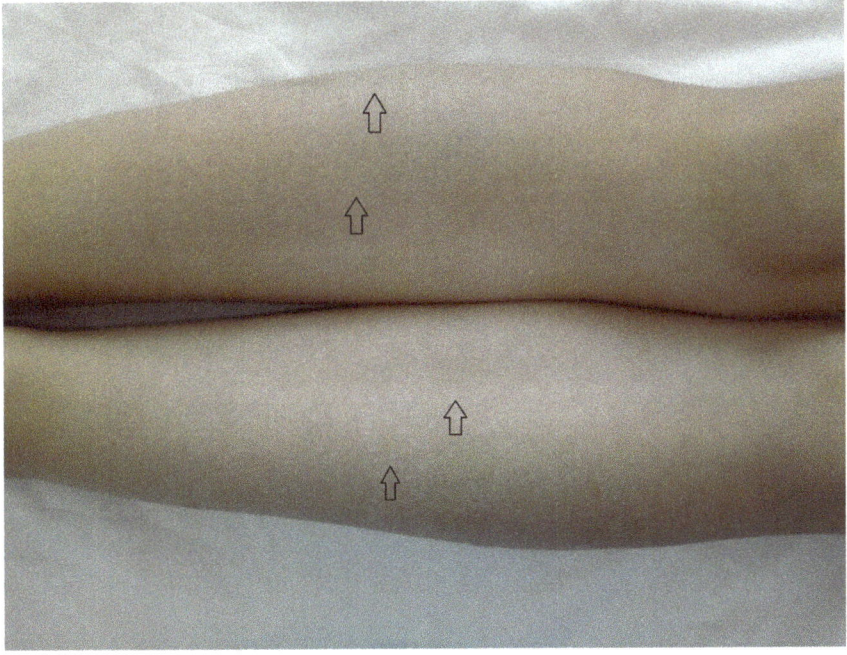

Figure 3. Confetti-like lesions on the legs.

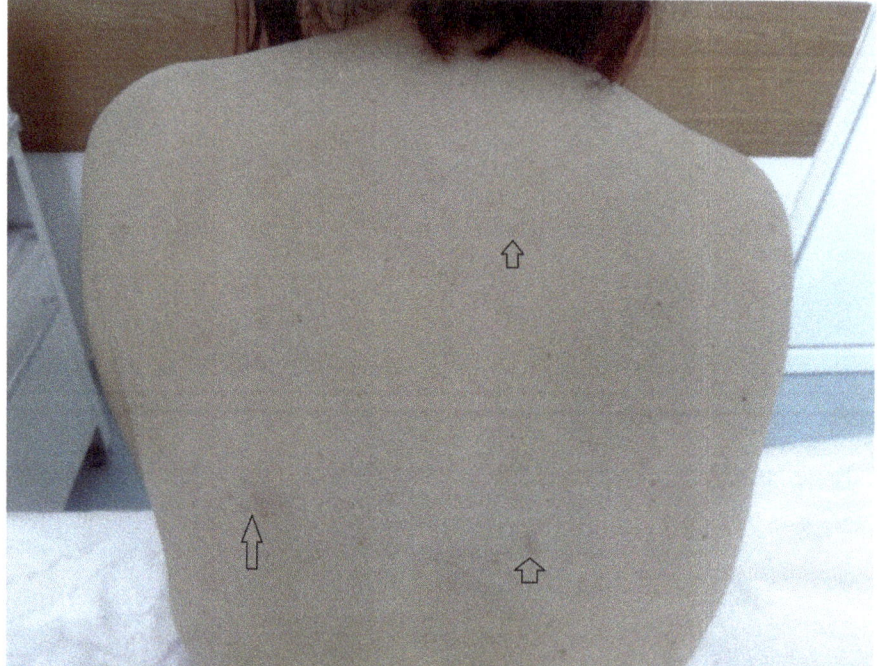

Figure 4. Small shagreen spots on the posterior hemithorax.

Neurological examinations showed reduced osteotendinous reflexes (bicipital and patellar), without other pathologic findings. The ultrasound examination showed liver with nonhomogeneous echo pattern, steatosis, possible homogeneous hyperechoic hemangiomas. Kidneys appeared with irregular contours difficult to delimit from the surrounding tissues, very much modified structure with multiple, well delimited nodular images with mixed structure, consistent with ultrasound findings of angiomyolipomas and mild pyelocaliceal dilatation, both suggestive of bilateral obstructive lithiasis, complicated by uretero-hydronephrosis. The echocardiography examination showed aortic aneurysm and ECG showed sinus arrhythmia.

The chest X-ray results were normal, but the computer tomography (CT) scan of the abdomen and pelvis evidenced irregular kidney contour layout, undifferentiated images between cortical and medullar structures, with non-homogenous round components, suggestive of bilateral kidney angiomyolipomas, renal cortical retention cysts (with diameters between 3–16 mm), with dilatatory secretion in the right side and conserved secretion and excretion on the left side. Images of a lithiasic component were also found on the middle right caliceal branches (size of 7.1/6.5 mm) and one of the left side with a smaller dimension, 2.5/2.5 mm (Figures 5–7). Similarly, the computer tomography scan of the abdomen and pelvis showed bilateral inflammatory infiltration in soft tissue surrounding the kidney and the entire surface of the ureters, as well as a small quantity of fluid in the right perirenal area—suggestive of pyelonephritis, periurethritis and angiomyolipomatosis. The computer tomography scan of the abdomen and pelvis revealed subcentimeter periaortic and intraortocaval lymph nodes. Moreover, the CT changes were represented by the evidence of the osteolytic lesions in the thoraco-lumbar and pelvic bones. The CT scan of the skull revealed the following changes: a subependymal giant cell astrocytoma (SEGA), with incipient hydrocephalus in the left lateral ventricle.

From the medical history, the clinical examination and diagnostic procedures, the final diagnosis was established: TSC, bilateral obstructive kidney stones with left acute pyelonephritis and acute periurethritis. The diagnosis of tuberous sclerosis is supported by renal, cerebral and cutaneous modifications. The renal modifications consist in multiple kidney angiomyolipomas. The cerebral modifications consist of SEGA with incipient hydrocephalus on the left. The cutaneous modifications are represented by facial angiofibromas on the nasal wings, cheek and chin, hypopigmented plaques on the lower limbs, confetti-like lesions on the legs and small shagreen spots on the posterior hemithorax. The patient needed specific urological treatment for the bilateral obstructive kidney stones and was admitted in the urology clinical department, where the obstructive pyelonephritis and other associated diseases were treated. The patient received antibiotic treatment in concordance with the antibiogram (amikacin and cefoperazone/sulbactam), which led to a decrease in body temperature to normal values, and almost remitted the infectious process. After the complete remission of the infectious process, the patient underwent flexible ureteroscopy with laser lithotripsy, as this method was the most appropriate for the treatment of the patient. The genetic test revealed mutations in the TSC2 gene at chromosome 16p13.3. Her family did not want to perform a genetic test. So far, the patient has not had history of epileptic seizures, but over time has had intellectual disability (concentration and learning disorders), with mild psychomotor developmental deficits. Upon discharge, the patient began treatment with an m-TOR inhibitor (Everolimus 5 mg 1 tb/day).

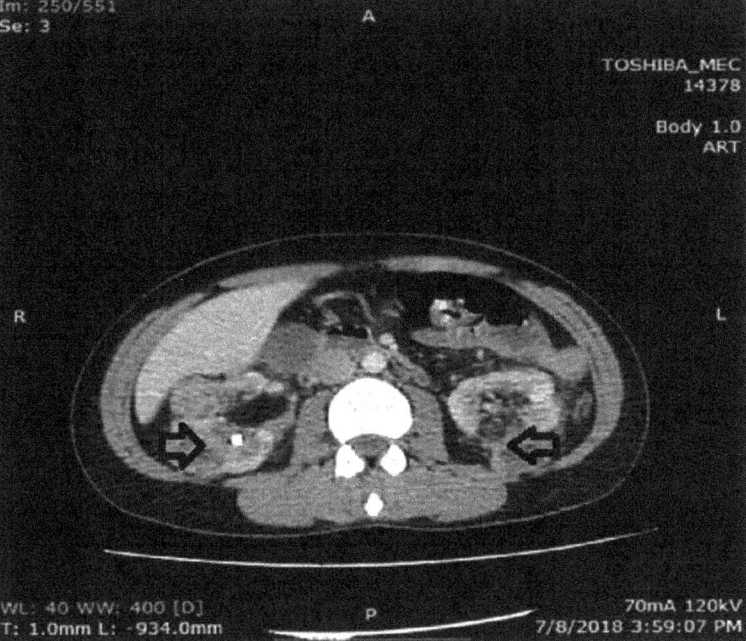

Figure 5. Axial computer tomography (CT) section with contrast substance. Kidneys with alteration of the physiological architecture with erasure of the cortico-medullary differentiation, by the presence on the entire bilateral renal surface of round oval formations, diffusely contoured with mixed component. The CT appearance pleads for angiomyolipomas.

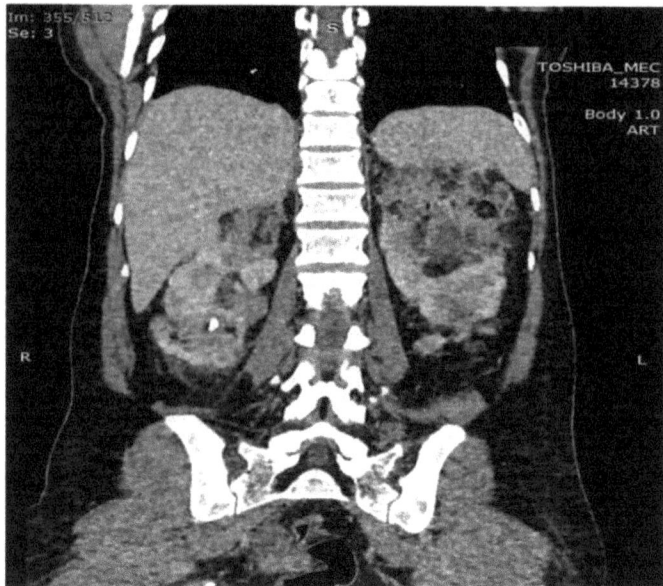

Figure 6. CT aspect of kidney modifications. Sagital CT section with contrast substance.

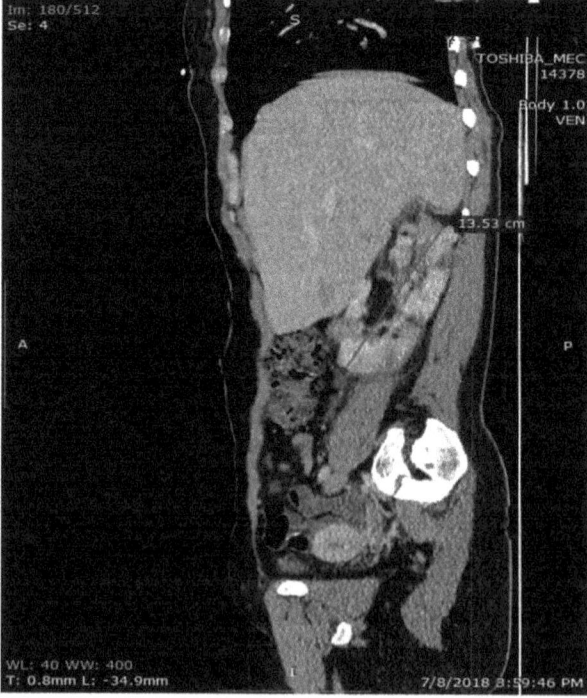

Figure 7. Coronal section examination CT. Kidneys enlarged in volume with the same changes in shape and structure by the presence of angiomyolipomatous formations that deform the renal contours without causing infiltration of proximity structures.

3. Discussion

The major features for the clinical diagnostic criteria of TSC are: hypopigmented macules (>3, at least 5-mm in diameter), angiofibromas (>3) or fibrous cephalic plaque, ungual fibromas (>2), shagreen patch, multiple retinal hamartomas, cortical dysplasia, subependymal nodules, subependymal giant cell astrocytoma, cardiac rhabdomyoma, lymphangioleiomyomatosis (LAM) and angiomyolipomas (>2). Minor features are: "confetti" skin lesions, dental enamel pits (>3), intraoral fibromas (>2), retinal achromatic patches, multiple renal cysts, non-renal hamartomas. Two major features or one major feature with >2 minor features lead to the final diagnosis. Either one major feature or >2 minor features lead to a possible diagnosis [1].

SEGA can also be detected prenatally or at birth and has an incidence of 5–15% in TSC [4]. It is benign and typically slow-growing, but can cause obstructive hydrocephalus. An important source of mortality and morbidity in TSC are renal manifestations [5]. Angiomyolipomas are benign tumors composed of smooth muscle, vascular and fatty tissue [6]. They are observed most commonly in the kidneys of TSC patients, but can also occur in other organs. In 80% of TSC patients, fat-containing angiomyolipomas were observed [7]. Renal angiomyolipomas can cause serious issues with bleeding, because of their vascular nature, and can lead to the need for dialysis, and even renal transplantation [8]. In the general population, multiple renal cysts are not commonly observed [9], but can be seen in TSC patients who have a TSC1 or TSC2 mutation or as part of a contiguous gene deletion syndrome involving the TSC2 and PKD1 genes [6]. In 10–25% of TSC patients, liver angiomyolipomas are reported [10].

Differential diagnosis includes other causes of epilepsy, renal tumors, intellectual disability, rash and benign hamartoma syndromes. Vigabatrin is first-line treatment recommended for spasms in TSC. Steroids are a typical second line treatment, with sodium valproate as the third line option. Ketogenic diet is a treatment used in epilepsy related to TSC [11]. A symptomatic SEGA requires urgent surgery, which may include a ventriculoperitoneal shunt. Even if they cease spontaneously, bleeding renal angiomyolipomas have a high risk of re-bleed. Percutaneous embolization is the first choice of management. Smaller angiomyolipomas do not usually cause symptoms, but lesions larger than 4 cm in diameter are associated with an increased risk of serious hemorrhage [3,12].

Cysts greater than 4 cm in diameter are more likely to be symptomatic, and might present with flank pain or gross hematuria or as a tender mass [13]. Autosomal dominant polycystic kidney disease (ADPKD) will develop in patients with a contiguous deletion of the *PKD1* gene, which is associated with flank pain, hypertension, pyelonephritis and progressive renal failure [14].

4. Conclusions

Treatment should be organ specific, symptomatic and directed to improve the patient's outcome and quality of life. Treatment and modern diagnostic imaging have improved both the life expectancy and the quality of life of patients with TSC. Quality of life and morbidity are largely determined by the neurologic manifestations, which include intellectual disability and seizures.

Author Contributions: P.T., O.D. and V.E.S. performed urological procedure; investigation, V.P., I.P., R.P., and D.D.; data curation, R.C.C., V.P., R.P., and A.R.M.; writing—original draft preparation, V.P., O.D., V.E.S., and R.P.; V.P., R.P., D.D. and R.C.C. performed literature data review; V.P. and I.P. finally reviewed the manuscript. All authors have read and agreed to the published version of the manuscript.

Funding: This research received no external funding.

Conflicts of Interest: The authors declare no conflict of interest.

References

1. Northrup, H.; Krueger, D.A. International Tuberous Sclerosis Complex Consensus Group. Tuberous sclerosis complex diagnostic criteria update: Recommendations of the 2012 international tuberous sclerosis complex consensus Conference. *Pediatr. Neurol.* **2013**, *49*, 243–254. [CrossRef]

2. Randle, S.C. Tuberous sclerosis complex: A review. *Pediatr. Ann.* **2017**, *46*, e166–e171. [CrossRef]
3. Roach, E.S.; Sparagana, S.P. Diagnosis of tuberous sclerosis complex. *J. Child Neurol.* **2004**, *19*, 643–649. [CrossRef]
4. Crino, P.; Mehta, R.; Vinters, H. Pathogenesis of TSC in the brain. In *Tuberous Sclerosis Complex: Genes, Clinical Features, and Therapeutics*; Kwiatkowsi, D., Whittemore, V., Thiele, E., Eds.; Wiley-Blackwell: Weinheim, Germany, 2010; pp. 285–309.
5. Shepherd, C.; Gomez, M.; Lie, J.; Crowson, C. Causes of Death in Patients with Tuberous Sclerosis. *Mayo Clin. Proc.* **1991**, *66*, 792–796. [CrossRef]
6. Bissler, J.; Henske, E. Renal manifestations of tuberous sclerosis complex. In *Tuberous Sclerosis Complex: Genes, Clinical Features, and Therapeutics*; Kwiatkowsi, D., Whittemore, V., Thiele, E., Eds.; Wiley-Blackwell: Weinheim, Germany, 2010.
7. Kozlowska, J.; Okon, K. Renal tumors in postmortem material. *Pol. J. Pathol.* **2008**, *59*, 21–25. [PubMed]
8. Bissler, J.; Kingswood, J. Renal angiomyolipomata. *Kidney Int.* **2004**, *66*, 924–934. [CrossRef] [PubMed]
9. Pei, Y. Practical genetics for autosomal dominant polycystic kidney disease. *Nephron Clin. Pract.* **2010**, *118*, c19–c30. [CrossRef] [PubMed]
10. Nakhleh, R.E. Angiomyolipoma of the Liver. *Pathol. Case Rev.* **2009**, *14*, 47–49. [CrossRef]
11. Youn, S.E.; Park, S.; Kim, S.H.; Lee, J.S.; Kim, H.D.; Kang, H.C. Long-term outcomes of ketogenic diet in patients with tuberous sclerosis complex-derived epilepsy. *Epilepsy Res.* **2020**, *164*, 106348. [CrossRef] [PubMed]
12. Henske, E.P. Tuberous sclerosis and the kidney: From mesenchyme to epithelium, and beyond. *Pediatr. Nephrol.* **2005**, *20*, 854–857. [CrossRef] [PubMed]
13. Cooper, C.S.; Elder, J.S. Renal angiomyolipoma. In *Pediatric Nephrology*; Avner, E.D., Harmon, W.E., Niaudet, P., Eds.; Lippincott Williams & Wilkins: Philadelphia, PA, USA, 2004; pp. 1120–1121.
14. Franz, D.N. Non-Neurologic Manifestations of Tuberous Sclerosis Complex. *J. Child Neurol.* **2004**, *19*, 690–698. [CrossRef] [PubMed]

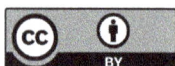

© 2020 by the authors. Licensee MDPI, Basel, Switzerland. This article is an open access article distributed under the terms and conditions of the Creative Commons Attribution (CC BY) license (http://creativecommons.org/licenses/by/4.0/).

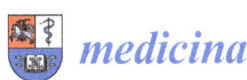

Review

Topical Corticosteroids a Viable Solution for Oral Graft versus Host Disease? A Systematic Insight on Randomized Clinical Trials

Arin Sava [1,†], Andra Piciu [2,†], Sergiu Pasca [3,†], Alexandru Mester [4,*] and Ciprian Tomuleasa [3]

1. Department of Oral Rehabilitation, University of Medicine and Pharmacy "Iuliu Hatieganu", 400012 Cluj-Napoca, Romania; arin_sava@yahoo.com
2. Department of Medical Oncology, University of Medicine and Pharmacy "Iuliu Hatieganu", 400012 Cluj-Napoca, Romania; piciuandra@gmail.com
3. Department of Hematology, University of Medicine and Pharmacy "Iuliu Hatieganu", 400012 Cluj-Napoca, Romania; pasca.sergiu123@gmail.com (S.P.); ciprian.tomuleasa@gmail.com (C.T.)
4. Department of Oral Health, University of Medicine and Pharmacy "Iuliu Hatieganu", 400012 Cluj-Napoca, Romania
* Correspondence: alexandrumester@yahoo.com
† These authors have equally contributed to the current manuscript.

Received: 20 June 2020; Accepted: 13 July 2020; Published: 14 July 2020

Abstract: *Background and Objectives:* This research attempts to provide a clear view of the literature on randomized clinical trials (RCTs) concerning the efficacy of topical dexamethasone, clobetasol and budesonide in oral graft versus host disease (GVHD). *Materials and Methods:* An electronic search of the PubMed, Web of Science and Scopus databases was carried out for eligible RCTs. Studies were included if they had adult patients with oral GVHD treatment with topical corticosteroids, and if the RCT study was published in English. The Cochrane Risk of Bias tool was used to assess the quality of these studies. Overall, three RCTs were included (an Open, Randomized, Multicenter Trial; a Randomized Double-Blind Clinical Trial; and an Open-Label Phase II Randomized Trial). *Results:* The trials involved 76 patients, of which 44 patients received topical dexamethasone, 14 patients received topical clobetasol and 18 patients received topical budesonide. Topical agents were most frequently used when oral tissues were the sole site of involvement. It appears that the best overall response is present for budesonide with no difference between the four arms, followed by clobetasol, and then by dexamethasone. The limitation of the current study is mainly represented by the fact that overall response was derived in two of the studies from other parameters. Moreover, both budesonide and clobetasol were used in only one study each, while two assessed dexamethasone. *Conclusions:* Based on the clinical trials, all three agents seem to be effective in treating oral GVHD and had a satisfactory safety profile. There is still a need for assessing high quality RCTs to assess the efficacy of these therapies on a larger cohort.

Keywords: oral graft versus host disease; topical corticosteroids; dexamethasone; clobetasol; budesonide

---

1. Introduction

Allogeneic hematopoietic cell transplantation (allo-HCT) is protocol treatment for hematological cancers and also for non-malignant disorders [1]. Graft versus host disease (GVHD), which is an important complication of allo-HCT is induced by the interactions of the host's immune system and transplanted donor cells. According to the time of appearance and clinical signs, GVHD is classified as acute or chronic [2,3]. Chronic GVHD (cGVHD), most frequently occurs ≥100 days after the transplant, affecting 25–40% of long-term HCT survivors [4]. cGVHD is classified as limited when single organs are involved, such as the skin or liver, and extensive when multiple affection occurs, in organs such as the skin, liver, eyes, salivary glands, oral mucosa and others [5–7].

Oral manifestations occur in about 80% of patients with extensive cGVHD. Most frequent oral lesions are erythema, atrophy of the mucosa, oral lichen planus, oral mucositis, xerostomia and oral infections [6,8,9]. Oral mucositis is an inflammatory reaction of the oral mucosa, often occurring after high doses of chemotherapy, radiation therapy and/or stem cell transplantation. In hematopoietic cell transplantation (HCT) patients, mucositis may often occur along the entire orodigestive tract. The prevalence of oral mucositis is stated to be at 30–70% after chemotherapy, up to 90% after HCT [10]. Oral lichen planus aspects may vary from white lacey patches to open sores, involving the tongue and inner surface of cheeks [10,11].

Oral involvement could represent the only manifestation of the cGVHD or could be comprised in a multitude of chronic symptoms. cGVHD may appear on the oral mucosa (e.g., oral verruciform xanthoma, erytroplakia), at the salivary glands (e.g., multiple mucoceles on the soft palate, hyposalivation, xerostomia, impairment in the quality of saliva, gland swelling) and in musculoskeletal apparatus disfunction [11–13].

Dysphagia is one of the most debilitating symptoms and is induced by the pain associated with oral mucositis [9]. Local palliation of the oral symptoms is achieved either by systemic therapy, or topical treatment, or both. In this light, the use of topical agents determines the reduction of the oral symptoms, determines the reduction of the systemic immunosuppressant doses, minimizes their side effects and increases the healing process [2,10].

Although topical corticosteroids are not specifically approved for treatment of oral cGVHD, they are used to treat these symptoms, based on previous experiences that prove their well accepted use in other mucosal conditions [13–15].

Given the availability of limited data, the present research attempts to provide a systematic approach of literature including randomized clinical trials (RCTs) concerning the efficacy of topical dexamethasone, clobetasol and budesonide in oral GVHD.

2. Materials and Methods

We conducted a systematic review using RCTs to compare topical dexamethasone, clobetasol and budesonide for oral GVHD. This study was in accordance with the PRISMA (Preferred Reporting Items for Systematic Reviews and Meta-Analyses) guidelines and the Cochrane Collaboration format [16,17].

Three databases (PubMed, Web of Science, Scopus) were searched to identify eligible articles from inception to February 2020, using keywords ("dexamethasone", "clobetasol", "budesonide", "topical corticosteroids", "corticosteroids", "oral graft versus host disease", "oral GVHD") combined with a Boolean term ("AND") as follows: "dexamethasone AND oral graft versus host disease"; "dexamethasone AND oral GVHD"; "clobetasol AND oral graft versus host disease"; "clobetasol AND oral GVHD"; "budesonide AND oral graft versus host disease"; "budesonide AND oral GVHD"; "topical corticosteroids AND oral graft versus host disease"; "topical corticosteroids AND oral GVHD"; "corticosteroids AND oral graft versus host disease"; and "corticosteroids AND oral GVHD". Articles were evaluated by their titles and abstracts. The contents of the articles were assessed in order to determine if the studies met the inclusion/exclusion criteria. The full texts of the potentially relevant studies were retrieved and assessed. The reference lists of the chosen articles were manually searched to identify any other relevant studies that have been missed out using the search strategy.

The inclusion criteria used in the article selection were adult (≥18 years) oral GVHD; treatment with topical corticosteroids (dexamethasone, clobetasol, budesonide); RCT; and human studies, published in English. All other articles that did not complete the upper criteria were excluded from our research.

Two independent reviewers assessed the articles for eligibility and extracted the data using a standardized data extraction form. All lack of concordance was solved by a third reviewer. The following data were taken out: author, year, country, study type, sample size, mean age, male: female ratio, oral GVHD at baseline, treatment design, clinical response, side effects, outcome.

The Cochrane Collaboration's "Risk of Bias" tool 2.0 was used to assess the quality of these studies [17]. For every RCT included, a risk of bias was provided for the following domains: random sequence generation, allocation concealment, blinding of outcome assessment, incomplete outcome data, selective reporting and other bias. These domains were judged by two reviewers and were evaluated as low, unclear or high, and a third reviewer was invited to solve all unclear results.

3. Results

The search strategy generated 1317 articles (Figure 1). After the exclusion of 584 articles, 733 articles were identified as eligible records. However, 723 articles were excluded because they did not fulfil all eligibility criteria. Therefore, 10 articles resulted as eligible, but 7 were excluded because they were prospective [18–21] or retrospective [22–24] studies. In the end, three RCTs were included [25–27].

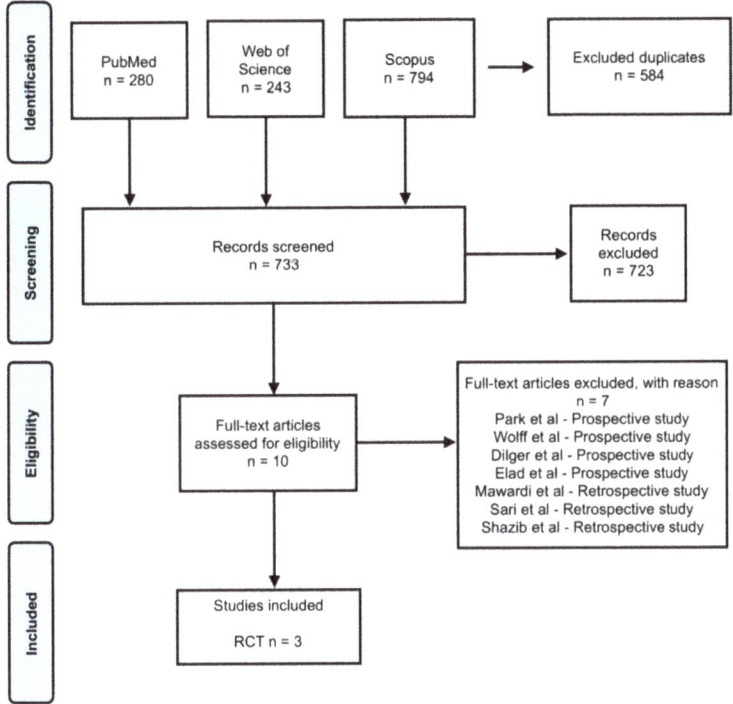

Figure 1. Flow chart of the study selection. RCT - randomized clinical trial.

The three RCTs included were an Open, Randomized, Multicentre Trial [25], a Randomized Double-Blind Clinical Trial [26] and an Open-Label Phase II Randomized Trial [27]. They were published between 2012 and 2016, involving a total of 76 patients, of which 44 patients received topical dexamethasone, 14 patients received topical clobetasol and 18 patients received topical budesonide. The studies were conducted in Israel/Germany [25], Brazil [26] and the USA [27]. The mean age of the participants varied from 43.8 to 55 years and the sex ratio was female dominant.

Oral GVHD diagnosis was done on different parameters across the included studies: WHO toxicity oral/gastrointestinal, modified oral mucosal rating scale (mOMRS), Oral Mucositis Assessment Scale (OMAS), National Institute of Health (NIH) oral cavity severity score, mucosal score and oral symptoms score. Oral lesions involved in GVHD were erythema, atrophy, ulcer, lichen, hyperkeratosis, pseudomembrane, edema and mucocele, appearing as a mucus cyst on the soft palate, on the labial and buccal mucosa. Clinical response to these agents were 61% for WHO toxicity oral/gastrointestinal, 50–61% for mOMRS, 69% for OMAS and 50% for NIH oral cavity response. Side effects reported were cheilitis, esophagitis, fungal infections, taste alteration, burning sensations and oral cavity pain. Additional data can be found in Table 1.

Figure 2 represents the overall response between the included studies. Red rectangles represent the proportion of patients that presented a response. Because of the heterogeneity of the studies, we considered for Elad et al. [25] the mOMRS any response, for Noce et al. [26] the symptomatic response and for Treister et al. [27] the overall response described by the authors. It appears that the best overall response is present for budesonide with no difference between the four arms, followed by clobetasol and then by dexamethasone. The limitation of the current study is mainly represented by the fact that the overall response was derived in two of the studies from other parameters. Moreover, both budesonide and clobetasol were used in only one study each, while two assessed dexamethasone.

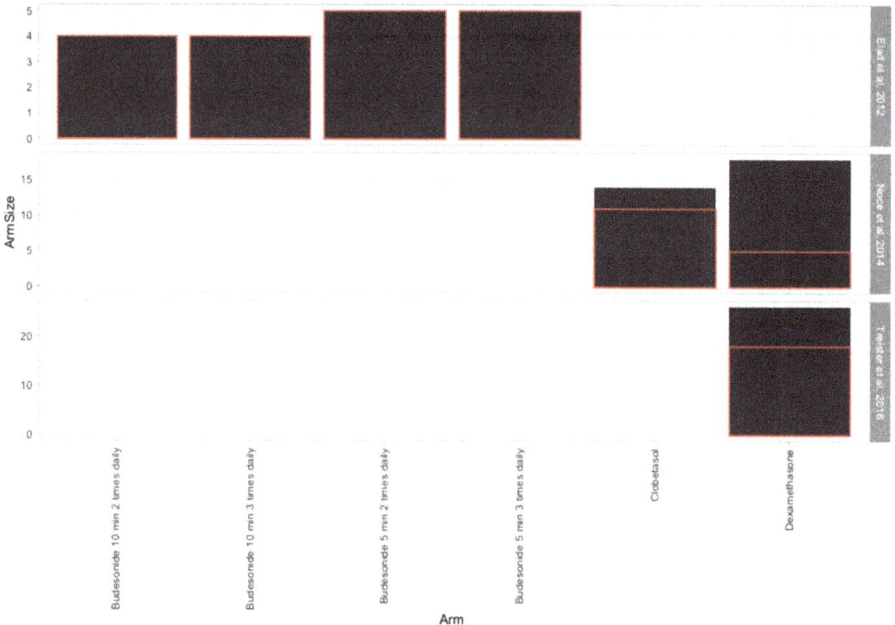

Figure 2. The overall response between the arms of the three studies included.

Overall, the three included RCTs were considered at "risk of bias" because of the lack of blinding of study participants, blinding of the outcome data and other bias. Figure 3 shows the analysis for the risk of bias for RCTs.

Table 1. Characteristics of the included randomized clinical trials (RCTs).

Author/Year/Country	Study Type	Sample Size	Oral GVHD at Baseline	Treatment Design	Clinical Response	Side Effects	Outcome
Elad et al., 2012, Israel/Germany	Open, Randomized, Multicenter	n = 18	Oral cGVHD WHO toxicity gastrointestinal/oral—grade 1 (n = 2)—grade 2 (n = 13)—grade 3 (n = 3) mOMRS (median)—26 OMAS (median)—1.9	Budesonide 3 mg/10 mL mouth rinse, for 8 weeks Arm A: 3 × 10 min daily Arm B: 3 × 5 min daily Arm C: 2 × 10 min daily Arm D: 2 × 5 min daily	WHO toxicity gastrointestinal/oral—61% mOMRS—61% OMAS—69%	Cheilitis, esophagitis, fungal infection, taste alteration	Topical budesonide in oral cGVHD has a safety profile. Safety analysis supports a dosing schedule of 3 mg of budesonide 3 times a day applied for 10 min in the form of a mouthwash.
Noce et al., 2014, Brazil	Randomized Double-Blind Clinical Trial	Clobetasol group n = 14 Dexamethasone group n = 18	Oral lesions of cGVHD Erythema (n = 29) Atrophy (n = 26) Ulcer (n = 22) Lichen (n = 21) Hyperkeratosis (n = 19) Pseudomembrane (n = 3) Edema (n = 2) Mucocele (n = 14)	Clobetasol: patients rinsed their mouths with 5 mL of a solution of clobetasol propionate 0.05% administered with nystatin 100000 IU/mL for 28 days. Dexamethasone: patients rinsed with 5 mL of a solution of dexamethasone 0.1 mg/mL administered with nystatin 100000 IU/mL for 28 days.	In 53.9% of the cases, the use of clobetasol resulted in an improvement of at least 50% in the mOMRS total score. For dexamethasone, this result was observed in 26.7% of the patients.	Clobetasol: burning sensation Dexamethasone: burning sensation	Topical clobetasol or dexamethasone was efficacious in the reduction of symptoms related to oral cGVHD. Clobetasol was significantly more effective than dexamethasone in the symptomatic and morphologic improvement of oral lesions.
Treister et al., 2016, USA	Open-Label Phase II Randomized Trial	n = 26	Oral cGVHD NIH oral cavity severity score NIH oral mucosal score NIH oral symptom scores Oral biopsies	Dexamethasone was dispensed as a commercially prepared 0.5 mg/5 mL solution; 4 rinses per day for at least 28 days.	Overall response—69% Oral Mucosal Score Response—PR (8%), NR (88%), PD (4%) NIH oral cavity response—50%	Oral cavity pain	Topical dexamethasone is safe and effective at reducing the symptoms of oral cGVHD. Dexamethasone should at present be considered for first-line topical therapy in patients with previously untreated and symptomatic oral cGVHD.

HCT, hematopoietic cell transplantation; mOMRS, modified oral mucosal rating scale; NIH, National Institute of Health; OMAS, Oral Mucositis Assessment Scale; PR, partial response; NR, no response; PD, progressive disease.

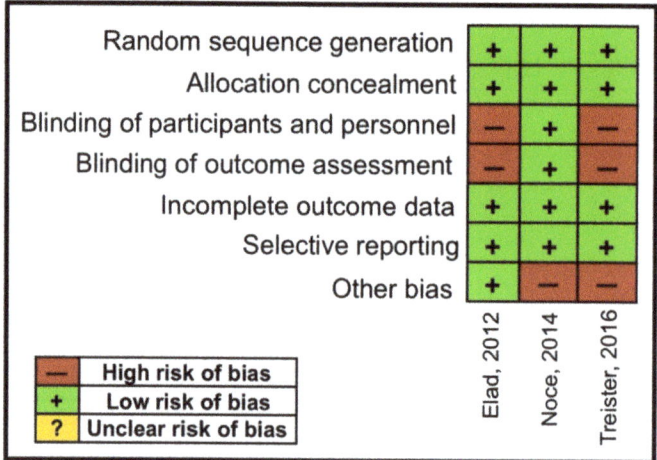

Figure 3. Risk of bias for the RCTs.

4. Discussion

Up to this moment, in the current literature, there are two systematic reviews trying to assess the benefits of using topical agents in oral GVHD [10,28]. Albuquerque et al. observed that there are a limited number of RCTs, and, therefore, the evidence sustaining the use of topical agents for the inflammatory lesions in oral GVHD is low [10]. The same authors have stated that there is still a need for quality RCTs to assess the efficacy of these agents in GVHD [10]. The paper of Elsaadany et al. reported moderate evidence for the efficacy of topical agents for oral GVHD, showing minimal side effects of clobetasol followed by budesonide [28]. Our systematic review had a homogenous selection of randomized clinical trials allowing a calculation of the Cochrane risk of bias and of the overall response, and, therefore, giving a clear recommendation for a better efficacy of budesonide, compared to clobetasol and then dexamethasone.

Another powerful parameter we have evaluated from the RCTs included in our review is the safety profile of the therapy. In the study of Elad et al. [25], the use of topical budesonide (3 mg/10 mL) showed that this corticosteroid had a satisfactory safety profile. Topical budesonide mouthwashes improved the oral condition when it was applied for 5–10 min, 2/3 times per day. Regarding the response in all treatment arms, Elad mentioned that it was the same, in any length of exposure to treatment and in any frequency. Safety analysis was performed at a dosing schedule of budesonide 3 mg, three times per day, for a period of 10 min, representing the most important exposure to the drug [25].

In the study of Noce et al. [26], a significant improvement in the symptoms appeared comparing to the baseline after the use of corticosteroids, but with a significantly greater response in the topical clobetasol group compared to dexamethasone. The authors stated that the limitations of their research were the low number of subjects and other confounding variables. They indicate that these variables in further studies should be taken into account, with a larger sample size and stratification of subjects [26].

Treister et al. [27] observed in their study that the patients with dexamethasone obtained a response of 58%. The overall global response rates were reported to reach up to 81% including responses such as much better. In total, 96% of the patients reported the dexamethasone rinses as being well tolerated and the taste being "very pleasant" or "tolerable". According to these results, the authors concluded that intensive topical therapy with this agent is efficient for managing oral chronic GVHD and should be used as a first line therapy [27].

Other topical therapies studied in the literature include triamcinolone, fluocinonide, betamethasone, tacrolimus and prednisolone, fluocinonide, halobetasol prepared as a gel or cream and topical platelet-rich gel, with various results. Because of their lack of availability in all countries we have used in our inclusion criteria only the studies mentioning the most common and used steroids: budesonide, clobetasol and dexamethasone [11].

Our research tried to do a systematic review and a meta-analysis. The second objective was not able to be fulfilled because of the heterogeneity of the articles included. The low number of RCTs included in this review represents a major limitation in concluding on the efficacy of topical corticosteroids in oral GVHD and establishing a therapy protocol. On the other hand, several weaknesses were observed within the studies included. First, a variation in assessing oral GVHD parameters before/after topical agents was observed. The adjustments of the oral GVHD parameters is required. Secondly, the sample sizes were too small; a larger sample size should be used in future studies. Third, all RCTs included only chronic GVHD patients, excluding the acute alarming manifestations. This research was made evaluating only three databases and included only articles written in English, leading to a possible exclusion of other important data.

5. Conclusions

The purpose of the oral GVHD treatment is to reduce symptoms, maintain or improve the quality of life and reduce complications. Topical corticosteroids are most frequently used when oral tissues are the sole site of involvement. Based on the clinical trials, all three agents seem to be effective in treating oral GVHD and have a satisfactory safety profile. More RCTs with larger cohorts are needed to assess the efficacy of this topical agents.

Author Contributions: Conceptualization, A.S., A.P., S.P. and A.M.; methodology, A.S., A.P., S.P. and A.M.; validation, C.T.; investigation, A.P., S.P. and A.M. writing—original draft, A.S., A.P., S.P. and A.M.; writing—review and editing, A.S., A.M. and C.T.; supervision, C.T. All authors have read and agreed to the published version of the manuscript.

Funding: This study did not receive funding.

Conflicts of Interest: The authors declare no conflict of interest.

References

1. Markey, K.A.; MacDonald, K.P.A.; Hill, G.R. Impact of cytokine gene polymorphisms on graft-vs-host disease. *Tissue Antigens* **2008**, *72*, 507–516. [CrossRef]
2. Imanguli, M.M.; Alevizos, I.; Brown, R.; Pavletic, S.Z.; Atkinson, J.C. Oral graft-versus-host disease. *Oral Dis.* **2008**, *14*, 396–412. [CrossRef] [PubMed]
3. Nicolatou-Galitis, O.; Kitra, V.; Van Vliet-Constantinidou, C.; Peristeri, J.; Goussetis, E.; Petropoulos, D.; Grafakos, S. The oral manifestations of chronic graft-versus-host disease (cGVHD) in paediatric allogeneic bone marrow transplant recipients. *J. Oral Pathol. Med.* **2001**, *30*, 148–153. [CrossRef] [PubMed]
4. Parkman, R. Chronic graft-versus-host disease. *Curr. Opin. Hematol.* **1998**, *5*, 22–25. [CrossRef] [PubMed]
5. Shulman, H.M.; Sullivan, K.M.; Weiden, P.L.; McDonald, G.B.; Striker, G.E.; Sale, G.E.; Hackman, R.; Tsoi, M.S.; Storb, R.; Thomas, E.D. Chronic graft-versus-host syndrome in man. A long-term clinicopathologic study of 20 Seattle patients. *Am. J. Med.* **1980**, *69*, 204–217. [CrossRef]
6. Filipovich, A.H.; Weisdorf, D.; Pavletic, S.; Socie, G.; Wingard, J.R.; Lee, S.J.; Martin, P.; Chien, J.; Przepiorka, D.; Couriel, D.; et al. National Institutes of Health consensus development project on criteria for clinical trials in chronic graft-versus-host disease: I. Diagnosis and staging working group report. *Biol. Blood Marrow Transplant.* **2005**, *11*, 945–956. [CrossRef]
7. Mester, A.; Irimie, A.; Oprita, L.; Dima, D.; Petrushev, B.; Lucaciu, O.; Campian, R.-S.; Tanase, A. Oral manifestations in stem cell transplantation for acute myeloid leukemia. *Med. Hypotheses* **2018**, *121*, 191–194. [CrossRef]
8. Mester, A.; Irimie, A.I.; Tanase, A.; Tranca, S.; Campian, R.S.; Tomuleasa, C.; Dima, D.; Piciu, A.; Lucaciu, O. Periodontal disease might be a risk factor for graft versus host disease. A systematic review. *Crit. Rev. Oncol. Hematol.* **2020**, *147*, 102878. [CrossRef]

9. Curtis, J.W.J.; Caughman, G.B. An apparent unusual relationship between rampant caries and the oral mucosal manifestations of chronic graft-versus-host disease. *Oral Surg. Oral Med. Oral Pathol.* **1994**, *78*, 267–272. [CrossRef]
10. Bollero, P.; Passarelli, P.C.; D'Addona, A.; Pasquantonio, G.; Mancini, M.; Condò, R.; Cerroni, L. Oral management of adult patients undergoing hematopoietic stem cell transplantation. *Eur. Rev. Med. Pharmacol. Sci.* **2018**, *22*, 876–887.
11. Elad, S.; Aljitawi, O.; Zadik, Y. Oral graft-versus-host disease: A pictorial review and a guide for dental practitioners. *Int. Dent. J.* **2020**. [CrossRef]
12. Fall-Dickson, J.M.; Pavletic, S.Z.; Mays, J.W.; Schubert, M.M. Oral Complications of Chronic Graft-Versus-Host Disease. *J. Natl. Cancer Inst. Monogr.* **2019**, *53*, lgz007. [CrossRef] [PubMed]
13. Capocasale, G.; Panzarella, V.; Tozzo, P.; Mauceri, R.; Rodolico, V.; Lauritano, D.; Campisi, G. Oral verruciform xanthoma and erythroplakia associated with chronic graft-versus-host disease: A rare case report and review of the literature. *BMC Res. Notes* **2017**, *10*, 63. [CrossRef] [PubMed]
14. Albuquerque, R.; Khan, Z.; Poveda, A.; Higham, J.; Richards, A.; Monteiro, L.; Jane-Salas, E.; Lopez-Lopez, J.; Warnakulasuriya, S. Management of oral Graft versus Host Disease with topical agents: A systematic review. *Med. Oral Patol. Oral Cir. Bucal* **2016**, *21*, e72. [CrossRef] [PubMed]
15. Mays, J.W.; Fassil, H.; Edwards, D.A.; Pavletic, S.Z.; Bassim, C.W. Oral chronic graft-versus-host disease: Current pathogenesis, therapy, and research. *Oral Dis.* **2013**, *19*, 327–346. [CrossRef] [PubMed]
16. Shamseer, L.; Moher, D.; Clarke, M.; Ghersi, D.; Liberati, A.; Petticrew, M.; Shekelle, P.; Stewart, L.A. Preferred reporting items for systematic review and meta-analysis protocols (PRISMA-P) 2015: Elaboration and explanation. *BMJ* **2015**, *350*, g7647. [CrossRef]
17. Higgins, J.P.T.; Altman, D.G.; Gotzsche, P.C.; Juni, P.; Moher, D.; Oxman, A.D.; Savovic, J.; Schulz, K.F.; Weeks, L.; Sterne, J.A.C. The Cochrane Collaboration's tool for assessing risk of bias in randomised trials. *BMJ* **2011**, *343*, d5928. [CrossRef]
18. Park, A.R.; La, H.O.; Cho, B.S.; Kim, S.J.; Lee, B.K.; Rhie, J.Y.; Gwak, H.S. Comparison of budesonide and dexamethasone for local treatment of oral chronic graft-versus-host disease. *Am. J. Health Syst. Pharm.* **2013**, *70*, 1383–1391. [CrossRef]
19. Wolff, D.; Anders, V.; Corio, R.; Horn, T.; Morison, W.L.; Farmer, E.; Vogelsang, G.B. Oral PUVA and topical steroids for treatment of oral manifestations of chronic graft-vs.-host disease. *Photodermatol. Photoimmunol. Photomed.* **2004**, *20*, 184–190. [CrossRef]
20. Dilger, K.; Halter, J.; Bertz, H.; Lopez-Lazaro, L.; Gratwohl, A.; Finke, J. Pharmacokinetics and pharmacodynamic action of budesonide after buccal administration in healthy subjects and patients with oral chronic graft-versus-host disease. *Biol. Blood Marrow Transplant.* **2009**, *15*, 336–343. [CrossRef]
21. Elad, S.; Or, R.; Garfunkel, A.A.; Shapira, M.Y. Budesonide: A novel treatment for oral chronic graft versus host disease. *Oral Surg. Oral Med. Oral Pathol. Oral Radiol. Endod.* **2003**, *95*, 308–311. [CrossRef] [PubMed]
22. Mawardi, H.; Stevenson, K.; Gokani, B.; Soiffer, R.; Treister, N. Combined topical dexamethasone/tacrolimus therapy for management of oral chronic GVHD. *Bone Marrow Transplant.* **2010**, *45*, 1062–1067. [CrossRef] [PubMed]
23. Sari, I.; Altuntas, F.; Kocyigit, I.; Sisman, Y.; Eser, B.; Unal, A.; Fen, T.; Ferahbas, A.; Ozturk, A.; Unal, A.; et al. The effect of budesonide mouthwash on oral chronic graft versus host disease. *Am. J. Hematol.* **2007**, *82*, 349–356. [CrossRef] [PubMed]
24. Shazib, M.A.; Muhlbauer, J.; Schweiker, R.; Li, S.; Cutler, C.; Treister, N. Long-Term Utilization Patterns of Topical Therapy and Clinical Outcomes of Oral Chronic Graft-versus-Host Disease. *Biol. Blood Marrow Transplant.* **2020**, *26*, 373–379. [CrossRef] [PubMed]
25. Elad, S.; Zeevi, I.; Finke, J.; Koldehoff, M.; Schwerdtfeger, R.; Wolff, D.; Mohrbacher, R.; Levitt, M.; Greinwald, R.; Shapira, M.Y. Improvement in oral chronic graft-versus-host disease with the administration of effervescent tablets of topical budesonide-an open, randomized, multicenter study. *Biol. Blood Marrow Transplant.* **2012**, *18*, 134–140. [CrossRef] [PubMed]
26. Noce, C.W.; Gomes, A.; Shcaira, V.; Correa, M.E.P.; Moreira, M.C.R.; Silva Junior, A.; Goncalves, L.S.; Garnica, M.; Maiolino, A.; Torres, S.R. Randomized double-blind clinical trial comparing clobetasol and dexamethasone for the topical treatment of symptomatic oral chronic graft-versus-host disease. *Biol. Blood Marrow Transplant.* **2014**, *20*, 1163–1168. [CrossRef]

27. Treister, N.; Li, S.; Kim, H.; Lerman, M.; Sultan, A.; Alyea, E.P.; Armand, P.; Cutler, C.; Ho, V.; Koreth, J.; et al. An Open-Label Phase II Randomized Trial of Topical Dexamethasone and Tacrolimus Solutions for the Treatment of Oral Chronic Graft-versus-Host Disease. *Biol. Blood Marrow Transplant.* **2016**, *22*, 2084–2091. [CrossRef]
28. Elsaadany, B.A.; Ahmed, E.M.; Aghbary, S.M.H. Efficacy and Safety of Topical Corticosteroids for Management of Oral Chronic Graft versus Host Disease. *Int. J. Dent.* **2017**, *2017*, 1908768. [CrossRef]

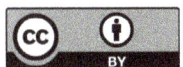

© 2020 by the authors. Licensee MDPI, Basel, Switzerland. This article is an open access article distributed under the terms and conditions of the Creative Commons Attribution (CC BY) license (http://creativecommons.org/licenses/by/4.0/).

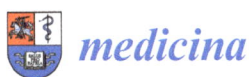

Article

Vaginal Reconstruction in Patients with Mayer–Rokitansky–Küster–Hauser Syndrome—One Centre Experience

Adelaida Avino [1,2], Laura Răducu [1,3,*], Adrian Tulin [4,5], Daniela-Elena Gheoca-Mutu [1,2], Andra-Elena Balcangiu-Stroescu [6,7], Cristina-Nicoleta Marina [1,2] and Cristian-Radu Jecan [1,3]

1. Department of Plastic and Reconstructive Surgery, "Prof. Dr. Agrippa Ionescu" Clinical Emergency Hospital, 011356 Bucharest, Romania; adelaida.avino@gmail.com (A.A.); mutu.danielaa@gmail.com (D.-E.G.-M.); cristina.cozma88@yahoo.com (C.-N.M.); jecan.radu@gmail.com (C.-R.J.)
2. Doctoral School, "Carol Davila" University of Medicine and Pharmacy, Faculty of Medicine, 020021 Bucharest, Romania
3. Department of Plastic and Reconstructive Surgery, Faculty of Medicine "Carol Davila" University of Medicine and Pharmacy, 020021 Bucharest, Romania
4. Department of General Surgery, "Prof. Dr. Agrippa Ionescu" Clinical Emergency Hospital, 011356 Bucharest, Romania; dr_2lin@yahoo.com
5. Department of Anatomy, Faculty of Medicine, "Carol Davila" University of Medicine and Pharmacy, 020021 Bucharest, Romania
6. Department of Dialysis, Emergency University Hospital, 050098 Bucharest, Romania; stroescu_andra@yahoo.ro
7. Discipline of Physiology, Faculty of Dental Medicine, "Carol Davila" University of Medicine and Pharmacy, 020021 Bucharest, Romania
* Correspondence: raducu.laura@yahoo.com; Tel.: +40-723-511-985

Received: 9 June 2020; Accepted: 30 June 2020; Published: 1 July 2020

Abstract: *Background and Objectives:* The Mayer–Rokitansky–Küster–Hauser syndrome is a congenital condition in which patients are born with vaginal and uterus agenesis, affecting the ability to have a normal sexual life and to bear children. Vaginal reconstruction is a challenging procedure for plastic surgeons. The aim of this study is to report our experience in the management of twelve patients with congenital absence of the vagina due to the MRKH syndrome. *Materials and Methods:* We performed a retrospective study on 12 patients admitted to the Plastic Surgery Department of the Clinical Emergency Hospital "Prof. Dr. Agrippa Ionescu", Bucharest, Romania, for vaginal reconstruction within a period of eleven years (January 2009–December 2019). All patients were diagnosed by the gynaecologists with vaginal agenesis, as part of the Mayer–Rokitansky–Küster–Hauser syndrome. The Abbe'–McIndoe technique with an autologous skin graft was performed in all cases. *Results:* The average age of our patients was 20.16 (16–28) years. All patients were 46 XX. The average surgical timing was 3.05 h (range 2.85–4h). Postoperative rectovaginal fistula was encountered in 1 patient. Postoperative average vaginal length was 10.4 cm (range 9.8–12.1 cm). Regular sexual life was achieved in 10 patients. *Conclusion:* Nowadays, there is no established standard method of vaginal reconstruction. In Romania, the McIndoe technique is the most applied. Unfortunately, even if the MRKH syndrome is not uncommon, less and less surgeons are willing to perform the procedure to create a neovagina.

Keywords: Mayer–Rokitansky–Küster–Hauser syndrome; primary amenorrhea; surgical management; vaginal reconstruction; plastic surgery

1. Introduction

The Mayer–Rokitansky–Küster–Hauser (MRKH) syndrome is considered to be the second most frequent cause of primary amenorrhea [1] being characterized by congenital absence of the uterus, and the upper part (2/3 proximal) of the vagina. The patients have a normal 46XX karyotype with a physiological growth of the secondary sexual features [2]. In the general population, the prevalence is up to 0.02% [3]. This syndrome is not linked with any racial predisposition. Even if it is a congenital disease, in most cases MRKH could not be diagnosed up to adolescence or at the beginning of adulthood [4].

There are two types described in the literature. The first one is characterised by solitary absence of the proximal two-thirds of the vagina [5] and agenesis of the uterus [4], although two symmetric rudimentary horns are present. They are linked by a peritoneal fold to the fallopian tubes, whereas the ovaries and the renal system have a normal development. This appears in almost 44% of all cases. There has been a reported growth of abnormalities of the caudal part of the Müllerian ducts. No other congenital malformations is detected, the patients are utterly asymptomatic and diagnosed during late adolescence due to primary amenorrhea [1]. Meanwhile, type II is associated with other congenital defects including vertebral, cardiac, auditory, renal and vertebral malformations [5]. This affects up to 56% of the patients, involving asymmetrical hypoplasia of one or two buds, with or without dysplasia of the fallopian tubes [1].

Precise history, clinical evaluation and transabdominal ultrasonography are used to diagnose the MRKH syndrome. After this, a check-up of the renal, skeletal, auditory and cardiac systems must be performed. Ovarian function can be analysed through the serum levels of the follicle stimulating hormone, luteinizing hormone, 17ß-oestradiol and androgens [6].

The optimal treatment is vaginal reconstruction in physically and psychologically mature women who are ready to start sexual intercourse [7]. In the literature, a variety of techniques have been presented, each with its advantages and disadvantages. Most commonly, the neovagina is created within the rectovesical space lined with skin (McIndoe Reed technique), peritoneum (Davydov procedure) or intestine. It is possible that in the future, vaginal mucosa-like engineered tissue will be used [8]. Moreover, an important step of therapeutic management is the psychosocial assistance not only for the patients, but also for their parents [9].

The aim of this study is to report our experience in the management of twelve patients with congenital absence of the vagina due to the MRKH syndrome.

2. Materials and Methods

We conducted a retrospective study on 12 patients admitted to the Plastic Surgery Department of the Clinical Emergency Hospital "Prof. Dr. Agrippa Ionescu", Bucharest, Romania, for vaginal reconstruction within a period of eleven years (January 2009–December 2019). Local ethical agreement and informed consent of the patients were obtained. The number of the document from the Ethical Commission of Clinical Emergency Hospital "Prof. Dr. Agrippa Ionescu" is 104663/10.04.2020. All patients were diagnosed by gynaecologists with vaginal agenesis, as part of the Mayer–Rokitansky–Küster–Hauser syndrome. All the data were taken from surgical operating files, medical letters and postoperative records. The data comprised demographic information, chromosomal analysis, surgery timing, preoperative and postoperative vaginal length, complications, postoperative treatment, but also other congenital malformations. The marital status was also evaluated. All cases underwent clinical examination and pelvic ultrasonography during preoperative evaluation. The surgical team included surgeons from the department of general surgery and plastic and reconstructive surgery. Preoperatively, a combination of amoxicillin and clavulanic acid was administered as a prophylactic antibiotic.

The Abbe'–McIndoe technique with an autologous skin graft was performed in all cases. The surgical procedure was performed on patients placed in the lithotomy position (Figure 1) and under general anaesthesia with urinary catheterization. The general surgeon initiated the intervention.

Through a Y-shaped incision in the perineum, a vesico-rectal cavity was created (Figure 2). The dissection was performed between the urethra, bladder and the rectum, the Douglas pouch being the upper and posterior limit. A careful haemostasis of the neovaginal cavity was the last manoeuvre performed by the general surgeon. A split-thickness skin graft was harvested from the anterior part of the thigh, using a Humby knife. The graft was placed on a vaginal stent with its inner surface, the dermal part facing towards the exterior and was sewn with non-absorbable sutures (Figure 3).

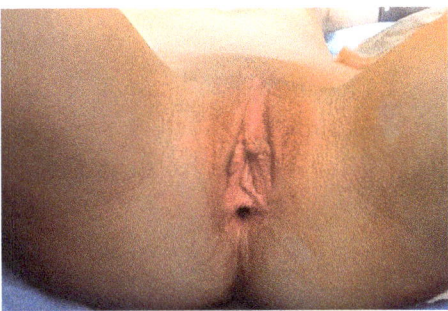

Figure 1. Preoperative photograph in a patient with vaginal agenesis.

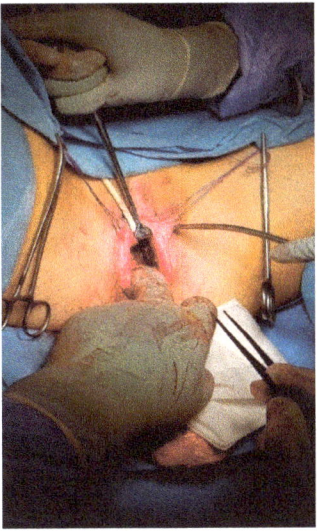

Figure 2. Y-shape incision in the perineum, creating a vesico-rectal cavity.

Afterwards, the stent was inserted into the preformed neovaginal space. The free margins of the skin graft were sutured to the borders of the incisions made in the perineum, creating this way the introitus of the neovagina. In all cases, the vaginal stent was made of silicone, having the shape of a cylinder with a channel inside it, in order to cleanse the neovagina. The patients were put on absolute bed rest and a special diet was given for the first 9 days. The neovagina was irrigated daily through the channel of the stent with diluted (1%) povidone-iodine solution and normal saline. After 9 days, the vaginal stent was removed and the neovagina was checked and cleansed. Elastic panties were worn in order to retain the stent. The sutures were eliminated after 14 days (Figure 4). In the first 3 months, the vaginal stent had to be kept permanently, except when using the toilet or while bathing, in order to prevent the contraction of the vagina. During this period, the patients irrigated the vagina with sodium bicarbonate solution, wormwood tea or a mixture of normal saline and povidone-iodine.

Patients were informed not to replace the vaginal stent into the vagina unless it had been washed with soap and hot water and they had applied cream with the free protein extract of calf blood or vitamin A oil. Subsequently, they were advised using the vaginal stent only during the night for the next 3 months. Six months after the surgery, the vaginal stent had to be used for 3 nights per week, until the patient had a stable partner and regular sexual intercourse (at least 3 times per week). In the case of the absence of regular sexual intercourse, the stent had to be used 3 nights per week to maintain the vaginal cavity open.

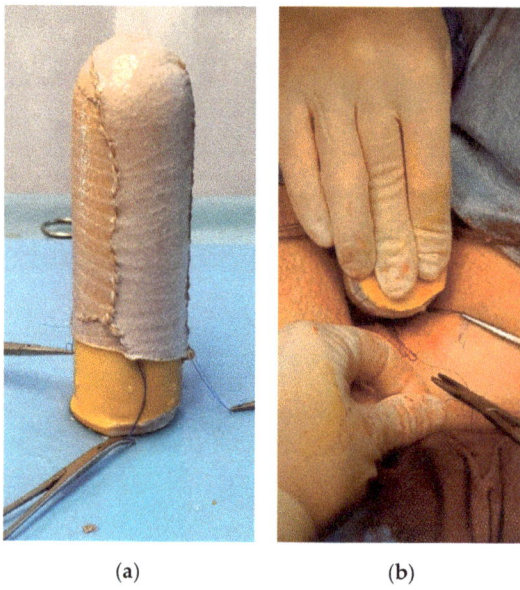

(a)   (b)

Figure 3. (a) The vaginal stent with the skin grafts. (b) The fixation of the vaginal stent in the neovaginal space.

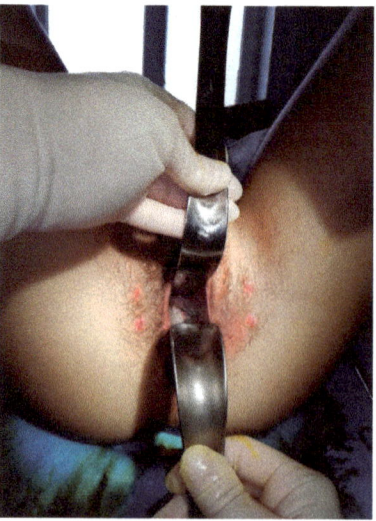

Figure 4. 20 days after vaginal reconstruction.

Postoperatively, all patients were followed up monthly in the first 6 months, respectively, 9 months and after that, once a year.

Local ethical agreement and informed consent of the patients were obtained.

3. Results

Twelve cases of vaginal reconstruction were performed throughout the period of the study. The average age of the patients undergoing surgery was 20.16 years (range 16–28 years). All the patients were living in an urban area and two of them were smokers. Preoperatively, one patient was engaged, and the others were single, but after the surgery ten patients found a stable partner and got married.

All patients presented primary amenorrhea at 14–15 years old. Upon clinical examination, external genitalia had a normal appearance in all patients. None of them presented a uterus, but only ovaries. The vagina was totally absent in all cases. According to chromosomal analysis, all patients were 46XX. One patient had an anorectal malformation and two interventions were performed by a paediatric surgeon during childhood. Moreover, she also presented mitral valve regurgitation. One patient, a 25-year-oldwoman came to our clinic with a neovagina of 3 cm, with the complaint that she could not have a normal sexual life with her future husband. Her first vaginal reconstruction was performed when she was 22. The modified McIndoe technique with full-thickness skin grafts harvested from the anterior part of the thigh was performed in all cases. The average surgical timing was 3.05 h (range 2.85–4 h). Postoperatively, the vaginal length varied from 9.8 to 12.1 cm, with a mean length of 10.4 cm.

Regarding acute postoperative complications, we would like to mention the acute bleeding of the donor site in one patient. Moreover, haemorrhage of the posterior wall was encountered in one case, 12 days after the surgery. The patient raised the skin graft from the posterior wall as a result of forcing the stent inside the neovagina after it slipped out during the night. Meticulous haemostasis was decided and re-epithelialization of the affected part was preferred from the integrated skin grafted margins. Silver dressings were used to cover the donor site for 10 days.

The surgical intervention performed for the patient with the neovagina of 3 cm was challenging. The space that was previously created became a fibrotic scar tissue, which was difficult to dissect. After one month postoperative, the patient presented rectovaginal fistula. Colostomy was decided before repairing the fistula. The colostomy was kept for 6 months, until the fistula was completely healed.

No early complications were seen in other cases, and all of them used a vaginal stent, as recommended. During the follow-up, 4 of them presented keloid scars on the donor site and recurrent urinary tract infections were detected in 9 patients. Psychosocial assistance was mandatory for all the patients.

4. Discussion

The Mayer–Rokitansky–Küster–Hauser syndrome is the most common cause of vaginal agenesis, known also as Müllerian agenesis, Müllerian aplasia or CAUV (congenital absence of the uterus and vagina) [10]. It is not considered a rare disease, but it is usually discovered in adolescence due to primary amenorrhea [11]. More than 2000 years ago, Hippocrates mentioned vaginal agenesis for the first time [12] as "membranous obstruction" (obstructed vagina), in his book "De la nature de la femme" (On the Nature of Women). Not until 1559 were the medical reports of Matteo Realdo Colombo, regarding the absence of both the uterus and vagina, first mentioned in literature. In 1572, he described the disease under the name "vulva rara". The medical eponym honours August Franz Josef Karl Mayer, Karl Freiherr von Rokitansky, Hermann Küster and Georges Andre Hauser thanks to their remarkable contributions towards the discovery of this congenital syndrome. In 1829, Mayer presented the anatomical abnormalities; in 1838 [10], Rokitansky documented the absence of the uterus and vagina in 19 adult autopsies [13], highlighting the importance of a classification system, based on cases of uterovaginal agenesis. In 1910, Hermann Küster outlined the association of renal and skeletal malformations with the uterovaginal agenesis and in 1961, Hauser presented his findings in 21 patients [10].

Initially, MRKH syndrome was considered to be sporadic, depending on exogenous factors (gestational diabetes) or exposure to teratogens (thalidomide). However, several epidemiological studies failed to identify any relationship between drug use, illness, or exposure to known teratogens during pregnancy and the birth of a child with MRKH [14].Despite many studies that have been conducted to discover the cause, the exact aetiology of the syndrome remains unclear. Defects during embryogenesis lead to malformations of the genitourinary system [4]. Specifically, during the end of the fourth week of fetal life, abnormalities of the intermediate mesoderm determine deficiency in the development of the blastema of the cervicothoracic somites and the pronephric ducts. These modifications affect the mesonephros and then the Wolffian and Müllerian ducts [2].The distal extremity of the Müllerian ducts creates the proximal 2/3rd parts of the vagina and uterine cervix, the intermediate part forms the uterine body, while the cranial segments open in the coelomic cavity (future peritoneal cavity), shaping the fallopian tubes. Meanwhile, the ovaries develop from the mesenchyme and from the epithelium of the genital crest of the intermediate mesoderm, this process is not associated with the mesonephros. Thus, in most cases, the defects of the Müllerian ducts are not linked to abnormalities of the ovaries [4]. The distal third of the vagina is developed from ectodermal cells, so it can create a shallow pouch in the perineum [13]. Regarding genetics, in literature there have been mentions of an association between the mutations of the WNT4 and TCF2 genes and MRKH syndrome [15].

In general, the patients with MRKH syndrome are first seen by a gynaecologist at age 14 to 18 years [16], when the absence of the menarche causes concern. Menstruation does not appear at the usual age because the uterus is absent, but ovulation occurs regularly [13]. However, the patients may be diagnosed at birth or during childhood due to other congenital malformations [16]. In our study, 11 patients were diagnosed at 14–15 years due to primary amenorrhea.

One patient presented a recto-vestibular fistula at birth, which was corrected by the paediatric surgeon. The final diagnosis, the MRKH syndrome, was confirmed during childhood after exploratory laparotomy. It revealed no uterus, but both ovaries were present and attached to a cord-like structure without any evidence of fallopian tubes. Anorectal malformations are exceptionally described as part of the MRKH syndrome, most commonly encountering recto-vestibular fistulae and cloacal malformations [10]. Wang et al. (2010) suggested a single-stage ano-recto-vaginoplasty in patients who had MRKH syndrome and recto-vestibular fistulae with imperforate anuses, to avoid the fibrosis and scarring created by repeated surgery. The surgical intervention should be performed later in life if the recto-vestibular fistula is asymptomatic or causes modest discomfort, and might be guided by dietary adjustments. If the single-stage procedure is performed before the age of 14, long-term postoperative dilation of the neovagina might be difficult for young girls. Therefore, treatment should be decided individually for each patient [17]. In addition, one patient presented a mild mitral valve insufficiency. Heart malformations are less frequent. Pittock et al. (2005) described in their study a mild mitral regurgitation and mitral valve prolapse with valvular regurgitation, but also other cardiac problems in patients with MRKH such as truncus arteriosus with complete repair in infancy and patent ductus arteriosus [18]. The most common heart defects linked to MRKH syndrome are aorto-pulmonary window, atrial septal defects, pulmonary valvular stenosis and tetralogy of Fallot [19].

The primary goal of vaginoplasty in patients with vaginal agenesis is to create a vagina of adequate length, diameter and with a stable lining for sexual intercourse. Several surgical procedures were presented in the literature, from serial dilation, Vecchietti's technique, sigmoid or ileal flaps, the gracilis flap, the Singapore flap to the expanded vulvar flap [20].

In our study, the McIndoe technique with autologous skin graft was used to create the neovagina. For a better approach, the general surgeon chose a Y-shaped incision in the perineum, instead of H-shaped incision (Bastu et al., 2012) [21]. Due to the fact that our patients presented vaginal agenesis, the surgical intervention was the only option for creating the neovagina.

In the last 20 years, alternatives of the McIndoe procedure have been proposed because of the permanent scars at the donor site. Lin et al. (2003) highlighted the possibility of covering the vaginal canal with autologous buccal mucosa. Starting from the idea that the autologous buccal mucosa has been used to substitute skin and bladder mucosa grafts in urethroplasty, the procedure was performed on 8 young patients. The results were encouraging, the patients had an adequate vaginal length, without strictures and with no deficiency in opening their mouth. The buccal mucosa was used due to its characteristics of being an easily accessible, non-hair-bearing material, with excellent cosmetic results [22]. Teng et al. (2019) used an autologous micromucosa graft harvested from the vulva and the buccal cavity. The mucosal patch was cut into particles, which were immersed in saline, and then manually adhered to a gauze mould. The 8 cm gauze vaginal stent was changed after 7 days with a 10 cm glass mould, with a satisfactory clinical outcome [23]. Hopefully, in the future, vaginal mucosa-like engineered tissue will be used to line the neovagina.

Baptista et al. (2016) created the neovagina using the laparoscopic modified Vecchietti technique, an intervention with good results that involves a single suprapubic ancillary trocar. This procedure eliminates the incision of the vesicorectal peritoneum [24]. Unfortunately, in our clinic this technique was never used.

In our study, the vaginal stent was removed after 9 days in all cases. The stent had a 4.5 cm diameter and a length of 13 cm. Seccia et al. (2002) presented their technique, where the removal of the mould was performed after 7 days [25]. Before the daily replacement of the vaginal stent, cream with free protein extract of calf blood was used. This promotes oxidative metabolism and shifts the redox-balance of cells to produce more oxidized substrates, leading to a faster healing [26]. The mean length of the neovagina was 10.4 cm. In the literature, there have been results that presented 7.8 cm [21] or 8.9 cm [20] in length. We did not change or improve the McIndoe procedure, but we used a bigger vaginal stent compared to those reported in the literature, creating in this way a neovagina of 10.4 cm.

Nowadays, more and more new dressings for wounds are created to reduce pain and local discomfort [27]. We used silver dressings for the donor site to accelerate the healing [28].

In the literature, postoperative complications have been recorded, such as rectovaginal fistula, vaginal stricture, bleeding, recurrent infections of the urinary system, urinary incontinence or rectocele [29–31]. In our study, the worst complication that we encountered in one patient was the rectovaginal fistula. All patients presented, years after the interventions, recurrent urinary tract infections.

Even if the patients could adopt a child, none of our patients did. In Romania there is not the possibility of surrogacy or uterine transplantation.

5. Conclusions

Based on our experience, the McIndoe procedure is the classic and optimal intervention procedure for vaginal reconstruction in cases of congenital vaginal agenesis. It is important to highlight the necessity of the proper management of using the vaginal stent postoperatively and of a monthly follow-up in the first 6 months. Moreover, psychosocial assistance is mandatory for all patients.

Author Contributions: Conceptualization, C.-R.J.; methodology, L.R.; software, D.-E.G.-M., A.-E.B.-S. and C.-N.M.; validation, A.T.; formal analysis, A.-E.B.-S. and C.-N.M.; investigation, A.A. and A.T.; resources, C.-R.J.; data curation, A.A. and D.-E.G.-M.; writing—original draft preparation, A.A.; writing—review and editing, L.R. and D.-E.G.-M.; visualization, A.-E.B.-S. and C.-N.M.; supervision, A.T.; project administration, L.R. and C.-R.J. All authors have read and agreed to the published version of the manuscript.

Funding: This research received no external funding.

Acknowledgments: Thank for your all contribution and support, Carmen-Florentina Caramitru.

Conflicts of Interest: The authors declare no conflict of interest.

References

1. Fontana, L.; Gentilin, B.; Fedele, L.; Gervasini, C.; Miozzo, M. Genetics of Mayer-Rokitansky-Küster-Hauser (MRKH) syndrome. *Clin. Genet.* **2017**, *91*, 233–246. [CrossRef]

2. Morcel, K.; Camborieux, L. Programme de Recherches sur les Aplasies Müllériennes, Guerrier D. Mayer-Rokitansky-Küster-Hauser (MRKH) syndrome. *Orphanet. J. Rare Dis.* **2007**, *2*, 13. [CrossRef]
3. Herlin, M.; Bjørn, A.M.; Rasmussen, M.; Trolle, B.; Petersen, M.B. Prevalence and patient characteristics of Mayer-Rokitansky-Küster-Hauser syndrome: A nationwide registry-based study. *Hum. Reprod.* **2016**, *31*, 2384–2390. [CrossRef]
4. Pizzo, A.; Laganà, A.S.; Sturlese, E.; Retto, G.; Retto, A.; De Dominici, R.; Puzzolo, D. Mayer-rokitansky-kuster-hauser syndrome: Embryology, genetics and clinical and surgical treatment. *ISRN Obstet Gynecol.* **2013**, *2013*, 628717. [CrossRef]
5. Soedjana, H.; Hasibuan, L.Y.; Septiani, G.A.; Davita, T.R. Case report in experience with neovaginal reconstruction using the inverted Y flap in Mayer-Rokitansky-Küster-Hauser syndrome and androgen insensitive syndrome: A pilot study. *Int. J. Surg. Open* **2018**, *15*, 46–50. [CrossRef]
6. Al-Mehaisena, L.; Amarina, Z.; Bani Hani, O.; Ziad, F.; Al-Kuranb, O. Ileum neovaginoplasty for Mayer–Rokitansky–Küster–Hauser: Review and case series. *Afr. J. Urol.* **2017**, *23*, 154–159. [CrossRef]
7. Mungadi, I.A.; Ahmad, Y.; Yunusa, G.H.; Agwu, N.P.; Ismail, S. Mayer-rokitansky-kuster-hauser syndrome: Surgical management of two cases. *J. Surg Tech. Case Rep.* **2010**, *2*, 39–43. [CrossRef] [PubMed]
8. Michala, L.; Cutner, A.; Creighton, S. Surgical approaches to treating vaginal agenesis. *BJOG* **2007**, *114*, 1455–1459. [CrossRef] [PubMed]
9. LeRoy, S. Vaginal reconstruction in adolescent females with Mayer-Rokitansky-Kuster-Hauser syndrome. *Plast. Surg. Nurs.* **2001**, *21*, 23–39. [CrossRef]
10. Patnaik, S.S.; Brazile, B.; Dandolu, V.; Ryan, P.L.; Liao, J. Mayer-Rokitansky-Küster-Hauser (MRKH) syndrome: A historical perspective. *Gene* **2015**, *555*, 33–40. [CrossRef]
11. Bean, E.J.; Mazur, T.; Robinson, A.D. Mayer-Rokitansky-Küster-Hauser Syndrome: Sexuality, Psychological Effects, and Quality of Life. *J. Pediatr. Adol. Gynec.* **2009**, *22*, 339–346. [CrossRef] [PubMed]
12. Dobroński, P.; Czaplicki, M.; Borkowski, A. History of vaginal reconstruction. *Ginekol Pol.* **2004**, *75*, 65–75. [PubMed]
13. Fiaschetti, V.; Taglieri, A.; Gisone, V.; Coco, I.; Simonetti, G. Mayer-Rokitansky-Kuster-Hauser syndrome diagnosed by magnetic resonance imaging. Role of imaging to identify and evaluate the uncommon variation in development of the female genital tract. *J. Radiol. Case Rep.* **2012**, *6*, 17–24. [PubMed]
14. Morcel, K.; Guerrier, D.; Watrin, T.; Pellerin, I.; Levêque, L. Le syndrome de Mayer-Rokitansky-Küster-Hauser (MRKH):clinique et génétique. *J. Gynecol. Obst. Bio. R.* **2008**, *37*, 539–546. [CrossRef] [PubMed]
15. Tiwari, C.; Shah, H.; Waghmare, M.; Khedkar, K. Mayer-Rokitansky-Kuster-Hauser syndrome associated with rectovestibular fistula. *Turk. J. Obstet. Gynecol.* **2017**, *14*, 70–73. [CrossRef]
16. Govindarajan, M.; Rajan, R.S.; Kalyanpur, A.; Ravikumar. Magnetic resonance imaging diagnosis of Mayer-Rokitansky-Kuster-Hauser syndrome. *J. Hum. Reprod. Sci.* **2008**, *1*, 83–85. [CrossRef]
17. Wang, S.; Lang, J.H.; Zhu, L. Mayer-Rokitansky-Küester-Hauser (MRKH) syndrome with rectovestibular fistula and imperforate anus. *Eur. J. Obstet. Gynecol. Reprod Biol.* **2010**, *153*, 77–80. [CrossRef]
18. Pittock, S.T.; Babovic-Vuksanovic, D.; Lteif, A. Mayer-Rokitansky-Küster-Hauser anomaly and its associated malformations. *Am. J. Med. Genet.* **2005**, *135A*, 314–316. [CrossRef]
19. Nguyen, B.T.; Dengler, K.L.; Saunders, R.D. Mayer–Rokitansky–Kuster–Hauser Syndrome: A Unique Case Presentation. *Mil. Med.* **2018**, *183*, e266–e269. [CrossRef]
20. Yogishwarappa, C.N.; Devi, P.; Vijayakumar, A. Surgical neovagina reconstruction in mullerian agenesis. *Int. J. Bio. Adv. Res.* **2016**, *7*, 175–180.
21. Bastu, E.; Akhan, S.E.; Mutlu, M.F.; Nehir, A.; Yumru, H.; Hocaoglu, E.; Gungor-Ugurlucan, F. Treatment of vaginal agenesis using a modified McIndoe technique: Long-term follow-up of 23 patients and a literature review. *Can. J. Plast. Surg.* **2012**, *20*, 241–244. [CrossRef]
22. Lin, W.C.; Chang, C.Y.; Shen, Y.Y.; Tsai, H.D. Use of autologous buccal mucosa for vaginoplasty: A study of eight cases. *Hum. Reprod.* **2003**, *18*, 604–607. [CrossRef] [PubMed]
23. Teng, Y.; Zhu, L.; Chong, Y.; Zeng, A.; Liu, Z.; Yu, N.; Zhang, W.; Chen, C.; Wang, X. The Modified McIndoe Technique: A Scar-free Surgical Approach for Vaginoplasty With an Autologous Micromucosa Graft. *Urology* **2019**, *131*, 240–244. [CrossRef] [PubMed]
24. Seccia, A.; Salgarello, M.; Sturla, M. Neovaginal reconstruction with the modified McIndoe technique: A review of 32 cases. *Ann. Plast. Surg.* **2002**, *49*, 379–384. [CrossRef] [PubMed]

25. Baptista, E.; Carvalho, G.; Nobre, C.; Dias, I.; Torgal, I. Creation of a Neovagina by Laparoscopic Modified Vecchietti Technique: Anatomic and Functional Results. *RBGO* **2016**, *38*, 456–464. [CrossRef]
26. Lee, P.Y.F.; Kwan, A.P.; Smith, P.M.; Brock, J.; Nokes, L. Actovegin Equals to Performance Enhancing Drug Doping: Fact or Fiction? *J. Tissue Sci. Eng.* **2016**, *7*, 3. [CrossRef]
27. Răducu, L.; Cozma, C.N.; Balcangiu Stroescu, A.E.; Avino, A.; Tănăsescu, M.D.; Balan, D.; Jecan, C.R. Our Experience in Chronic Wounds Care with Polyurethane Foam. *Rev. Chim.* **2018**, *69*, 585–586. [CrossRef]
28. Avino, A.; Jecan, C.R.; Cozma, C.N.; Balcangiu Stroescu, A.E.; Balan, D.G.; Ionescu, D.; Mihai, A.; Tanase, M.; Raducu, L. Negative Pressure Wound Therapy Using Polyurethane Foam in a Patient with Necrotizing Fasciitis. *Mater. Plast.* **2018**, *55*, 603–605. [CrossRef]
29. Hojsgaard, A.; Villadsen, I. McIndoe procedure for congenital vaginal agenesis: Complications and results. *Br. J. Plast. Surg.* **1995**, *48*, 97–102. [CrossRef]
30. Tiglis, M.; Neagu, T.P.; Elfara, M.; Diaconu, C.C.; Bratu, O.G.; Vacaroiu, I.A.; Grintescu, I.M. Nefopam and its role in modulating acute and cronic pain. *Rev. Chim.* **2018**, *69*, 2877–2880. [CrossRef]
31. Laslo, C.; Pantea Stoian, A.; Socea, B.; Paduraru, D.; Bodean, O.; Socea, L.; Neagu, T.P.; Stanescu, A.M.A.; Marcu, D.; Diaconu, C. New oral anticoagulants and their reversal agents. *J. Mind Med. Sci.* **2018**, *5*, 195–201. [CrossRef]

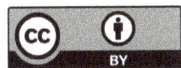

© 2020 by the authors. Licensee MDPI, Basel, Switzerland. This article is an open access article distributed under the terms and conditions of the Creative Commons Attribution (CC BY) license (http://creativecommons.org/licenses/by/4.0/).

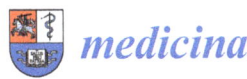

Article

Patterns and Factors Associated with Self-Medication among the Pediatric Population in Romania

Petruța Tarciuc [1], Ana Maria Alexandra Stanescu [2], Camelia Cristina Diaconu [2,3], Luminita Paduraru [4,*], Alina Duduciuc [5] and Smaranda Diaconescu [4]

1. Family Medicine, University of Medicine, Pharmacy, Science and Technology "Emil Palade", 540142 Târgu Mures, Romania; petrutatarciuc@yahoo.com
2. Department of Internal Medicine, University of Medicine and Pharmacy "Carol Davila", 020021 Bucharest, Romania; alexandrazotta@yahoo.com (A.M.A.S.); drcameliadiaconu@gmail.com (C.C.D.)
3. Internal Medicine Clinic, Clinical Emergency Hospital of Bucharest, 014461 Bucharest, Romania
4. Mother and Child Department, "Grigore T. Popa" University of Medicine and Pharmacy, 700115 Iasi, Romania; turti23@yahoo.com
5. Faculty of Communication and Public Relations, National University of Political Science and Public Administration, 012104 Bucharest, Romania; alina.duduciuc@comunicare.ro
* Correspondence: luminita.paduraru@gmail.com; Tel.: +40-745631053

Received: 26 April 2020; Accepted: 23 June 2020; Published: 25 June 2020

Abstract: *Background and objectives:* Self-medication is a global phenomenon in both developed and emerging countries. At present, data regarding the practice, patterns, and factors associated with self-medication in Romanian patient groups of various ages and health are relatively scarce. A pilot study that uses a questionnaire was conducted to observe the attitudes as well as the behaviors of a group of Romanian parents related to self-medication, specifically their beliefs and perceived risks of the administration of medicine to their children without medical advice, frequency of self-medications, symptoms, and types of medications most commonly used without medical advice. *Materials and Methods:* The questionnaire was sent via e-mail or WhatsApp link on a mobile phone using the existing data at the general practitioner's office together with the protection of data form and the informed consent form; some participants completed the questionnaire when they came for a regular visit at the general practitioner's office. Of 246 applied questionnaires, we had a rate of responses of 98%. *Results:* We found a high percentage (70%) of parents who self-medicate their children. The data reveals a significant relation between parents' beliefs on self-medication and their tendency to administrate drugs to their children without medical advice. A significant relation was also found between the likelihood of parental self-medication for their children and the number of illnesses experienced by their children over the six-month period prior to the survey. Even when parents have a correct understanding of self-medication risks, these are not aligned with actual behavior; therefore, parents continue to administer drugs to their children without medical advice. *Conclusions:* Our study helps to describe the patterns of parents' decisions about self-medicating their children and to identify parents who are more predisposed to administering self-medication to their children.

Keywords: children; self-medication; risks; beliefs

1. Introduction

Self-medication is defined as "the taking of drugs, herbs or home remedies on one's own initiative, or on the advice of another person, without consulting a doctor" [1] or by "the use of medicinal products by the individual to treat self-recognized disorders or symptoms" [2]. In the 1990s, the first worldwide reports of this phenomenon were made, and in 2000, the WHO published "guidelines for the regulatory assessment of medicinal products for use in self-medication" [3]. In pediatrics, self-medication means that medications for various disorders are administered by the caretakers of children without medical consultation. In addition, various reports highlight the fact that teenagers self-medicate on their own [4,5]. Economic, political, and cultural factors are responsible for the prevalence of, and increase in self-medication practices worldwide. These factors include the wide availability of drugs, improper advertising, parental education level, socioeconomic status, and access to healthcare services [2]. Studies reveal an increased prevalence of self-medication among pediatric populations worldwide: Germany 25.2%, China 62%, Italy 69.2%, and France 96% [6,7]. Studies in Pakistan showed that almost half of parents self-medicated children between ages 1 and 5 years, and one-third self-administered medication to children aged 5–12 years [8]. In Romania, it is estimated that 10% of the systemic antibiotics sold at pharmacies are sold without a prescription, and in our country, sales of self-prescribed medications were 488.8 million Euro in 2017; this amount included 103.1 million Euro sales in analgesics and 145.3 million Euro sales in cough and cold products [9,10]. Other studies report that Romanian pharmacists are influenced by the socioeconomic condition of the patient and are more likely to sell antibiotics without a medical prescription to socially vulnerable persons [11,12].

Despite these facts, in a study from Mureș County, Romania, the majority of respondents had good knowledge of antibiotic usage and the risks of self-prescribed antibiotics [13]. A study from another region of Romania regarding self-medication with analgesics showed that 84.8% of 461 adults aged 20–90 years used this type of medicine, both in rural and urban areas, with a predominance of females (75.5%) and young adults (70.1%) [14]. Data regarding self-medication in children by their parents or self-medication of teenagers are scarce in Romania. One study from the western part of the country reported a high prevalence of self-medication in children under 12 years old (81.0%); young mothers (30–39 years old) who were highly educated were most likely to administer medication to their children using the family pharmacy kit (83.6%) for fever, pain, and cough [15]. In our country, the few existing studies report regional data, address different age groups (mainly adults), and focus on specific categories of medication.

This study aimed to identify the individuals' attitudes and behaviors in regards to self-medication, particularly parents' beliefs and perceived risks in terms of administering certain treatments to their children without seeking medical advice. We tried to identify behavior patterns connected to medication and self-medication, the types of symptoms that most frequently lead to self-medication, the categories of administered substances, and the relevant context thereof (for instance, outside the hometown).

2. Materials and Methods

Data collection: The survey was conducted online, between August and October 2019, using the databases of four family medicine offices in the metropolitan area of Bucharest. The respondents (parents) were also recruited when they came to the doctor's office for their own medical problems.

Inclusion criteria: Adults enrolled in one of the four family medicine offices with whom the coordinator of the study collaborated with; adults with at least one child aged 0–18 years registered at the same office.

Exclusion criteria: Adults without children; adults with all children older than 18 years.

The study sample comprised a total of 241 adults from various regions of Romania; their children were born in different maternity hospitals, and at the time of the study, they all lived in Bucharest together with their parents.

Instrument questionnaire. The survey questionnaire consisted of 25 questions (Supplementary Text S1) that gathered the opinions of parents on topics related to pediatric self-medication as follows: Frequency of medication without medical advice (measured on a three-point scale, where 3 = often, 2 = sometimes, 1 = never), types of symptoms in which self-medication was given (multiple-choice question), types of medicines parents used for their children (multiple-choice question), the type of online or offline source of medical information (multiple-choice question), and the perceived risks of self-medication (closed question). The beliefs of parents on pediatric self-medication were measured through a question where patients expressed their agreement on a three-point scale (where 3 = disagree, 2 = agree, 1 = don't know/can't answer) with a set of statements reproducing beliefs on self-medication derived from literature research.

Categorical data, such as socio-demographics (age, gender, education level, employment, number of children), were also collected during the study.

The questionnaire was sent via e-mail or WhatsApp link on a mobile phone using the existing data at the general practitioner's office together with the protection of data form and the informed consent form; some participants completed the questionnaire when they came for a regular visit at the general practitioner's office.

The respondents received the link on WhatsApp or e-mail so as to respond to the survey instrument (the questionnaire) according to their willingness. The respondents were informed that our study did not collect personal data of patients (such as name, address, email, or current state of health). The questionnaire was administered online, i.e., patients received the link with the questionnaire and were solicited to answer the questions therein. As participation in the study was voluntary, the respondents could exit the questionnaire if they did not wish to complete it. The study was approved by the ethics committee of the Romanian Academy of Medical Sciences (no. 2 SNI/27.02.2019).

Statistical analysis was conducted using SPSS 20 software, including descriptive (frequency and percentage) and cross-data (Fisher's Exact Test) statistics, when applicable. As our study was a preliminarily one and the sample was homogeneous in terms of categorical variables (Table 1), we chose to analyze the overall data, looking at the occurrence of self-medication in general. Fisher's exact test was performed to determine associations between the frequency of self-medication and the parents' beliefs regarding medication of their children without medical advice. Furthermore, we used Fisher's exact test to observe if the likelihood of parental self-medication is related to the number of illnesses experienced by their children over the six-month period prior to the survey.

Table 1. Socio-demographic characteristics of the sample ($N = 241$).

		N	%
Age	18–25 years	7	3
	26–33 years	112	46
	34–41 years	101	42
	41–48	19	8
	+49	2	1
	Total	241	100
Gender	Male	26	11
	Female	215	89
	Total	241	100
Marital Status	Married	235	97
	Unmarried	4	2
	Divorced	2	1
	Total	241	100
Number of Children Per Family	1 child	144	59
	2 children	90	37
	3 children or more	7	3
	Total	241	100
Education	Baccalaureate	29	12
	University degree	162	67
	PhD or postgraduate studies	50	21
	Total	241	100

3. Results

The subjects of the current study were 241 adults from an urban area (Bucharest, Romania) whose children were registered in the databases of four family physician offices in Bucharest. Of the 246 applied questionnaires, 241 parents gave their consent to answer the questionnaire. Only 5 parents from 246 declined the questionnaire (response rate 98%).

The socio-demographic characteristics of the sample are presented in Table 1.

Prevalence and Characteristics of Self-Medication Practices

The majority of parents were members of an online group for medical discussions (62%). The majority of respondents (70%) resorted to self-medication often (9%) or sometimes (61%).

Of the total sample, 73 persons (30%) reported never having given their children any medicine without prior medical advice (Figure 1).

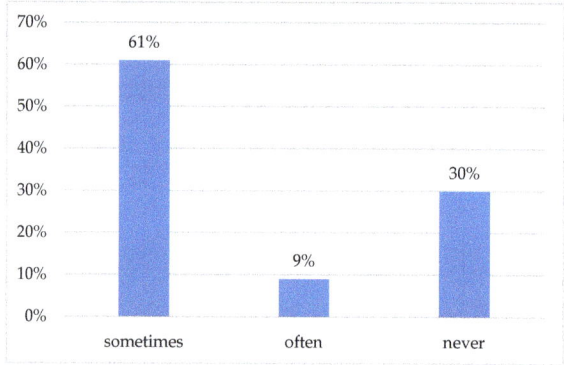

Figure 1. The frequency of self-medication administered to children ($N = 241$ parents).

Parents most often chose to treat their children's medical issue on their own during the night (53%), when they were unable to access healthcare services (61%), when they were out of their hometown (47%), and during weekends (28%).

When their children are ill, a large proportion of our respondents said they call their doctor ($N = 211$; 88%); only 24 (10%) of the respondents rarely phone the doctor while 6 (2%) of them have never done so (see question 10 from Supplementary Text S1). Some parents (40%) request and receive a medical visit. Among them, there are parents that resort to self-medication using medicines, homeopathic preparations, or plant extracts (phytotherapy) based on personal experience (30%), or that use previous doctor-recommended treatment schemes (35%). Their children's illness also leads some parents to seek medical information online using Google's search engine (54%), online parent groups, or medical websites for parents (43%) (Figure 2).

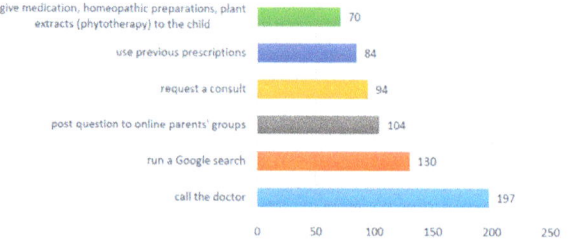

Figure 2. Number of parents that resort to certain solutions when their child is ill.

The results revealed that, in general, respondents are aware that self-medication is undesirable and most (82%) believe that administering certain treatments to their children without a medical consult is only allowed in the case of minor symptoms. Most respondents disagree with the following statements: "Self-medication is cheaper than medical consults" (88%) and "self-medication is a solution when you lack time" (62%). However, around one in three respondents (32%) found self-medication more efficient when medical consults are difficult to access (32%), and 13 respondents (5%) found self-medication to be less expensive than medical consultation (Figure 3).

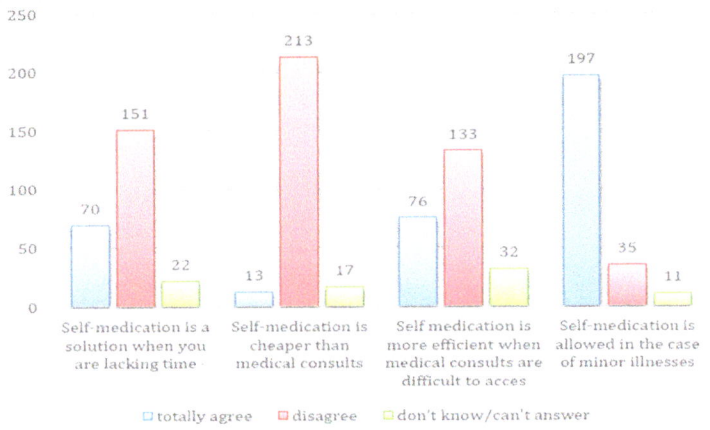

Figure 3. Number of parents that agree or disagree with statements on self-medication.

In our study, we were interested to see if there is a statistically significant association between beliefs regarding self-medication and associated behaviors, as well as whether the incidence of self-medication is higher among parents dealing more often with their children's health issues. For this purpose, we performed Fisher's exact test to determine whether the frequency of parents toward self-medication correlated with the frequency of their children's health issues over the last six months. The results revealed a significant relation between the likelihood of parental self-medication for their children and the number of the children's health issues ($p = 0.004$) (Table 2), that is, parents that were confronted with more than two medical issues of their children tend to give them drugs without medical advice compared with those who experienced less than two health issues.

Table 2. Self-medication distribution across the frequency of children's health issues.

Number of Children Health Issues In the Last 6 Months	How Many Times Did You Give Drugs to Your Children without Medical Advice?			Total	p * Value
	Often	Sometimes	Never		
less than 2	14 (7%)	126 (61%)	67 (32%)	207 (100%)	0.004
more than 2	8 (25%)	19 (59%)	5 (16%)	32 (100%)	
Total	22 (9%)	145 (61%)	72 (30%)	239 (100%)	

* Fisher's Exact Test.

We were also interested to see if there is a significant association between the frequency of self-medication and parents' beliefs regarding medication of their children without medical advice. The Fisher's exact test values indicated that there is a statistically significant association ($p = 0.000$); specifically, parents who agreed that self-medication is allowed in the case of minor illnesses were the ones that resorted more often to self-medication when dealing with their children's diseases (Table 3).

Table 3. Self-medication likelihood among parents who believe self-medication is allowed in case of minor health issues.

		Self-Medication Is Allowed in Case of Children's Minor Health Issues			
		Agree	Disagree	Total	p * Value
Parental medication of children without medical advice	yes	146 (92%)	12 (8%)	158 (100%)	
	no	49 (70%)	21 (30%)	70 (100%)	0.000
Total		195 (85%)	33 (15%)	228 (100%)	

* Fisher's Exact Test.

We also found that parents who often resort to self-medication of their children were those that believed that self-medication is a solution when health services are difficult to access ($p = 0.000$) and when they do not have enough time ($p = 0.020$) compared with those that do not self-medicate their children (Tables 4 and 5).

Table 4. Self-medication likelihood among parents who believe self-medication is allowed in case of minor health issues.

		Self-Medication Is a Solution When Health Services Are Difficult to Access			
		Agree	Disagree	Total	p * Value
Parental medication of children without medical advice	yes	63 (44%)	79 (66%)	142 (100%)	
	no	13 (19)	54 (81%)	67 (100%)	0.000
Total		76 (36%)	133 (64%)	209 (100%)	

Table 5. Self-medication likelihood among parents who believe self-medication is a solution when you do not have enough time.

		Self-Medication Is a Solution When You Do Not Have Enough Time			
		Agree	Disagree	Total	p * Value
Parental medication of children without medical advice	yes	55 (37%)	93 (63%)	148 (100%)	
	no	15 (21%)	56 (79%)	71 (100%)	0.02
Total		70 (32%)	149 (68%)	219 (100%)	

* Fisher's Exact Test.

Further, in our study, we tested the relation between self-medication beliefs and ways of purchasing medicine. Considering the descriptive data (Table 6), parents who agreed that self-medication is allowed in the case of minor health conditions are inclined to purchase medicine directly from the pharmacy ($N = 189; 81\%$) while parents that disagreed procure the medicine using previous prescriptions ($N = 33; 20\%$). We also performed a Fisher's exact test, which indicates there is no significant difference between those that agree or disagree with the statements regarding self-medication and their means to procure medicine.

The majority of respondents ($N = 171; 74\%$) said that they administer drugs when they are familiar with symptoms, a quarter of them ($N = 61; 25\%$) when the first symptoms occur, and 34 of the parents (14%) when they notice a worsening of the child's general condition.

Table 6. Source of the drugs administered to the children among parents who believe that self-medication is allowed in the case of minor health issues.

When Choosing to Handle Things on Your Own, How Do You Procure the Medicine?	Self-Medication Is Allowed in the Case of Minor Health Issues				Total
	System Missing	Agree	Disagree	Don't Know/Don't Answer	
directly from the pharmacy	1 (0.4%)	189 (81%)	32 (14%)	11 (5%)	22 (100%)
from acquaintances/relatives	1 (33%)	2 (67%)	0 (0%)	0 (0%)	146 (100%)
from previous prescriptions	0 (0%)	4 (80%)	1 (20%)	0 (0%)	73 (100%)
Total	2 (0.8%)	195 (81%)	33 (14%)	11 (5%)	241 (100%)

Respondents were aware of the risks of administering medication without a medical prescription. The majority believed that administration errors may occur in terms of both the preparation (77%) and the dosage (60%). Varying numbers of respondents were aware of the possibility of side effects from the medications (51%), the fact that self-medication can mask the symptoms of a severe condition (64%), the likelihood of drug interactions with the onset of adverse effects (38%), and that delay in seeking medical consultation entails risks (38%).

Symptoms that lead parents to treat their children without a medical consult include fever (80%), cough (50%), minor trauma (41%), diarrhea (31%), vomiting (16%), and abdominal pain (12%) (Figure 4).

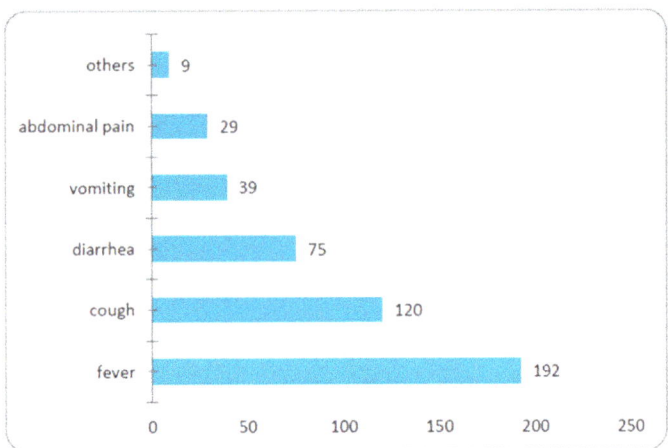

Figure 4. Number of parents that resort to self-medication when they observe the symptomatology of children.

The medications with which respondents most frequently self-medicate their children are analgesics (94%), antitussives (36%), and antidiarrheals (30%); only 1% of respondents admitted to self-administering antibiotics to their children (Figure 5). The majority of parents ($N = 233$; 95%) stated they purchase medication "directly from the pharmacy," while others resort to previous prescriptions ($N = 5$; 2%) or to their friends ($N = 3$; 1%).

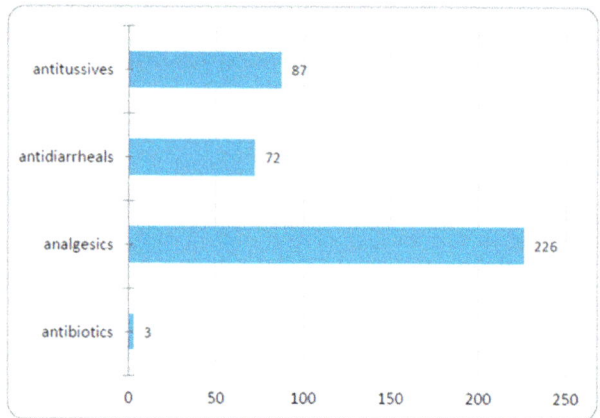

Figure 5. Number of parents that give certain medicine to their children without medical advice.

Our research also explored whether there is a relevant association of self-medication to the use of media versus interpersonal sources of communication for medical purposes. Our results revealed that "traditional" medical sources continue to be frequently accessed by parents to retrieve medical information, namely doctors (98%) and pharmacists (37%). Only 5% reported relying on friends for medical information. Online resources have become increasingly accessible with the large-scale use of new Internet-connected devices. Respondents reported using medical websites (19%), Google (9%), and online parent groups and forums (4%).

The majority of respondents (67%) believed that online healthcare-related information assisted them to some extent in solving their children's health issue, while approximately one-fifth (19%) of the respondents considered they found a solution for their medical issue using online sources (Figure 6).

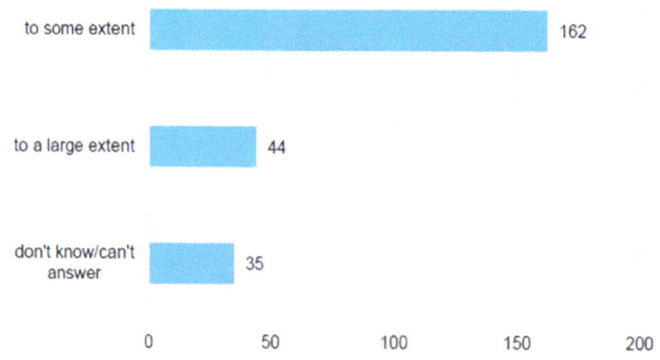

Figure 6. Number of parents that perceived the efficiency of online medical information.

When searching online sources, the majority of respondents (78%) sought information on the most frequent symptoms of common pediatric diseases. Approximately half of the subjects searched for information on therapeutic options for various common pathologies (47%). More than half of the respondents (60%) expressed their interest in homeopathic preparations or plant extracts (phytotherapy), while half of the participants (50%) were interested in other parents' online descriptions of their experiences with their children's health issues.

4. Discussions

In our study, we found that married urban females with higher university or post-graduate education who join online groups for medical discussions were more likely to self-medicate their children. The high percentage of current Romanian respondents (70%—as 61% who sometimes self-medicated their children and 9% that did the same often) we found who medicate their children without professional medical input is consistent with previous studies conducted in Italy and Pakistan but higher than those in France, Germany, and Spain [6–8,16,17]. This variability can be explained by the data collection methods, cultural factors, availability of pediatric services, the costs of healthcare services, and respondents' socioeconomic status [17–19].

The large majority of parents in our study (88%) declared that they call their child's doctor when the child has an illness (as the responses to question 10 indicate, see Supplementary Text S1). Moreover, when we measured their beliefs regarding self-medication, we found that parents, in a close percentage (82%), believed that self-medication is used only for minor complaints of the children (as the responses to question 20 indicate, see Supplementary Text S1). The certain responses we obtained in our study—the high likelihood of self-medication of children by their parents (70%) and in contrast, a high percentage (82%) who declared they call the doctor when their children are ill—could be explained by the social desirability effect as public health campaigns have lately been run in Romania to discourage self-medication.

The symptoms we found for which parents medicated their children were similar to those reported in other studies, i.e., fever, coughing, abdominal pain, and diarrhea [4,15,20].

The data of our research also showed that parents who administrate medicine without medical advice are mostly those who think medical services are difficult to access and whose children commonly have more than two health issues during the previous half-year. This result could be related to Romanian health care particularities, where primary care is under-used [21].

Our results are consistent with those of other authors showing that the most frequently parentally administered medicines are analgesics, antitussives, and antidiarrheals [4,15,22]. Recent studies conducted in adults show that medications for the musculoskeletal and nervous systems rank at the top (NSAIDs and other analgesics despite the risk of gastrointestinal complications), followed by medications for digestive, respiratory, and cardiovascular symptoms [17,23–26]. Parental reports of antibiotic self-administration to their children were not common in our study, despite the fact that the consumption of antibiotics in Romania is very high in the community; among the most used antibiotics are penicillins, cephalosporins, and quinolones [27]. We considered two possible explanations for the low rate of reported antibiotic self-medication to children. First, our parent group was highly educated, and they may recognize the risks of antibiotic overuse. Second, recognizing the societal harm from overuse of antibiotics, they may not have been fully honest in their responses to this question.

The high access to online information, as well as online healthcare communication sources, has not diminished parents' focus on primary information sources, i.e., doctors and pharmacists, as highlighted by most studies [4,8,15]. The World Health Organization has acknowledged the importance and role of pharmacists in patients' self-medication and self-care. The pharmacists' role has become essential for responsible self-medication [28].

Accessing online sources to obtain medical information is becoming common practice among parents. Studies show that parents seeking information on their children's symptoms and treatment via Google tend to be distrustful of medical assessment, requesting a second opinion, which often results in delayed diagnosis. Considering this aspect, they can also request a second opinion, but most importantly, they should discuss with the doctor the information they obtained from the internet. On the other hand, pediatricians should encourage parents to share their concerns in order to obtain answers about alternate diagnoses. Doctors' knowledge of this approach, and its use thereof, during discussions with parents boosts the latter's confidence level and subsequently the quality of the medical care [29].

This study provided insight into the pediatric self-medication patterns and beliefs among urban Romanian parents, an area for which little information was previously available in the published literature. This study reports on parental self-medication practices in a region of Romania that was not included in previous studies. Nevertheless, the present study has a number of limitations. The respondents are homogenous in respect to socio-demographic characteristics (age, education, residence, employment, number of children). Furthermore, other variables should be taken into account in order to achieve an integrated explanatory model on pediatric self-medication in a larger sample and assess the reliability of the questionnaire used in this study.

5. Conclusions

In Romania, we are still faced with a high incidence of self-medication, even within the pediatric population. The study highlighted the perceived risks of self-medication, as well as the beliefs and knowledge of this topic, and identified some determinants of parental predisposition to self-medication of their children. Implementing educational measures focused on parent communities is essential in our country.

Supplementary Materials: The following are available online at http://www.mdpi.com/1010-660X/56/6/312/s1, Text S1: Questionare for self-medication among the pediatric population.

Author Contributions: Conceptualization, P.T. and S.D.; methodology, A.M.A.S.; software, L.P.; validation, C.C.D., A.D. and N.B.; formal analysis, P.T.; investigation, A.M.A.S.; resources, L.P.; data curation, A.D. and S.D.; writing—original draft preparation, P.T.; writing—review and editing, P.T., C.C.D., A.M.A.S.; visualization, L.P. and A.D.; supervision, C.C.D.; project administration, L.P. All authors have read and agreed to the published version of the manuscript.

Funding: This research received no external funding.

Acknowledgments: We acknowledge the support of Edward F. Bell from University of Iowa, USA, for proofreading the article.

Conflicts of Interest: The authors declare no conflict of interest.

References

1. Hernandez-Juyol, M.; Job-Quesada, J.R. Dentistry and self-medication: A current challenge. *Med. Oral.* **2002**, *7*, 344–347. [CrossRef]
2. Bennadi, D. Self-medication: A current challenge. *J. Basic Clin. Pharm.* **2013**, *5*, 19–23. [CrossRef]
3. Geneva: WHO 2000. Guidelines for the Regulatory Assessment of Medicinal Products for Use in Self-Medication. Available online: https://apps.who.int/iris/bitstream/handle/10665/66154/WHO_EDM_QSM_00.1_eng.pdf (accessed on 1 October 2019).
4. Naaraayan, A.S.; Rathinabalan, I.; Seetha, V. Self-medication pattern among children attending a tertiary hospital in South India: A cross-sectional study. *Int. J. Contemp. Pediatr.* **2016**, *3*, 1267–1271. [CrossRef]
5. Gualano, M.R.; Bert, F.; Passi, S.; Stillo, M.; Galis, V.; Manzoli, L.; Siliquini, R. Use of self-medication among adolescents: A systematic review and meta-analysis. *Eur. J. Public Health* **2014**, *25*, 444–450. [CrossRef]
6. Du, Y.; Knopf, H.C. Self-medication among children and adolescents in Germany: Results of the National Health Survey for Children and Adolescents (KiGGS). *Br. J. Clin. Pharmacol.* **2009**, *68*, 599–608. [CrossRef]
7. Garofalo, L.; Di Giuseppe, G.; Angelillo, I.F. Self-Medication Practices among Parents in Italy. *BioMed Res. Int.* **2015**, *2015*, 1–8. [CrossRef] [PubMed]
8. Gohar, U.F.; Khubaib, S.; Mehmood, A. Self-Medication Trends in Children by Their Parents. *J. Dev. Drugs* **2017**, *6*. [CrossRef]
9. Safrany, N.; Monnet, D.L. Antibiotics obtained without a prescription in Europe. *Lancet Infect. Dis.* **2012**, *12*, 182–183. [CrossRef]
10. Sales in the Self-Medication Market in Selected European Countries in 2017. Available online: https://www.statista.com/statistics/417589/self-medication-market-sales-in-europe/ (accessed on 1 April 2020).

11. Lescure, D.; Paget, J.; Schellevis, F.; Van Dijk, L. Determinants of Self-Medication with Antibiotics in European and Anglo-Saxon Countries: A Systematic Review of the Literature. *Front. Public Health* **2018**, *6*, 370. [CrossRef] [PubMed]
12. Ghiga, I.; Lundborg, C.S. 'Struggling to be a defender of health' -a qualitative study on the pharmacists' perceptions of their role in antibiotic consumption and antibiotic resistance in Romania. *J. Pharm. Policy Pract.* **2016**, *9*, 10. [CrossRef] [PubMed]
13. Voidăzan, S.; Moldovan, G.; Voidăzan, L.; Zazgyva, A.; Moldovan, H. Knowledge, Attitudes and Practices Regarding The Use Of Antibiotics. Study on The General Population of Mureş County, Romania. *Infect. Drug Resist.* **2019**, *12*, 3385–3396. [CrossRef] [PubMed]
14. Alexa, D.I.; Pancu, A.G.; Morosanu, I.A.; Ghiciuc, C.M.; Lupuşoru, C.; Prada, G.I.; Cepoi, V. The impact of self-medication with NSAID/analgesics in a north-eastern region of Romania. *Farmacia* **2014**, *62*, 1164–1170.
15. Cristescu, C. Study Regarding the Parents' Use of Self–Medication Among Children Under 12 Years Old. *Farmacia* **2018**, *66*, 811–819. [CrossRef]
16. Escourrou, B.; Bouville, B.; Bismuth, M.; Durrieu, G.; Oustric, S. Self-medication in children by parents: A real risk? A cross-sectional descriptive study. *Rev. Prat.* **2010**, *60*, 27–34.
17. Ortiz, M.V.; Ruiz-Cabello, F.J.S.; Uberos, J.; Ros, A.F.C.; Ortiz, C.V.; Morales, M.C.A.; Muñoz-Hoyos, A. Self-medication, self-prescription and medicating "by proxy" in paediatrics. *Anales de Pediatría* **2017**, *86*, 264–269. [CrossRef]
18. Sontakke, D.S.; Magdum, A.; Jaiswal, K.; Bajait, C.; Pimpalkhute, S.; Dakhale, G. Evaluation of parental perception about self-medication and other medicine use practices in children. *Eur. J. Pharm. Med. Res.* **2015**, *2*, 179–185.
19. Chrissini, M.; Sifaki-Pistolla, D.; Tzanakis, N.; Tsiligianni, I. Family and individual dietary and lifestyle habits as predictors of BMI and KIDMED score in Greek and immigrant preschoolers. *Arch. Balk. Med. Union* **2019**, *54*, 659–671. [CrossRef]
20. Alele, P.M.; Musoke, P.; Nicollette, N. Self-medication practices by caretakers for children under five years in a rural district of eastern Uganda. *IIJMMS* **2015**, *2*, 165–171.
21. Available online: https://ec.europa.eu/health/sites/health/files/state/docs/2019_chp_romania_english.pdf (accessed on 25 May 2020).
22. Mande, B.G.; Tebandite, K.E.; Marini, R.; Alworonga, O. Determinants of Self-medication of Children by Their Parents at Kisangani. *Asian J. Res. Med. Pharm. Sci.* **2018**, *4*, 1–8. [CrossRef]
23. Negovan, A.; Iancu, M.; Moldovan, V.; Sàrkàny, K.; Bataga, S.M.; Mocan, S.; Ţilea, I.; Banescu, C. The contribution of clinical and pathological predisposing factors to severe gastro-duodenal lesions in patients with long-term low-dose aspirin and proton pump inhibitor therapy. *Eur. J. Intern. Med.* **2017**, *44*, 62–66. [CrossRef]
24. De Oliveira, S.B.V.; Barroso, S.C.C.; Bicalho, M.A.C.; Reis, A.M.M. Profile of drugs used for self-medication by elderly attended at a referral center. *Einstein (São Paulo)* **2018**, *16*, 1–7. [CrossRef] [PubMed]
25. Tilea, I.; Petra, D.; Voidazan, S.; Ardeleanu, E.; Varga, A. Treatment adherence among adult hypertensive patients: A cross-sectional retrospective study in primary care in Romania. *Patient Prefer. Adherence* **2018**, *12*, 625–635. [CrossRef] [PubMed]
26. Gheorghe, G.; Stoian, A.P.; Gaman, M.-A.; Socea, B.; Neagu, T.P.; Stanescu, A.M.A.; Bratu, O.G.; Mischianu, D.L.D.; Suceveanu, A.I.; Diaconu, C.C. The Benefits and Risks of Antioxidant Treatment in Liver Diseases. *Rev. Chim.* **2019**, *70*, 651–655. [CrossRef]
27. Summary of the Latest Data on Antibiotic Consumption in the European Union, ESAC-Net Surveillance Data November 2017. Available online: https://www.ecdc.europa.eu/sites/portal/files/documents/Final_2017_EAAD_ESAC-Net_Summary-edited%20-%20FINALwith%20erratum.pdf (accessed on 11 November 2019).

28. The Role of the Pharmacist in Self-Care and Self-Medication. In *Report of the 4th WHO Consultative Group on the Role of the Pharmacist*; World Health Organization: The Hague, The Netherlands, 26–28 August 1998; Available online: https://apps.who.int/medicinedocs/en/d/Jwhozip32e/ (accessed on 24 November 2019).
29. Sood, N.; Jimenez, D.; Pham, T.B.; Cordrey, K.; Awadalla, N.; Milanaik, R. Paging Dr. Google: The Effect of Online Health Information on Trust in Pediatricians' Diagnoses. *Clin. Pediatr.* **2019**, *58*, 889–896. [CrossRef]

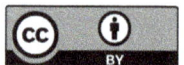

© 2020 by the authors. Licensee MDPI, Basel, Switzerland. This article is an open access article distributed under the terms and conditions of the Creative Commons Attribution (CC BY) license (http://creativecommons.org/licenses/by/4.0/).

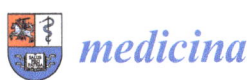

Article

Reasons for and Facilitating Factors of Medical Malpractice Complaints. What Can Be Done to Prevent Them?

Bianca Hanganu [1], Magdalena Iorga [2,3,*], Iulia-Diana Muraru [2] and Beatrice Gabriela Ioan [1]

1. Legal-Medicine Department, Faculty of Medicine, "Grigore T. Popa" University of Medicine and Pharmacy of Iasi, 700115 Iasi, Romania; bianca-hanganu@umfiasi.ro (B.H.); beatrice.ioan@umfiasi.ro (B.G.I.)
2. Behavioral Sciences Department, Faculty of Medicine, "Grigore T. Popa" University of Medicine and Pharmacy Iasi, 700115 Iasi, Romania; diana.muraru@umfiasi.ro
3. Faculty of Psychology and Education Sciences, "Alexandru Ioan Cuza" University of Iasi, 700554 Iasi, Romania
* Correspondence: magdalena.iorga@umfiasi.ro

Received: 3 May 2020; Accepted: 25 May 2020; Published: 27 May 2020

Abstract: *Background and objectives.* Medical malpractice is an increasing phenomenon all over the world, and Romania is not spared. This matter is of concern as it has a significant impact on the physicians and the patients involved, as well as on the health care system and society in general. The purpose of our study was to perform an insight analysis on the reasons for medical malpractice complaints as well as the factors that facilitate the complaints to identify specific ways to prevent them and, implicitly, to improve the medical practice. *Materials and Methods.* The authors conducted a retrospective study of the medical malpractice complaints registered in the period 2006–2019 at the Commission for monitoring and professional competence for malpractice cases in the region of Moldova, Romania, collecting data on both the patients and the medical professionals involved. *Results.* The authors analyzed 153 complaints directed against 205 medical professionals and identified 15 categories of reasons for complaints, the most significant being related to the occurrence of complications, and to the doctor–patient interaction (e.g., communication, behavior, informed consent). The most frequently reported medical specialties were obstetrics and gynecology, emergency medicine, general surgery, and orthopedics and traumatology. Emergency medicine was often involved in complaints suggesting an over utilization of this department in our country and the need for health policies, which could divert the large number of patients accessing emergency medicine towards primary care. *Conclusions.* Regarding the dysfunctions in the doctor–patient relationship frequently claimed by patients, the authors concluded that doctors need special undergraduate training and periodic updating during their practice for them to be able to adequately address the challenges of interacting with their patients.

Keywords: medical malpractice; doctor–patient relationship; communication; complications; diagnostic error; preventive measures; retrospective study

---

1. Introduction

The medical practice has been regulated throughout its entire historical evolution by specific legal and ethical norms, which are aimed at carrying out the medical act in optimal conditions, protecting the patients, and sanctioning the doctors who violate the norms of good practice [1]. Medicine and science, in general, enjoy quasi-constant advancements, which bring multiple benefits through their wide applicability [2]. Nonetheless, by increasing public expectations, emphasizing the publicity of patient rights [1,3] and the marketing of medicine [3], the progress in technology places a greater burden on the shoulders of the doctors, which often leads patients to have unrealistic expectations and causes them to sanction any mistake or any result that does not coincide with their expectations [4]. This, in turn, leads to tensions in the doctor–patient relationship [2]. Thus, the current medical practice risks being dominated by fear of potential malpractice complaints and their consequences on the medical staff.

The increasing number of medical malpractice complaints represents an alarming reality worldwide, with reports from various health services in Europe, the United States of America, and Australia confirming it [5,6]. Thus, Jena et al. (2011) showed that in the United States of America, 7.4% of medical professionals are accused of malpractice each year [7]. Likewise, a 2009 study showed that about 4% of the 108,000 physicians insured by a German insurance company faced a medical malpractice accusation each year [8]. In the United Kingdom, the number of complaints against general practitioners (GP) increased more than two-fold during a period of 5 years, between 2007 and 2012 [6]. In Romania, the malpractice complaints submitted to the court annually increased from 8 in 2008 to 65 in 2017, with a total of 331 in the period 2007–2018, 62 (18.73%) of these being registered in the eight counties included in our study [9].

The increase in the number of malpractice complaints is a burden for both the doctors and the medical system through their impact on the medical practice, as it can lead to the approach to the medical act in a defensive manner, as well as through the judicial procedure which usually lasts for a long time and involves significant costs for physicians and medical institutions [2,6].

Defensive medicine involves requesting more medical tests, more medical opinions, prescribing more drugs, more referrals to specialized examinations, refusing to perform certain high-risk procedures, or even refusing to assist patients with severe illnesses. These practices are not always for the benefit of the patients; on the contrary, they subject them to unnecessary and sometimes risky interventions, increase the costs of medical care, and decrease the level of satisfaction among physicians [2].

To reduce the negative impact of the judicial process for the resolution of malpractice complaints on doctors and patients, an extrajudicial procedure (e.g., no-fault system, mediation) has been introduced in many countries alongside the judiciary system. This extrajudicial procedure has a number of advantages for both the patient and the doctor and the medical system in general. In out-of-court settlements, complaints are resolved more quickly and efficiently, with lower costs compared to judicial resolution. An out-of-court settlement promotes the disclosure of medical practice incidents, which can increase patients' trust in physicians and can improve the physician–patient relationship, thus being preventive, and increases patient safety by improving the quality of medical care [10–12]. Likewise, resolving the complaints out-of-court decreases the level of psychological stress to which the doctor and the patient are subjected, and the doctor can continue or resume his/her professional activity without fear or pressure resulting from the complaint being made in court or released in the press. These latter aspects are particularly important as after the disclosure of the complaints in the press and the presentation in court, even if the doctor is exonerated, the associated psychological stress could irreversibly damage his/her professional life [12].

In Romania, the out-of-court procedure for resolving medical malpractice complaints was legislated in 2006, when the Commissions on monitoring and professional competence for malpractice cases were created. These Commissions carry out their activity at the level of the Public Health Directorates (PHD) in each county and in Bucharest, and their composition is mixed, covering the activity of physicians, dentists, nurses, midwives, and pharmacists. The working procedure of these commissions provides that patients who consider themselves harmed as a result of the medical act, or their family members (in the case of deceased or incompetent patients), may submit complaints accompanied by documents certifying the harm. The complaints are analyzed with the support of medical experts in the targeted medical specialty to determine whether or not the patients have suffered as a result of malpractice. The medical experts who analyze the complaints belong to various medical specialties and are included in a list available nationwide. They are designated randomly, by drawing lots, and their fee is paid by the plaintiff. To prove an act of malpractice, four criteria must be met cumulatively: (a) the existence of a deed produced during a prevention, diagnosis, or treatment activity; (b) the deed is causing patrimonial or non-patrimonial (moral) damage to the patient; (c) the guilt of the medical professional; (d) the causal relationship between the deed and the prejudice [13].

This study aimed to analyze the reasons for the complaints of medical malpractice submitted to the commissions at the PHDs in the region of Moldova, as well as the factors that facilitate the complaints, to identify ways to prevent the complaints and, implicitly, to improve the medical practice. Moldova is a large territory located in the northeast and partially the southeast of Romania, between the Carpathians Mountains and the Prut River, and includes 8 counties out of the total of 41, plus the capital city, Bucharest (Bacau, Botosani, Galati, Iasi, Neamt, Suceava, Vaslui, and Vrancea), with a total surface of about 46,000 km^2 and around 4 million people.

To our knowledge, this research is the first of its kind in Romania.

This study is part of a broader doctoral research, which aims to identify methods to prevent the complaints of medical malpractice submitted by patients and to reduce their impact on the medical staff.

2. Materials and Methods

2.1. Data Collection

The authors conducted a retrospective multi-centric study of malpractice complaints registered in the period 2006–2019 at the Commissions on monitoring and professional competence for malpractice cases in the region of Moldova, which includes 8 counties (Bacau, Botosani, Galati, Iasi, Neamt, Suceava, Vaslui, Vrancea). Data were collected from complaints submitted by patients who were treated in either public ($n = 26$) or private ($n = 14$) medical institutions or their family members and from decisions made by the commissions in each case. The collection, storage, and processing of data were done with respect for the confidentiality of personal data of doctors and plaintiffs.

The collected data concerned, on the one hand, the reasons for the complaints and, on the other hand, the persons who made the complaints (patients or family members) and the doctors who were involved in the respective cases. More specifically, the data regarding the persons who filed the complaints concerned the following aspects: the socio-demographic characteristics of the patients (gender, age, residence area); the existence of multiple pathologies; if the patient died or not; the petitioner who filed the complaint (the patient or their family members); the number of days of hospitalization; the existence of multiple hospitalizations. The data about the doctors concerned: medical specialty, professional degree, and gender.

The analysis of the reasons underlying the complaints led to the identification of 15 categories, depending on the central, essential elements mentioned in the complaints. For identifying the categories of reasons, the authors used an inductive approach. All authors read the reasons as stated by the complainants multiple times, and to ensure rigor, they met several times to analyze them. In this way, the authors identified 15 categories related to aspects of the medical act itself or to the doctor–patient relationship and decided together on the inclusion of each reason in one of the established categories.

2.2. Ethical Approval

The research was approved by the Research Ethics Commission of the "Grigore T. Popa" University of Medicine and Pharmacy of Iasi, Romania, No. 16434 / July 30, 2019.

2.3. Statistical Analysis

The collected data were analyzed using IBM SPSS Statistics, version 23. Percentages, means, and standard deviations were used for the descriptive analysis. The independent samples *t*-Test was used in the case of variables where there were two independent groups to determine if there were any statistically significant differences between the means of these groups. The Chi-square test was used to test the association between categorical variables.

3. Results

We analyzed 153 complaints directed against 205 medical professionals (physicians, nurses, physiotherapists, and dentists). In 12 cases, the plaintiff also complained about the hospital. Of the people who filed complaints, 82 (53.6%) were male, and 71 (46.4%) were female. Their ages ranged from 0 (new-born) to 90 (M = 37.21, SD = 24.38); however, the analyzed documents did not specify the age of the plaintiffs in 12 cases. Close to half of the patients were deceased (43.8%). Most of the plaintiffs live in urban areas (67.3%), and most of them filed the complaints in Iasi (30.1%) and Galati (28.1%) counties. In more than half of the cases, the plaintiffs were members of the patient's family (in case of deceased or incompetent patients). All the data related to the socio-demographic characteristics of the plaintiffs are presented in Table 1.

Table 1. Socio-demographic characteristics of the plaintiffs.

Variables		N (%)
Gender	Male	82 (53.6)
	Female	71 (46.4)
County	Iasi	46 (30.1)
	Vaslui	9 (5.9)
	Botosani	13 (8.5)
	Suceava	16 (10.5)
	Galati	43 (28.1)
	Neamt	8 (5.2)
	Bacau	8 (5.2)
	Vrancea	10 (6.5)
Deceased	Yes	67 (43.8)
Residence area	Rural	42 (27.5)
	Urban	103 (67.3)
	Missing data	8 (5.2)
Plaintiff	Patient	63 (41.2)
	Patient's family	90 (58.8)
Multiple hospitalizations	Yes	57 (37.3)
	Missing	8 (5.2)
New-born	Yes	8 (5.2)
Age (M ± SD)		37.21 (±24.38)
Hospitalization days (M ± SD)		14.86 (±18.86)

The medical specialties in which most complaints were found were (1) obstetrics and gynecology, with 24 (15.7%) claims against 29 physicians (14.14%), (2) emergency medicine, with 18 (11.8%) claims against 20 physicians (9.75%), (3) general surgery with 16 (10.5%) claims against 20 physicians (9.75%), and (4) orthopedics and traumatology with 12 (7.8%) claims involving 19 physicians (9.26%).

We identified 15 categories of reasons for complaints. Categories, examples of specific reasons for each category and the most involved specialties in each category are shown in Table 2.

Table 2. Categories of reasons.

Category	Examples of Reasons Mentioned by Patients and Family Members in Proxy Position	No of Cases	No of Physicians	Most Involved Specialties *
I. Reasons Related to Technical Aspects of the Medical Activity				
Complications	Injuries produced while admitted to the hospital and during surgical intervention Infection of the surgical incision Post-surgery complication Retained foreign object	59 38.6%	75 36.58%	OG GS OT

Table 2. Cont.

Category	Examples of Reasons Mentioned by Patients and Family Members in Proxy Position	No of Cases	No of Physicians	Most Involved Specialties *
Treatment errors	Total hysterectomy instead of myomectomy Wrong maneuver leading to dislocation of the prosthesis Wrong epidural injection	45 29.4%	66 32.19%	OG Dentist GS
Negligence	Patient left unsupervised Superficial clinical examination Overlooking important findings Failure to recommend/refer for additional examinations Failure to hospitalize the patient	40 26.1%	45 21.95%	EM
Diagnostic errors	Small cell carcinoma vs. large cell carcinoma Establishing diagnosis without performing all the necessary tests Intestinal obstruction vs. botulism	19 12.4%	28 13.65%	Pediatrics OT OG
Delay	In diagnosis In transferring the patient In examining the patient (waiting too long in the waiting room) In performing investigation In child delivery In treatment	18 11.8%	20 9.75%	GS EM Pediatrics
Lack of competence/ Professionalism	Incompetence Lack of knowledge Insufficient medical knowledge	13 8.5%	19 9.26%	OG EM Pediatrics
Lack of diagnosis	Missed the bone fissure on the X-ray Missed the injury of the left ear Missed the nuchal cord Missed the rupture of the aortic aneurism	8 5.2%	11 5.36%	GS OT Pediatrics
Deficiencies in filling out the medical file	Failure to mention all the information in the medical file Mentioning more diagnoses than the patient actually had Replacing the medical file, etc.	7 4.6%	8 3.90%	OG GS
Administrative	Improper functioning of the emergency system	3 2.0%	4 1.95%	OT
II. Reasons Related to the Relationship between Patients and Medical Staff				
Lack of information/informing deficiency	Failure to mention the risks Failure to offer explanations Failure to provide information about the diagnosis	24 15.7%	30 14.63%	GS Pediatrics OG EM
Inappropriate behavior of the physician	Insufficient interaction Expecting monetary incentive Arrogance Distant attitude Disrespect	14 9.2%	18 8.78%	EM PS OH
Inappropriate language	Allusion to ethnicity Inappropriate tone of voice Offensive words	14 9.2%	19 9.26%	OG EM Pediatrics
Suggestion made by other doctors	Blaming the late transfer on the previous doctor Blaming the patient's previous doctor for brutal procedures Blaming the patient's previous doctor for errors in treatment in open discussions with fellow colleagues Inciting the patient to legal proceeding against previous doctors and medical units	14 9.2%	13 6.34%	GS EM Ophthalmology
Failure in obtaining informed consent	Apical resection without obtaining the patient's consent Removing the ovarian adherences detected during the surgery to prepare the ovaries for IVF, against patient's expressed refusal of IVF Failure to follow the previously established therapeutic plan and proceeding to change without prior informing the patient	10 6.5%	18 8.78%	OG Dentist
Inappropriate communication among medical team members	Failure to inform fellow doctors about the special technique he was performing/about the surgical intervention Lack of communication between physicians who were treating the patient	3 2.0%	5 2.43%	Ophthalmology

* OG—obstetrics and gynecology, OT—orthopedics and traumatology, GC—general surgery, EM—emergency medicine, PS—plastic surgery, OH—oncology and hematology.

We tested the association between the reasons mentioned above and some of the study variables concerning the plaintiff (residence area, gender, if the patient was deceased, if the plaintiff was the patient or a family member, if the patient was hospitalized multiple times, if the patient was a new-born) and we found several statistically significant results. Six of the reasons for complaint (treatment errors, reasons suggested by colleagues, inappropriate communication among team members, administrative reasons, legal reasons, and lack of competence/professionalism) were not associated with any of the aforementioned variables. The other nine had associations with the study variables in various ways as showed below.

3.1. Reasons Related to Technical Aspects of the Medical Activity

3.1.1. Complications

"Complications" as a reason for complaint was associated with:

- Whether the patient was deceased or not: $\chi2(1) = 20.913$, $p < 0.001$; Phi coefficient = −0.371, $p < 0.001$, indicating a small size effect; more specifically, "complications" was more likely to be a reason for complaint in cases where the patients did not die (54.7%) compared with the cases where they did (18.2%);
- Gender: $\chi2(1) = 7.929$, $p = 0.005$; Phi coefficient = 0.228, $p = 0.005$, indicating a small size effect; more concretely, "complications" was more likely to be a reason for complaint in the cases of female patients (50.7%) compared to male patients (28.4%);
- Whether the plaintiff was the patient or a family member: $\chi2(1) = 10.402$, $p = 0.001$; Phi coefficient = −0.262, $p = 0.001$, indicating a small size effect; in this case, patients were more likely to complain about the occurrence of complications (54.0%) than their relatives (28.1%);
- Whether the patient had multiple hospitalizations: $\chi2(1) = 4.370$, $p = 0.037$; Phi coefficient = 0.174, $p = 0.037$, indicating a small size effect; specifically, patients with multiple hospitalizations were more likely to complain about complications (49.1%) compared to those without multiple hospitalizations (31.8%).

In addition, there was a statistically significant difference in number of hospitalization days between patients who complained about complications and those who did not: $t(128) = -4.824$, $p < 0.001$; the patients from the former category had a higher mean of hospitalization days (M = 24.85) compared to the latter (M = 8.71).

3.1.2. Negligence

"Negligence" as a reason for complaint was associated with whether the plaintiff was the patient or a family member: $\chi2(1) = 4.351$, $p = 0.037$; Phi coefficient = 0.169, $p = 0.037$, indicating a small size effect. In this case, relatives were more likely to complain about negligence (32.6%) than the patient (17.5%).

There was a statistically significant difference in number of hospitalization days between patients who complained about negligence and those who did not: $t(128) = 2.900$, $p = 0.004$. Patients who complained about negligence had a higher mean of hospitalization days (M = 8.94) compared to those who did not (M = 17.12).

3.1.3. Diagnostic Errors

"Diagnosis errors" as a reason for complaint was associated with whether the patient had multiple hospitalizations: $\chi2(1) = 4.094$, $p = 0.043$; Phi coefficient = 0.168, $p = 0.043$, indicating a small size effect. Patients with multiple hospitalizations were more likely to complain about diagnosis errors (19.3%) compared to those without multiple hospitalizations (8.0%).

3.1.4. Delay (in Examination, in Diagnosis, in Treatment)

"Delay" as a reason for complaint was associated with:

- Whether the patient was deceased or not: $\chi 2(1) = 13.239, p < 0.001$; Phi coefficient = $0.295, p < 0.001$, indicating a small size effect; delay was more likely to be a reason for complaint in cases where the patients died (22.7%) compared to the cases where they did not (3.5%);
- Whether the plaintiff was the patient or a family member: $\chi 2(1) = 5.166, p = 0.023$; Phi coefficient = $0.184, p = 0.023$, indicating a small size effect; delay was more likely to be a reason for complaint by family members (16.9%) compared to patients (4.8%).

3.1.5. Lack of Diagnosis

"Lack of diagnosis" as a reason for complaint was associated with gender: $\chi 2(1) = 7.402, p = 0.007$; Phi coefficient = $-0.221, p = 0.007$, indicating a small size effect. More concretely, lack of diagnosis was more likely to be a reason for complaint in the cases of male patients (9.9%) compared to female patients (0.0%).

3.2. Reasons Related to the Relationship between Patients and Medical Staff

3.2.1. Lack of Information/Informing Deficiency

"Lack of information/informing deficiency" as a reason for complaint was associated with:

- Whether the plaintiff was the patient or a family member: $\chi 2(1) = 7.212, p = 0.007$; Phi coefficient = $0.218, p = 0.007$, indicating a small size effect; lack of information/informing deficiency was more likely to be a reason for complaint for family members (22.5%) compared to patients (6.3%);
- Whether the patient was deceased or not: $\chi 2(1) = 4.223, p = 0.040$; Phi coefficient = $0.167, p = 0.040$, indicating a small size effect; lack of information/informing deficiency was more likely to be a reason for complaint in cases where the patients died (22.7%) compared to those cases in which the patients did not die (10.5%);
- Whether the patient was newborn or not: $\chi 2(1) = 13.857, p < 0.001$; Phi coefficient = $0.302, p < 0.001$, indicating a medium size effect; in cases where patients were newborn, lack of information/informing deficiency was more likely to be a reason for complaint (62.5%) compared to those in which the patients were not newborn (13.2%).

3.2.2. Inappropriate Language

"Inappropriate language" as a reason for complaint was associated with whether the patient was newborn or not: $\chi 2(1) = 8.082, p = 0.004$; Phi coefficient = $0.231, p = 0.004$, indicating a small size effect. In cases where patients were newborn, inappropriate language was more likely to be a reason for complaint (37.5%) compared to those in which the patients were not newborn (7.6%).

3.2.3. Informed Consent

"Informed consent" as a reason for complaint was associated with whether the patient was newborn or not: $\chi 2(1) = 4.662, p = 0.031$; Phi coefficient = $0.175, p = 0.031$, indicating a small size effect. In cases where the patients were newborn, informed consent was more likely to be a reason for complaint (25.0%) compared to those in which the patients were not newborn (5.6%).

3.2.4. Inappropriate Behavior

"Inappropriate behavior" as a reason for complaint was associated with the residence area (rural or urban): $\chi 2(1) = 4.296, p = 0.038$; Phi coefficient = $0.172, p = 0.038$, indicating a small effect size. In cases where patients lived in rural areas, inappropriate behavior was more likely to be a reason for complaint (16.7%) compared to those who lived in urban areas (5.8%).

4. Discussion

This study allowed the analysis of data gathered during 14 years of activity of the Commissions on monitoring and professional competence for cases of malpractice in the Moldova region of Romania. Our results showed several findings that could be the starting point for formulating prevention methods designed to the reduction in the number of malpractice claims.

Our study showed that the ground for complaints are both reasons related to technical aspects of the medical activity and reasons related to the relationship between patients and medical staff, these results are consistent with literature data [14]. The analysis of these reasons is important so as to improve the medical practice by identifying various prevention methods that target both the medical practice and the doctor–patient relationship, to improve medical services provided to patients, and to protect the medical staff from complaints [2].

In our study we found that over half of the complaints were registered in two counties (Iasi and Galati). The large number of cases in these two counties (compared to the other counties included in the research) is due, most likely, to the fact that Iasi and Galati are university centers, with clinical hospitals, which can provide a higher level of medical services and can treat more severe cases, and where many patients from other counties in Moldova are referred from smaller hospitals. Likewise, many patients request on their own initiative a referral by the general practitioners to specialists working in university centers, sometimes contrary to their recommendation [15].

Literature data show that there are no medical specialties spared by malpractice complaints, but some specialties have a higher risk compared to others [16].

In our study, the most frequently reported medical specialties are obstetrics and gynecology, emergency medicine, general surgery, and orthopedics and traumatology. These results are partly consistent with those of other studies. Obstetrics and gynecology, general surgery, and orthopedics and traumatology also occupy the first places in studies conducted in other countries, such as the United Kingdom, China or the United States of America [4,7,17].

The increased risk of certain medical specialties for malpractice claims is mainly due to the particularities of the medical services provided and the patients treated. Physicians in obstetrics and gynecology, for example, treat not only one patient, but often at least two (mother and child) or even three, if we take into account the concerns of the future father, while by taking care of the reproductive system of the woman, it also deals with potential future patients, the reproduction of the human species, thus becoming a specialty of the entire family [4]. Patients accessing obstetrics and gynecology services often expect for more than what a doctor can actually do, asking for flawless results of the medical interventions, such as safe labor when the child is to be given birth [18]. Becoming a parent can be an overwhelming issue, and the perinatal period is characterized by plenty of emotions related to the health status of the newborn. As such, this emotional burden on the parents may become a trigger for complaints against professionals in this field when the newborn is not healthy [19].

Physicians in orthopedics and traumatology are at high risk because they have to take care of patients' work capacity [4], which may have significant social and professional implications.

The increased risk for complaints of malpractice in surgical specialties is underlined by Jena et al. (2011), who showed that allegations of medical malpractice occur quite frequently in this specialty. Those authors found that 88% of physicians in at-risk surgical specialties (neurosurgery, thoracic and cardiovascular surgery, general surgery) had one complaint against them until the age of 45, and the number increased to 99% by the age of 65 [7]. Patients who need surgery usually suffer from severe diseases for which they expect doctors to work miracles. As the medical procedures are more complex, the associated risks increase in a directly proportional manner [4].

A peculiar result of our study was the fact that emergency medicine was the second most claimed specialty in terms of the number of complaints, and the third most claimed specialty in terms of the number of doctors involved, which is in contradiction with other studies that found a small number of complaints against the medical personnel who work in emergency medicine units, patients and the general public taking into account that physicians in this specialty work in critical conditions [20]. However, a similar result was reported in the study conducted by Hwang et al. (2018) in Taiwan, where this specialty occupied the third place, with 8.5% of complaints, after obstetrics and orthopedics [18]. Furthermore, unlike various studies published in the literature in which there is an increased number of complaints against general practitioners [21–23], in our study family medicine (which in Romania is equivalent to general practice) was involved in only one complaint against doctors from several specialties.

Our finding that the ratio between the number of complaints in Emergency Medicine and that in family medicine was reversed compared to other studies finds its explanation in the fact that Romanian patients use emergency medicine unit services excessively, to the detriment of primary health care services [15,24]. Patients often shunt the family doctors, abusively calling emergency medical services, even in non-life-threatening situations. This overuse of emergency medicine to the detriment of family medicine (which is underused) is also demonstrated by the fact that many ambulance requests, especially during regular working hours, are resolved at the patients' homes, representing situations that could have been solved by the family doctor [15]. An essential reason for patients requesting excessive consultations from emergency services is the possibility to be seen by a doctor without a referral from the family medicine physician or in case they do not have health insurance. Although health insurance is mandatory for all Romanian citizens, European Commission reports show that in 2017, 11% of the population did not have it [25]. There are certain diseases (e.g., genetic diseases, diabetes, tuberculosis, myasthenia gravis, increased obstetrical risk in pregnant women, peptic ulcer, mental illnesses) [15,26] which can be assessed or followed up by a specialist physician directly in the outpatient department, without a referral from the family doctor [24], which could further explain the lower number of complaints to the latter, by the lower addressability. Moreover, the primary health care system in Romania is not accessible to everyone, about 2.5% of the population do not have access to a family doctor [27].

In our study, 9.2% of the patients complained about the doctors' inappropriate language, 9.2% complained about their inappropriate behavior, and 15.7% complained about the lack of information or the deficiency in offering information. These issues raise an alarm about how doctors approach and relate to their patients and the fact that deficiencies in the doctor–patient relationship can lead to a malpractice complaint.

Our study highlights that individuals from rural areas were more likely to report inappropriate behavior compared to those from urban areas. In rural areas, the relationship between the doctors and their patients is much closer [28,29]. This closer relationship might result in the patient preferring to wait a long time (sometimes even a few hours) to be examined by their own doctor when the latter is very busy, or even to postpone a consultation if their doctor is not available, instead of contacting another physician [28]. Interpersonal relationships are generally closer in rural areas, where communities are small, people communicate more with each other (for example, they usually all greet even if they do not know each other), they live in communion. The rural environment is characterized by greater social integration, with friendly and neighborly support and involvement by the community, compared to the urban environment [30]. The rural patient, accustomed to close interpersonal relationships in their area of residence, both with the community and with the physician, is disturbed when urban physicians, with less time allocated to patients, interact less with the patient, behave more distantly and sometimes arrogantly, as some patients in our study pointed out. These issues become more relevant when the outcome of the medical intervention is not in line with the patient's expectations.

Data from the literature show that in addition to the actual harm caused to the patient, as an independent reason, an important role in formulating the complaint has a series of triggers, especially related to the relationship between doctor and patient [31], to how the patient is approached by the doctor [5], and to the fact that the doctor often leaves the patient without explanations as to the reasons for the failure of the medical act [32]. At the same time, there are studies showing that despite the occurrence of harm to the patient, the proper way in which physicians have related to their patients contributed to the patients' decision to not complain about the medical act [33].

The ability of inter-human relationships, in the form of communication and the attitude of the doctor towards the patient [5], strongly influences the medical practice. Communication failure often predisposes the occurrence of adverse events [34]. Moreover, patients are more likely to complain about the doctor after the occurrence of an adverse event if the doctor–patient relationship is dysfunctional [3]. Thus, the study conducted by Veerman et al. (2019) showed that at least 10% of patients were disappointed in how their doctors behaved and communicated with them, in the sense that their problems were not given due consideration and that their doctors were too busy to discuss with them [5].

A study conducted in the United States of America that analyzed the malpractice complaints in general surgery showed that 34% of complaints were related to poor communication [35].

Doctor–patient communication triggers complaints of malpractice also from the perspective of obtaining the medical history. Failure to obtain an accurate medical history predisposes to misdiagnosis and treatment errors, which generates patient dissatisfaction and subsequent malpractice complaint [36]. On the other hand, a good communication may prevent the patient from making a malpractice complaint even if the result of the medical act is not as expected, because the level of communication between doctor and patient allows the latter to understand the situation and accept the result [37]. Regarding the starting point of conflicts, both family members and physicians recognize the implications of poor communication [38]. Doctors who disregard their patients' feelings and concerns, who provide little information, who do not have the patience to listen to or are not open with their patients are more likely to be reported, compared to their colleagues who communicate more efficiently with patients [3].

Our study showed that the lack or deficiency in communication was more likely to be reported by the family than by the patient, rather when the patient had died and when the patient was a newborn. These elements suggest the need of the family to be informed in difficult moments, such as the unexpected death of a family member or the health condition of their children. Moreover, when death occurs in a child, the need for the parents to receive information and explanations is even higher, given that usually a child is not supposed to die from natural causes [20]. Communicating bad news can be a difficult task for doctors, with a great emotional load on both sides. To provide it in an appropriate way, the doctors need specific training and protocols [39]. In general, the perinatal period is associated with a strong emotional load [19], and as the reality of a newborn's health problem adds significant a degree of vulnerability [40], it can strongly upset the new parents, some of them perhaps experiencing parenthood for the first time. Therefore, the need for realistic, accurate information about the medical situation becomes essential [38,40]. Moreover, it is necessary that the doctor–parent interaction be grounded on clear, prompt, and compassionate communication by doctors [38,40].

In our study, inadequate informed consent or lack thereof was reported in 6.5% of cases. This result is closely related to the results of other studies, such as one conducted in Australia, which showed that 5% of negligence claims and conciliated complaints were related to the process of obtaining the informed consent [32]. Obtaining the informed consent is an important part of the process of communicating with the patient. Agarwal et al. (2018) identified aspects related to professionalism and inadequate informed consent as factors favoring the initiation of malpractice complaints in cases involving spine surgery [41].

Our results showed a higher probability of complaining about the lack of consent in cases where patients were newborns. This result was related to another result of our study indicating that the lack or deficiency of communication was a more common reason for complaint by the patient's family (when the patient died, or the patient was a newborn or incompetent). Data from the literature indicate the need for a family-centered approach in the medical settings for the care of newborns, requiring the adequate approach of the parents [40,42,43]. In a family-centered approach, the parents and the doctor form a partnership in which the parents are offered the opportunity to actively participate in the care of their child [42,43]. Sarin and Maria (2019) reported that parents often show distress, frustration, and alienation when they are not involved in caring for their own child [42], thus creating the premises for complaints when the evolution of the case is not favorable.

Patients who complain about their doctors for the damage they suffered as a result of a misdiagnosis or treatment error [2] may want to obtain compensation, to find out what happened [3], to get an explanation, or they may want the doctor to admit their mistake [3,31] and express their regret [31]. Patients may also want to prevent the occurrence of similar incidents in the future or for justice to be done, i.e., those responsible for the mistake to be held accountable [3,44].

Our results showed that in 59 (38.5%) cases the reason for complaints was the occurrence of a complication of the medical act, the complaints being directed towards 75 (36.58%) physicians. The most frequently claimed specialties for this reason were obstetrics and gynecology (15 complaints, 19 doctors), general surgery (6 complaints, 10 doctors) and orthopedics and traumatology (7 complaints, 9 doctors), all of them major surgical specialties, which, by their nature, involve an intrinsic risk of the occurrence of additional harm during surgical interventions which are often complex [4]. Some of the complications are related to the complexity of the disease, but others are related to errors that could have been prevented [45]. Our results show that women were more likely to claim complications than men and for the complaint to be made by the patients rather than their relatives, probably because the patient is the one who endures the physical suffering associated with the occurrence of a complication and the subsequent necessary treatments. The complaint for the occurrence of a complication of the medical act was associated with a greater number of hospitalization days and with multiple hospitalizations because the occurrence of a complication requires additional medical or surgical treatment.

The diagnostic error was a reason for complaint identified in 19 (12.4%) cases, involving a number of 28 (13.65%) individual physicians, the three most involved specializations for this reason being pediatrics (4 complaints, 6 doctors), obstetrics and gynecology (2 complaints, 3 doctors), and orthopedics and traumatology (2 complaints, 5 doctors). This was a more likely reason for complaint for patients with multiple hospitalizations. The lack of diagnosis was a reason for complaint in 8 (5.22%) cases, involving 11 (5.36%) doctors, the most involved specialty for this reason being general surgery (2 complaints, 4 physicians). Although the literature data most often refer to diagnosis errors in general (lack of diagnosis, misdiagnosis, and delay in diagnosis), the results of our study showed a lower percentage compared to those reported in other studies. For example, 32.1% complaints related to diagnosis were reported by Gupta et al. (2018), 38.8% of them concerning hospitalized patients [46]. Gupta et al. (2018) observed a decrease in this percentage during the 13 years of the study period (January 1, 1999-December 31, 2011), an aspect that can be explained by the increasing accessibility of the diagnosis techniques, especially in the medical imaging field [46]. The diagnostic errors in outpatients were estimated at 5.1% of the cases [46]. Schaffer et al. (2017) showed that diagnostic errors were the most reported reason in cases of paid claims, being found in 31.8% of these cases [47]. Diagnostic errors were the most common cause of complaint in the study performed by Saber Tehrani et al. (2013), which showed that diagnostic errors were accompanied by the highest costs and the highest degree of danger for patients [48].

Misdiagnosis is often associated with mistreatment and may require multiple re-admissions in the hospital, increasing morbidity and the associated costs [46]. Agarwal et al. (2018) found 31.6% claims for delayed diagnosis and 32.7% claims for failure to provide appropriate treatment, which may underline that acute patients need prompt and appropriate care [41].

In our study the lack of diagnosis was reported by men rather than women, a similar result being obtained by Gupta et al. (2018) [46]. According to the empathizing-systemizing theory, proposed by Baron-Cohen and cited by Zaidi (2010), men tend to systematize, seek solutions, understand, and build different systems, going to the root of the problems, so that everything becomes clear to them. Therefore, male patients are dissatisfied by the lack of a clear explanation for their health problems and start their own search for solutions or answers [49].

The consequences of diagnosis errors have been analyzed by several studies. For example, Zwaan et al. (2010) identified a 6.5% death rate in a hospital due to adverse events [50]. Gupta et al. (2018) showed that diagnosis errors result in 47.4% of deaths and 33.9% of disabilities [46]. In our study, diagnosis errors were not significantly associated with the patient's death, this being reported only in 10.6% ($n = 7$) of the deceased patients. A reason for complaint strongly associated with the patient's death in our study was the delay of the medical act. The most involved specialties for claiming delay in the medical act were general surgery (4 complaints, 5 physicians) and emergency medicine (4 complaints, 4 physicians). Delay as a reason for medical malpractice claim in emergency medicine is again associated with the overutilization of the emergency services where the waiting time to receive medical care is inversely proportional to the severity of the emergency.

In cases when the patient is deceased or incompetent (i.e., by age, by physical or psychical disability), the complaint is submitted by a family member. In our study, this occurred in more than half of the cases (i.e., 58.8%). This aspect has multiple facets. Except for the already mentioned reason regarding the stress and emotions surrounding the perinatal period, the parents of an injured child might be preoccupied by the future of their offspring in case of disability [19]. Likewise, the death of a loved one may cause a great deal of distress, with material or moral prejudice, the family thus being entitled to ask for explanation and compensation in case of the physician's malpractice leading to the misfortunate event [1]

Strengths and Limitations

This study has several strengths and limitations. Regarding the strengths, this study is the first of its kind to be conducted in Romania and covered a significant geographic part of the country, Moldova being one of the largest Romanian regions. Therefore, the results offer an image of the situation for about 20% of the country's entire population and can represent the starting point for studies in the other regions, to have a national perspective on this subject. Second, the research analyzed complaints registered for 14 years, offering an objective data analysis. Third, the results are discussed and explained in opposition with other medical systems showing the most vulnerable medical specialties in Romania compared to other countries.

The limitation of the study stems from the fact that some of the cases had missing data regarding the socio-demographic characteristics of the plaintiffs and some of the claims did not contain precise information on the number of doctors involved. This limitation was the result of the fact that the patients gave a personal account of the events, instead of having access to a default form with specific items for each category of information.

5. Conclusions

Complaints of medical malpractice continue to follow an ascending trend worldwide, and their consequences are multifaceted, affecting both the medical staff and patients and society in general. Therefore, it becomes significantly necessary to identify solutions meant to reduce the number of complaints, a goal that could be met by conducting studies aimed at formulating recommendations in this regard.

The results of our study showed that the most frequently involved specialties were obstetrics and gynecology, emergency medicine, general surgery, and orthopedics and traumatology. Particularly in this list was the presence of the emergency medicine, a result explained by the overuse of these services in our country and the underutilization of primary health care services. Therefore, health policies are needed to divert the large number of patients accessing emergency medicine to primary care.

Many of the aspects the plaintiffs complained about were represented by deficiencies in the interaction between doctor and patient or his/her family (lack of or deficiency in information, the doctor's inappropriate behavior or language, failure to obtain informed consent). Based on this finding, we consider that doctors need special training during their undergraduate medical studies, as well as periodic updating during their career to meet the challenges of communication and relationships with patients and their families.

Author Contributions: All authors had equal contributions. Conceptualization, B.H. and B.G.I.; methodology, B.H., B.G.I., and M.I.; software, I.-D.M. and B.H.; validation, B.H., B.G.I., and M.I.; formal analysis, I.-D.M. and

B.H.; investigation, B.H. and B.G.I.; resources, B.H., B.G.I., M.I., and I.-D.M.; data curation, B.H. and B.G.I.; writing—original draft preparation, B.H.; writing—review and editing, B.H., B.G.I., M.I., and I.-D.M.; supervision, B.G.I. and M.I.; project administration, B.G.I. All authors have read and agreed to the published version of the manuscript.

Funding: This research received no external funding.

Conflicts of Interest: The authors declare no conflict of interest.

References

1. Ioan, B.G.; Nanu, A.C.; Rotariu, I. *Răspunderea Profesională în Practica Medicală*; Junimea: Iasi, Romania, 2017. (In Romanian)
2. Dolz-Guerri, F.; Gomez-Duran, E.L.; Martinez-Palmer, A.; Castilla Cespedes, M.; Arimany-Manso, J. Clinical safety and professional liability claims in Ophthalmology. *Arch. Soc. Esp. Oftalmol.* **2017**, *92*, 528–534. [CrossRef] [PubMed]
3. Chiu, Y.C. What drives patients to sue doctors? The role of cultural factors in the pursuit of malpractice claims in Taiwan. *Soc. Sci. Med.* **2010**, *71*, 702–707. [CrossRef]
4. Li, H.; Wu, X.; Sun, T.; Li, L.; Zhao, X.; Liu, X.; Gao, L.; Sun, Q.; Zhang, Z.; Fan, L. Claims, liabilities, injuries and compensation payments of medical malpractice litigation cases in China from 1998 to 2011. *BMC Health Serv. Res.* **2014**, *14*, 390. [CrossRef]
5. Veerman, M.M.; van der Woude, L.A.; Tellier, M.A.; Legemaate, J.; Scheltinga, M.R.; Stassen, L.P.S.; Leclercq, W.K.G. A decade of litigation regarding surgical informed consent in the Netherlands. *Patient Educ. Couns.* **2019**, *102*, 340–345. [CrossRef] [PubMed]
6. Bourne, T.; Vanderhaegen, J.; Vranken, R.; Wynants, L.; De Cock, B.; Peters, M.; Timmerman, D.; Van Calster, B.; Jalmbrant, M.; Van Audenhove, C. Doctors' experiences and their perception of the most stressful aspects of complaints processes in the UK: An analysis of qualitative survey data. *BMJ Open* **2016**, *6*, e011711. [CrossRef] [PubMed]
7. Jena, A.B.; Seabury, S.; Lakdawalla, D.; Chandra, A. Malpractice risk according to physician specialty. *N. Engl. J. Med.* **2011**, *365*, 629–636. [CrossRef]
8. Gao, P.; Li, X.; Zhao, Z.; Zhang, N.; Ma, K.; Li, L. Diagnostic errors in fatal medical malpractice cases in Shanghai, China: 1990–2015. *Diagn. Pathol.* **2019**, *14*, 8. [CrossRef]
9. Dumitrescu, R.M. Litigious side of the medical malpractice in Romania. *Mod. Med.* **2019**, *26*, 197–211. [CrossRef]
10. Essinger, K. Medical liability alternative ways to court procedures. In Proceedings of the European Conference "The Ever-Growing Challenge of Medical Liability: National and European Responses", Strasbourg, France, 2–3 June 2008.
11. Watson, K.; Koltenhagen, R. Patients' right, medical error and harmonization of compensation mechanisms in Europe. *Eur. J. Health Law* **2018**, *25*, 1–23. [CrossRef]
12. Lee, D.W.H.; Lai, P.B.S. The practice of mediation to resolve clinical, bioethical, and medical malpractice disputes. *HongKong Med. J.* **2015**, *21*, 560–564. [CrossRef]
13. Legea nr. 95/2006 privind reforma în domeniul sănătății, publicată în Monitorul Oficial al României, Partea I, nr. 372 din 28 aprilie 2006, In Romanian. [Law no 95/2006 on healthcare reform, published in the Official Gazette of Romania, Part One, No 372/April, 28th, 2006].
14. Charles, S.C.; Gibbons, R.D.; Frisch, P.R.; Pyskoty, C.E.; Hedeker, D.; Singha, N.K. Predicting risk for medical malpractice claims using quality-of-care characteristics. *West. J. Med.* **1992**, *157*, 433–439. [PubMed]
15. Vlădescu, C.; Scîntee, S.G.; Olsavszky, V.; Hernández-Quevedo, C.; Sagan, A. Romania: Health system review. *Health Syst. Transit.* **2016**, *18*, 1–170. [PubMed]
16. Ferrara, S.D.; Baccino, E.; Bajanowski, T.; Boscolo-Berto, R.; Castellano, M.; De Angel, R.; Pauliukevičius, A.; Ricci, P.; Vanezis, P.; Vieira, D.N.; et al. Malpractice and medical liability. European Guidelines on Methods of ascertainment and criteria of evaluation. *Int. J. Legal. Med.* **2013**, *127*, 545–557. [CrossRef] [PubMed]
17. Bark, P.; Vincent, C.; Olivieri, L.; Jones, A. Impact of litigation on senior clinicians: Implications for risk management. *Qual. Health Care* **1997**, *6*, 7–13. [CrossRef] [PubMed]
18. Hwang, C.Y.; Wu, C.H.; Cheng, F.C.; Yen, Y.L.; Wu, K.H. A 12 year analysis of closed medical malpractice claims of the Taiwan civil court. *Medicine* **2018**, *97*, 237. [CrossRef]

19. Domino, J.; McGovern, C.; Chang, K.W.C.; Carlozzi, N.E.; Yang, L. Lack of physician-patient communication as a key factor associated with malpractice litigation in neonatal brachial plexus palsy. *J. Neurosurg. Pediatrics* **2014**, *13*, 238–242. [CrossRef]
20. Casali, M.B.; Mobilia, F.; Del Sordo, S.; Blandino, A.; Genoveze, U. The medical malpractice in Milan-Italy. A retrospective survey on 14 years of judicial autopsies. *Forensic. Sci. Int.* **2014**, *242*, 38–43. [CrossRef]
21. Studdert, D.M.; Bismark, M.M.; Mello, M.M.; Singh, H.; Spittal, M.J. Prevalence and characteristics of physicians prone to malpractice claims. *N. Engl. J. Med.* **2016**, *374*, 354–362. [CrossRef]
22. Cunningham, W.; Crump, R.; Tomlin, A. The characteristics of doctors receiving medical complaints: A cross-sectional survey of doctors in New Zealand. *N. Z. Med. J.* **2003**, *116*, U625.
23. Wallace, E.; Lowry, J.; Smith, S.M.; Fahey, T. The epidemiology of malpractice claims in primary care: A systematic review. *BMJ Open* **2013**, *3*, e002929. [CrossRef]
24. OECD/European Observatory on Health Systems and Policies. *State of Health in the EU. Romania: Profilul Sănătății în 2017*; OECD Publishing: Paris, France; European Observatory on Health Systems and Policies: Brussels, Belgium, 2017. [CrossRef]
25. OECD/European Union. *Health at a Glance: Europe 2018: State of Health in the EU Cycle*; OECD Publishing: Paris, France, 2018. [CrossRef]
26. Casa Nationala de Asigurari de Sanatate (CNAS). LISTA Cuprinzând Afecțiunile Care Permit Prezentarea Direct la Medicul de Specialitate din Ambulatoriul de Specialitate. (In Romanian). Available online: http://www.cnas.ro/casmb/media/pageFiles/AFECTIUNI%20CU%20PREZENTARE%20DIRECTA%20IN%20AMBULATORIU%20CLINIC%2001.04.2018_%20ANEXA_13%20.pdf (accessed on 4 April 2020).
27. Federația Națională a Patronatelor Medicilor de Familie (FNPMF). *Harta Accesului Cetățenilor Români la Serviciile de Asistență Medicală Primară Oferite de Cabinetele de Medicina Familiei*; Federația Națională a Patronatelor Medicilor de Familie (FNPMF): Bucuresti, Romania, 2020. (In Romanian)
28. Pohontsch, N.J.; Hensen, H.; Schafer, I.; Schere, M. General practitioners' perception of being a doctor in urban vs. rural regions in Germany- a focus group study. *Fam. Pract.* **2018**, *35*, 209–215. [CrossRef]
29. Nielsen, M.; D'Agostino, D.; Gregory, P. Addressing rural health challenges head on. *Mo. Med.* **2017**, *114*, 363–366.
30. Burholt, V.; Naylor, D. The relationship between rural community type and attachment to place for older people living in North Wales, UK. *Eur. J. Ageing* **2005**, *2*, 109–119. [CrossRef]
31. Fountain, T.R. Ophthalmic malpractice and physician gender: A claims data analysis (an American ophthalmological society thesis). *Trans. Am. Ophtalmol. Soc.* **2014**, *112*, 38–49.
32. Posner, K.L.; Severson, J.; Domino, K.B. The role of informed consent in patient complaints: Reducing hidden health system costs and improving patient engagement through shared decision making. *J. Healthc. Risk. Manag.* **2015**, *35*, 38–45. [CrossRef]
33. Fishbain, D.A.; Bruns, D.; Disorbio, J.M.; Lewis, J.E. What are the variables that are associated with the patient's wish to sue his physician in patients with acute and chronic pain? *Pain Med.* **2008**, *9*, 1130–1142. [CrossRef] [PubMed]
34. Boyll, P.; Kang, P.; Mahabir, R.; Bernard, R.W. Variables that impact medical malpractice claims involving plastic surgeons in the United States. *Aesthet Surg J.* **2018**, *38*, 785–792. [CrossRef] [PubMed]
35. Griffen, F.D.; Stephens, L.S.; Alexander, J.B.; Bailey, R.; Maizel, S.E.; Sutton, B.H.; Posner, K.L. Violations of behavioral practices revealed in closed claims reviews. *Ann. Surg.* **2008**, *248*, 118–124. [CrossRef] [PubMed]
36. Hanganu, B.; Manoilescu, I.S.; Velnic, A.A.; Ioan, B.G. Physician-patient communication in chronic diseases. *Med. Surg. J.* **2018**, *122*, 417–422.
37. Hanganu, B.; Ioan, B.G. Malpraxisul medical: Cauze și consecințe asupra personalului medical. In *Psihologie Medicala. Studii Clinice*; Iorga, M., Roșca, C., Eds.; Editura Universitară: București, Romania, 2019; pp. 183–188. (In Romanian)
38. Boss, R.D.; Urban, A.; Barnett, M.D.; Arnold, R.M. Neonatal critical care communication (NC3): Training NICU physicians and nurse practitioners. *J. Perinatol.* **2013**, *33*, 642–646. [CrossRef]
39. Monden, K.R.; Gentry, L.; Cox, T.R. Delivering bad news to patients. *Proc. (Bayl. Univ. Med. Cent.)* **2016**, *29*, 101–102. [CrossRef] [PubMed]
40. Wigert, H.; Blom, M.D.; Bry, K. Parents' experiences of communication with neonatal intensive-care unit staff: An interview with neonatal intensive-care unit staff: An interview study. *BMC Pediatr.* **2014**, *14*, 304. [CrossRef] [PubMed]

41. Agarwal, N.; Gupta, R.; Agarwal, P.; Matthew, P.; Wolfrez, R., Jr.; Shah, A.; Adeeb, N.; Prabhu, A.V.; Kanter, A.; Okonkwo, D.; et al. Descriptive analysis of state and federal spine surgery malpractice litigation in the United States. *Spine* **2018**, *43*, 984–990. [CrossRef]
42. Sarin, E.; Maria, A. Acceptability of family-centered newborn care model among providers and receivers of care in a Public Health Setting: A qualitative study from India. *BMC Health Serv. Res.* **2019**, *19*, 184. [CrossRef]
43. Lv, B.; Gao, X.; Sun, J.; Li, T.; Liu, Z.; Zhu, L.; Latour, J.M. Family-centered care improves clinical outcomes of very-low-birth-weight infants: A quasi-experimental study. *Front. Pediatr.* **2019**, *7*, 138. [CrossRef] [PubMed]
44. Renkema, E.; Broekhuis, M.; Ahaus, K. Conditions that influence the impact of malpractice litigation risk on physicians' behavior regarding patient safety. *BMC Health Serv. Res.* **2014**, *14*, 38. [CrossRef]
45. Taghizadeh, Y.; Pourbakhtiar, M.; Ayimi, K.; Ghadipasha, M.; Soltani, K. Claims about medical malpractices resulting in neonatal and maternal impairment in Iran. *J. Forensic. Leg. Med.* **2019**, *66*, 44–49. [CrossRef]
46. Gupta, A.; Snyder, A.; Kachalia, A.; Flanders, S.; Saint, S.; Chopra, V. Malpractice claims related to diagnostic errors in the hospital. *BMJ Qual. Saf.* **2017**, *27*, 53–60. [CrossRef]
47. Schaffer, A.C.; Jena, A.B.; Seabury, S.A.; Singh, H.; Chalasani, V.; Kachalia, A. Rates and characteristics of paid malpractice claims among US physicians by specialty, 1992–2004. *JAMA Int. Med.* **2017**, *177*, 710–718. [CrossRef]
48. Saber Tehrani, A.S.; Lee, H.; Mathews, S.C.; Shore, A.; Makary, M.A.; Pronovost, P.J.; Newman-Toker, D.E. 25-Year summary of US malpractice claims for diagnostic errors 1986–2010: An analysis from the National Practitioner Data Bank. *BMJ Qual. Saf.* **2013**, *22*, 672–680. [CrossRef]
49. Zaidi, Z. Gender differences in human brain: A review. *Open Anat. J.* **2010**, *2*, 37–55. [CrossRef]
50. Zwaan, L.; de Bruijne, M.; Wagner, C.; Thijs, A.; Smits, M.; van der Wal, G.; Timmermans, D.R.M. Patient record review of the incidence, consequences, and causes of diagnostic adverse events. *Arch. Intern. Med.* **2010**, *170*, 1015–1021. [CrossRef] [PubMed]

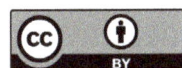

© 2020 by the authors. Licensee MDPI, Basel, Switzerland. This article is an open access article distributed under the terms and conditions of the Creative Commons Attribution (CC BY) license (http://creativecommons.org/licenses/by/4.0/).

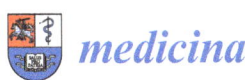

Article

Inherited Risk Factors of Thromboembolic Events in Patients with Primary Nephrotic Syndrome

Gener Ismail [1,2], Bogdan Obrișcă [1,2,*], Roxana Jurubiță [1,2], Andreea Andronesi [1,2], Bogdan Sorohan [1,2] and Mihai Hârza [2,3]

[1] Department of Nephrology, Fundeni Clinical Institute, Bucharest 022328, Romania; gener732000@yahoo.com (G.I.); roxana_jurubita@yahoo.com (R.J.); andreea.andronesi@yahoo.com (A.A.); bogdan.sorohan@yahoo.com (B.S.)
[2] Department of Uronephrology, "Carol Davila" University of Medicine and Pharmacy, Bucharest 020021, Romania; mihai.harza@gmail.com
[3] Center of Uronephrology and Renal Transplantation, Fundeni Clinical Institute, Bucharest 022328, Romania
* Correspondence: obriscabogdan@yahoo.com; Tel.: +40-721-256-797

Received: 23 April 2020; Accepted: 16 May 2020; Published: 19 May 2020

Abstract: *Background and objectives.* Venous thromboembolic events (VTEs) are among the most important complications of nephrotic syndrome (NS). We conducted a study that aimed to determine the prevalence of inherited risk factors for VTE in NS and to identify which factors are independent predictors of VTE. *Materials and Methods.* Thirty-six consecutive patients with primary NS that underwent percutaneous kidney biopsy between January 2017 and December 2017 were enrolled in this retrospective, observational study. VTEs were the primary outcome. Baseline demographic and biochemical data were collected from medical records, and genetic testing was done for polymorphisms of Factor V, PAI, MTHFR, and prothrombin genes. *Results.* The incidence of VTE was 28%, and the median time to event was 3 months (IQR: 2–9). The prevalence of inherited risk factors was 14% for Factor V Leiden mutation, 5.6% for prothrombin G20210A, 44.5% for PAI, and 27.8% for each of the two polymorphisms of the MTHFR gene. On multivariate analysis, the presence of at least two mutations was independently associated with the risk of VTE (HR, 8.92; 95% confidence interval, CI: 1.001 to 79.58, $p = 0,05$). *Conclusions.* These findings suggest that genetic testing for inherited thrombophilia in NS could play an important role in detecting high-risk patients that warrant prophylactic anticoagulation.

Keywords: nephrotic syndrome; thrombosis; inherited risk factors; mutation; anticoagulation

1. Introduction

Venous thromboembolic events (VTEs) are serious complications of nephrotic syndrome (NS), associated with significant morbidity and mortality [1]. The reported incidence varies widely (5–50%), due primarily to the retrospective nature of most studies and the lack of an accurate screening method that eludes an important number of asymptomatic cases [1–4]. Current clinical guidelines have inadequate evidence to support prophylactic anticoagulation, taking into account only serum albumin level and proteinuria over 24 h as markers of VTE risk [5].

VTEs must be viewed as a multifactorial disorder with the underlying pathogenesis being a complex interplay of inherited and acquired risk factors [6]. Hemostasis imbalance secondary to the NS [7], chronic inflammation associated with certain glomerulonephritis [1], a genetic background [1,6], when associated, can trigger a VTE. Usually, an inherited thrombophilia does not result in a spontaneous VTE, until an acquired hypercoagulable state (nephrotic syndrome) determines the clinical expression of the prothrombotic tendency [6]. With past clinical trials focusing mainly on serum albumin or proteinuria to define the VTE risk [3,8–10], the magnitude of additional risk factors has been evaluated only in small series, with conflicting results [2,11–14]. Additionally, polymorphisms associated with inherited thrombophilia seem to be relatively prevalent in the general population, and screening for these disorders remains debatable [2,6,15–17].

We conducted a retrospective, observational study that sought to identify the prevalence of inherited risk factors for VTEs in a population of NS patients and to define the risk of VTEs in such patients.

2. Materials and Methods

2.1. Study Patients' Characteristics

All consecutive patients with primary NS admitted to our department between January 2017 and December 2017 were considered for inclusion, and only those with a histopathological diagnosis were further included in the study. NS was defined as a level of proteinuria over 3.5 g/day and hypoalbuminemia. Exclusion criteria were age under 18 years, presence of known secondary causes of NS (diabetes, hepatitis B or C virus infection, HIV infection, systemic lupus erythematosus), a previous VTE, disorders that interfere with the synthesis of hemostasis-related factors (severe hepatic impairment) and therapy that influences hemostasis (antiplatelet drugs, anticoagulants).

Baseline demographics and biochemical data collected included age at presentation, gender, proteinuria over 24 h, serum albumin, and creatinine level. Glomerular filtration rate (GFR) was estimated using the Chronic Kidney Disease Epidemiology Collaboration (CKD-EPI) equation. The genetic testing panel included the assessment for polymorphisms of Factor V gene (G1691A, T1250C, Cambridge and Hong-Kong mutations), PAI gene (plasminogen activator inhibitor—4G/5G mutation), methylene tetrahydrofolate reductase (MTHFR) gene (C677T and A1298C mutations) and prothrombin gene (G20210A mutation). Genetic testing was performed using a real-time polymerase chain reaction method (RT-PCR).

The study was conducted in accordance with the Declaration of Helsinki, and the protocol was approved by the Ethics Committee of Fundeni Clinical Institute (No. 20638/30 March 2020).

2.2. Diagnosis of Venous Thromboembolic Events

VTEs were suspected on clinical grounds (unilateral limb pain or edema, cough, dyspnea, hemoptysis, loin pain, hematuria) and, additionally, were screened by D-dimers level to identify asymptomatic events. The D-dimers level was determined every 3 months and considered elevated if the level was over 2 mcg/mL. VTEs were confirmed by imaging studies: deep vein thrombosis (DVT) by Doppler ultrasound, renal vein thrombosis (RVT) by Doppler ultrasound followed by contrast spiral computed tomography (CT), pulmonary embolism (PE) by spiral CT. The ultrasonographic criteria for diagnosis of venous thrombosis (deep vein, renal vein) were direct visualization of thrombi and absent venous flow. Additionally, in the case of RVT, a confirmatory CT scan was undertaken to document filling defects during the venous phase following intravenous contrast.

2.3. Statistical Analysis

Data distribution was evaluated with the Jurque–Bera test. Normally distributed variables were expressed as means and standard deviations, while the non-normally distributed variables were expressed as a medians and interquartile ranges (IQRs). Categorical variables were expressed as numbers and frequencies. For continuous data, differences between groups were assessed using the Student t-test and univariate ANOVA, depending on the level of the independent variable. For categorical data, differences between groups were evaluated using the χ^2 test. To determine the relationship between the studied parameters and the primary endpoint (occurrence of VTE), univariate and multivariate Cox proportional hazard regression was performed. All p values were two-tailed, and all p values less than 0.05 were considered statistically significant. The time to event was measured from the baseline to the moment of documented VTE. The probability of event-free survival was assessed using a Kaplan–Meyer curve. The statistical analysis was performed using SPSS 17.0 (SPSS Inc., Chicago, IL, USA).

3. Results

3.1. Patient Characteristics

The study cohort included 36 patients with the baseline characteristics shown in Table 1. Four patients were excluded from the study due to the absence of histopathological diagnosis or identification of a secondary cause for the nephrotic syndrome (amyloidosis). Membranous nephropathy (MN) was the most common type of glomerulopathy found on kidney biopsy (38.9%), followed by IgA nephropathy (IgAN) (27.8%), minimal-change disease (MCD) (19.4%) and focal and segmental glomerulosclerosis (FSGS) (13.9%).

Table 1. Characteristics of the Study Population.

Variable	Overall	MN	MCD	FSGS	IgAN	*p*-Value
Number of patients	36	14	7	5	10	
Number of VTEs	10	5	2	1	2	0.827
Age (y)	43.4 ± 14.2	47.7 ± 14	40.5 ± 19.8	44.4 ± 12.4	39.2 ± 11	0.52
Serum albumin (g/dL)	2.58 ± 0.62	2.75 ± 0.52	2.2 ± 0.64	2.52 ± 1	2.66 ± 0.48	0.28
Proteinuria (g/day)	7.29 ± 2.4	6.2 ± 1.42	10.1 ± 0.7	7 ± 2.1	7 ± 3	0.002
Serum creatinine (mg/dL)	1.5 ± 0.9	1.37 ± 0.9	1.71 ± 1.2	1.07 ± 0.25	1.75 ± 0.88	0.48
Estimated GFR (mL/min/1.73 m^2)	66.2 ± 32.7	75.2 ± 38.1	63.4 ± 30.1	70.8 ± 20.6	53.3 ± 30.5	0.44

Abbreviations: VTE, venous thromboembolic events; GFR, glomerular filtration rate. For continuous data, differences between groups were assessed using univariate ANOVA, and for categorical data, differences between groups were evaluated using the χ^2 test.

The baseline 24-h proteinuria and serum albumin were 7.29 ± 2.4 g/day and 2.58 ± 0.62 g/dL, respectively. Additionally, 11 patients (30.5%) were over 50 years old, while three of them were over 65 years old. The average 24-h proteinuria differed across the four types of glomerulopathies ($p = 0.002$). Patients with minimal-change disease (MCD) had higher proteinuria levels than those with membranous nephropathy ($p < 0.001$) and IgA nephropathy ($p = 0.02$), respectively. Additionally, all patients with MCD had severe nephrotic syndrome with proteinuria levels over 8 g/day. The mean baseline estimated glomerular filtration rate (eGFR) was 66.2 ± 32.7 mL/min/1.73 m^2, and although MCD and IgA nephropathy patients seemed to have lower eGFR, it did not reach statistical significance ($p = 0.44$). The median follow-up time was 24 months (IQR 9–36). In terms of risk factors for VTE, five patients (13.9%) were obese, four patients (11.1%) were current or previous smokers, one patient had a previous history of VTE, and one patient had a diagnosis of antiphospholipid syndrome. Moreover, two patients had a history of other autoimmune disorders (ulcerative colitis and ankylosing spondylitis). There was no family history of VTE in the study cohort.

The prevalence of the inherited risk factors for VTE is depicted in Figure 1. Almost 3% of the patients were homozygous and 11% heterozygous for the Factor V mutation G1691A, while none had the Cambridge, Hong-Kong, or T1250C mutations. The prothrombin G20210A mutation was encountered in 5.6% of the patients. The two polymorphisms of the methylene tetrahydrofolate reductase gene and the mutation of the PAI gene were highly prevalent in the study cohort (28% and 45%, respectively). Additionally, 12 patients (33%) had at least two of the studied mutations (Table 2).

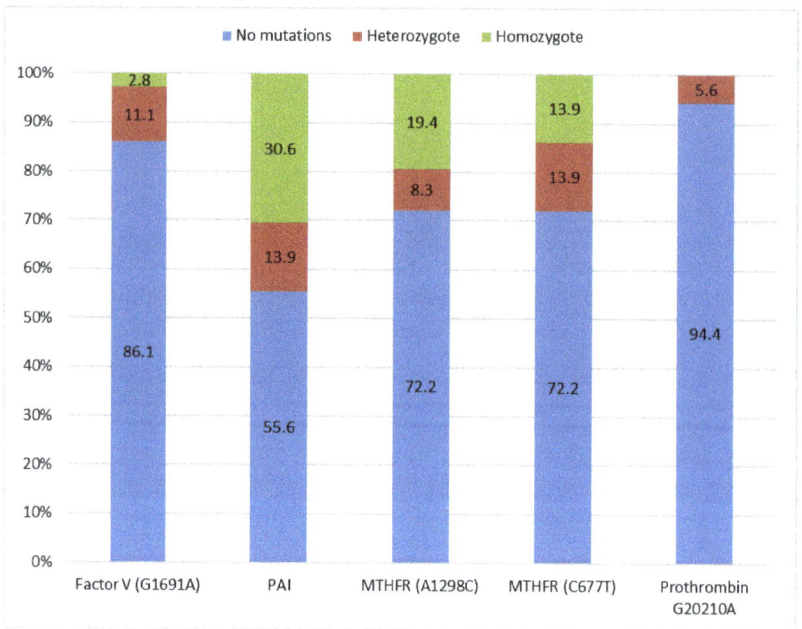

Figure 1. Prevalence of the inherited risk factors for VTEs in the study cohort.

Table 2. Type of mutations in patients with at least two associated mutations.

Patient	Factor V (G1691A)	PAI 4G/5G	MTHFR (A1298C)	MTHFR (C667T)	Prothrombin G20210A
1	Homozygote	-	-	-	Heterozygote
2	Heterozygote	Heterozygote	-	Homozygote	-
3	Heterozygote	Homozygote	Homozygote	-	-
4	-	Homozygote	Homozygote	-	-
5	Heterozygote	Homozygote	-	-	-
6	-	Homozygote	Heterozygote	Heterozygote	-
7	-	Homozygote	Homozygote	Homozygote	-
8	-	Heterozygote	-	Homozygote	-
9	-	Homozygote	Homozygote	Homozygote	-
10	-	Heterozygote	Homozygote	-	-
11	-	Homozygote	Homozygote	-	-
12	Heterozygote	Homozygote	-	-	-

Abbreviations: MTHFR, methylene tetrahydrofolate reductase; PAI, plasminogen activator inhibitor.

3.2. Venous Thromboembolic Events: Frequency

Ten VTEs were diagnosed in the study population (28%). The median time to VTE was 3 months (IQR 2–9), with 80% and 100% of VTE occurring during the first 6 months and the first year of follow-up, respectively. The vast majority of the thrombotic events were unilateral RVT (70%), followed by bilateral RVT, DVT, and PE, each being diagnosed in one patient. The majority of VTEs were asymptomatic, except in the cases of PE, DVT, and bilateral RVT. The asymptomatic events (unilateral RVT) were diagnosed by a confirmatory imaging method following the suspicion triggered by an increase in D-dimers level. There were no significant differences in terms of VTE frequency across the different types of glomerulopathies ($p = 0.827$).

3.3. Venous Thromboembolic Events: Risk Factors

The results of the univariate analysis in order to identify clinical and biochemical risk factors for the development of VTE are shown in Table 3. Patients that developed a VTE had higher levels of proteinuria ($p = 0.045$) and lower serum albumin ($p = 0.002$) than those event-free. Additionally, patients that developed a VTE had more frequent polymorphisms of the Factor V gene (G1691A), MTHFR gene (C677T), or the 4G/5G mutation of PAI gene than those event-free. Moreover, the association of at least two of the abovementioned mutations was encountered more frequently in those that developed a VTE. The percentage of patients with obesity ($p > 0.99$), that were older than 50 years of age ($p = 0.45$) or that were current or previous smokers ($p > 0.99$) did not differ between those that developed a VTE or not. Additionally, the patients with a previous history of VTE developed a pulmonary embolism, while the patients with a previous diagnosis of antiphospholipid syndrome developed an asymptomatic unilateral renal vein thrombosis. On multivariate Cox proportional hazard regression, only the association of at least two mutations was independently associated with the risk of VTE (HR, 8.92; 95% confidence interval, CI: 1.001 to 79.58, $p = 0.05$) (Table 4), these patients having a significantly lower probability of remaining VTE-free than those with no associated mutations ($p < 0.001$) (Figure 2).

Table 3. Patients characteristics at baseline.

Parameter	With VTE	Without VTE	p-Value
Age (years)	41.9 ± 18	44 ± 12.8	0.742
Proteinuria (g/day)	8.62 ± 2.27	6.78 ± 2.29	0.045
Serum Albumin (g/dL)	2 ± 0.6	2.8 ± 0.48	0.002
Serum creatinine (mg/dL)	1.56 ± 0.9	1.48 ± 0.92	0.808
eGFR (mL/min)	66.5 ± 37.61	66.1 ± 3.44	0.978
MTHFR (A1298C) (%)	50%	19.2%	0.1
MTHFR (C677T) (%)	60%	15.4%	0.01
Factor V (G1691A) (%)	60%	3.8%	0.015
Prothrombin G20210A (%)	10%	3.8%	0.48
PAI 4G/5G mutation (%)	80%	30.8%	0.011
Association of two mutations (%)	80%	15.4%	0.001

Abbreviations: eGFR, estimated glomerular filtration rate; MTHFR, methylene tetrahydrofolate reductase; PAI, plasminogen activator inhibitor. For continuous data, differences between groups were assessed using the Student t-test, and for categorical data, differences between groups were evaluated using the χ^2 test.

Table 4. Risk factors for venous thromboembolic events in patients with primary nephrotic syndrome (Cox proportional hazards model).

Variable	Univariate Analysis		Multivariate Analysis	
	Hazard Ratio (95% CI)	p-Value	Hazard Ratio (95% CI)	p-Value
Serum Albumin (for each 1 g/dL)	0.25 (0.11–0.58)	0.001	0.43 (0.1–1.89)	0.27
24-h proteinuria (for each 1 g/day)	1.33 (1.009–1.75)	0.04	1.14 (0.79–1.64)	0.46
MTHFR (A1298C) (presence vs. absence)	2.91 (0.84–10.11)	0.09	0.49 (0.07–3.11)	0.45
MTHFR (C677T) (presence vs. absence)	4.51 (1.27–16.02)	0.02	1.38 (0.23–8.36)	0.72
Factor V (G1691A) (presence vs. absence)	6.4 (1.77–23.08)	0.005	0.92 (0.12–6.83)	0.94
Prothrombin G20210A (presence vs. absence)	2.68 (0.33–21.38)	0.35	3.23 (0.26–39.9)	0.36
Association of two mutations (presence vs. absence)	10.51 (2.21–49.92)	0.003	8.92 (1.001–79.58)	0.05

Abbreviations: MTHFR, methylene tetrahydrofolate reductase.

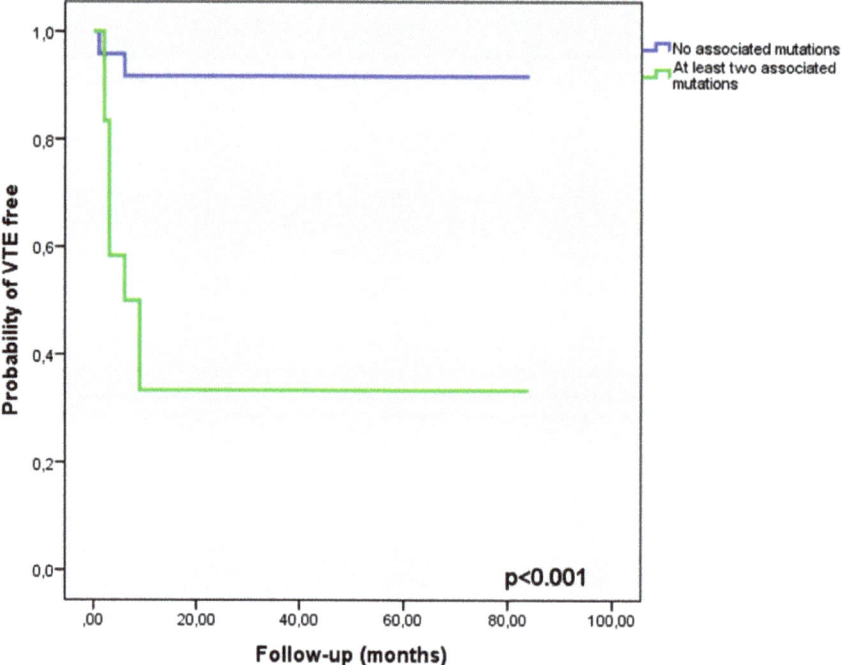

Figure 2. The risk of VTEs over time in patients with at least two associated mutations.

4. Discussion

VTEs are an important cause of morbidity and mortality among patients with nephrotic syndrome [18], with an incidence rate that varies greatly between different clinical trials [1]. Our study confirms the high prevalence of VTE (28%) in patients with primary nephrotic syndrome, with the vast majority of VTE being unilateral RVT (70%). The large variability in terms of VTE prevalence is mainly due to differences in methods used to diagnose VTE [1]. Although the frequency distribution of VTE appears to have changed over time—past clinical trials report RVT as the most common type of VTE [1,19–21], while more recent papers show a higher prevalence of PE and DVT [7,10]—caution must be employed when interpreting these results. Studies conducted in the 1980s and 1990s used renal venography as a screening method for RVT [19–22], capturing many asymptomatic events and thereby accounting for the higher prevalence of RVT, while the more recent retrospective studies focused mainly on symptomatic events [2,9,10]. Chronic RVT is usually asymptomatic and tends to occur more in older patients (mean age 40 years) than acute RVT (mean age 20 years) [1,2]. Our study population had a mean age of 43.4 ± 14.2 years, and we used a screening method for VTE detection (D-dimers levels), thereby explaining the higher prevalence of RVT in our cohort. The significance of screening asymptomatic events is debatable, but the presence of asymptomatic RVT determines an increased risk of PE, and a screening method could be undertaken at least in high-risk patients [23]. The predilection for RVT in nephrotic syndrome, and especially in MN, supposedly involves local disturbances in hemostasis, with generation of thrombin, and fibrinolysis, but this remains unproven [1,2,19].

Currently, the risk assessment of VTE in NS relies mainly on serum albumin, proteinuria level, and histological diagnosis [2,5]. Controversy exists regarding the cut-off limit for serum albumin, below which a high VTE risk could be defined [2,3]. Although most studies identified hypoalbuminemia (serum albumin below 2.5 g/dL) as an independent risk factor for VTE [3,7–9,20], others did not show significant differences between patients with or without VTE [3,21]. Our study did not identify serum albumin or proteinuria as independent risk factors for VTE. Despite the fact that most of our patients had severe hypoalbuminemia, we detected VTE even in patients with only a modest reduction in serum albumin (3 g/dL). As previously stated by other papers [2,3], it seems that hypoalbuminemia is a risk factor for VTE, but it is not mandatory for the development of these complications. In terms of histopathological diagnosis, MN is universally recognized as being associated with the highest risk for VTE development [2,8,24], although other studies did not confirm this predilection [10].

Uncertainties exist about which patients with idiopathic GN, other than MN, or with less severe NS would benefit from prophylactic anticoagulation, and identification of these high-risk patients still remains a challenge. The pathogenesis of thromboembolic complications in NS is multifactorial, with a complex interplay of acquired and inherited factors [1,6]. Although hemostasis derangements with a shift towards a prothrombotic state is well recognized in NS, studies linking these disturbances to VTE development are somewhat lacking [1]. Antithrombin III (AT III) deficiency is encountered in up to 80% of patients with NS [3]. Despite the fact that AT III deficiency reflects the severity of NS, as it is being correlated with the degree of hypoalbuminemia and proteinuria, not all studies confirmed the association between AT III deficiency and VTE [3]. Previous work of our group identified ionized calcium and a lower AT III activity as being independent predictors of VTE [7].

While most studies over the past decades evaluated mainly acquired risk factors for VTE in NS (serum albumin, proteinuria, hemostasis parameters) [8–10], few have addressed inherited risk factors with conflicting results [2,11–14].

Genetic mutations associated with inherited thrombophilia are frequently encountered in the general population [2,6,16,17,25–27]. Despite that the presence of these polymorphisms determines from a 3-fold increased risk (for prothrombin G20210A) to up to an 80-fold increased risk (for factor V Leiden homozygote) [6], the incidence of thrombotic events in susceptible individuals is highly variable, with many of them never developing VTE [17]. Although our study enrolled consecutive patients, we identified a higher prevalence of Factor V G1691A, prothrombin G20210A, and MTHFR polymorphisms than those encountered in the general population [6,28]. Additionally, 33% of our patients had at least two mutations, while the reported prevalence of heterozygosity for Factor V and prothrombin is 0.1%, and other associations have not been evaluated [6]. In univariate analysis, the presence of polymorphisms for the Factor V gene (G1691A), MTHFR gene (C677T), and the 4G/5G mutation of the PAI gene, and in addition, the presence of at least two mutations was associated with VTE. In multivariate analysis, only the combination of at least two mutations was identified as an independent predictor of VTE. Many studies over the past years have evaluated the risk of initial and recurrent VTE in patients carrying a single mutation [29,30]. Although the presence of polymorphisms for Factor V and prothrombin appears to increase the risk of initial VTE, most of the studies showed similar rates of VTE recurrence among carriers and non-carriers of thrombophilic mutations [29,31]. The general agreement exists that, in this setting, screening for these thrombophilias should not be undertaken because it can misguide the clinical decision on appropriate anticoagulation treatment duration [32]. Nevertheless, patients with double heterozygosity for factor V and prothrombin had, in one study, a 2.6-fold higher risk for VTE recurrence compared to those heterozygous only for factor V [33]. Despite not being supported by all studies [31], patients with coexistent thrombophilias may warrant prolonged anticoagulation [28]. Altough based on a small number of patients, the results of this study outline several important concepts. First of all, we confirmed that VTE is a multigenic disorder by the observation that the combination of two mutations confers an increased risk of VTE, as compared to the presence of either one alone [6]. The presence of these polymorphisms must be viewed as a risk factor for VTE, whose clinical expression is determined by acquiring the hemostasis disturbances associated with the NS [17]. Taken together, an increased level of Factor V associated with NS [1] in conjunction with inherited resistance to inactivation by protein C, coexistent mutations that cause higher plasma prothrombin levels, or hyperhomocysteinemia could explain why only some patients develop VTE in the setting of similar NS severity. Despite the fact that controversy still exists regarding the risk of coexistent thrombophilias for initial and recurrent VTE, none of those studies have addressed this concern in the setting of NS, and none of them have evaluated associations other than Factor V-prothrombin [29–31,33,34]. Since the majority of VTE in our study occurred during the first 6 months of follow-up, thereby confirming that the highest risk is within this time frame [7,9], early identification of high-risk patients for prophylactic anticoagulation is mandatory, and screening for thrombophilic defects might be of value in this setting (Table 5). Additionally, other studies have proposed the use of monitoring the D-dimers level as a screening method for VTE [7] that could reliably predict the risk of VTE recurrence, suggesting a possible role in tailoring anticoagulation treatment in these patients [35]. However, our study has some limitations (retrospective study, a small number of patients) that prevents the generalizability of the results. As such, larger, prospective, multicenter cohorts are needed to fully validate these findings.

Table 5. Evaluation of the risk factors for VTE in patients with NS.

History	Age, smoking history, previous or family history of VTE, pregnancy, prolonged immobilization, surgery, review of concomitant medication, neoplasia, chronic heart of pulmonary disorders, presence of central venous catheters, presence of inflammatory conditions
Laboratory predictors of VTE	Serum albumin level, 24-h proteinuria, D-dimers level, complete blood cell count, serum ionized calcium
Hemostasis-related protein disturbances	Coagulation parameters (prothrombin time, activated partial thromboplastin time, serum fibrinogen, antithrombin III, protein C and S, assessment of individual coagulation and fibrinolytic factors)
Genetic background	Protein C and S deficiency, antithrombin III deficiency, screening for polymorphisms of Factor V gene, PAI gene, methylene tetrahydrofolate reductase (MTHFR) gene and prothrombin gene (G20210A mutation).
Other inherited or acquired hypercoagulable states	Antiphospholipid syndrome (lupus anticoagulant, anticardiolipin antibodies, anti-β2-glycoprotein 1 antibodies), screening for other autoimmune or connective tissue disorders associated with an increased risk for VTE depending on the clinical scenario (e.g., inflammatory bowel disease).

Therefore, in the view that thromboembolic complications of NS are multifactorial in origin [1], one could not accurately predict the risk of VTE in NS while taking into account only serum albumin and proteinuria as risk stratifying markers. A risk score that would encompass serum albumin, hemostasis parameters (such as AT III), and the presence of these polymorphisms could better stratify these patients, but it needs to be validated in large clinical trials.

5. Conclusions

In summary, the association of two genetic mutations confers an independent risk for VTE in NS. Therefore, genetic testing for inherited thrombophilia in NS could play an important role in detecting high-risk patients that warrant prophylactic anticoagulation.

Author Contributions: Conceptualization, G.I., B.O., R.J., B.S. and A.A.; methodology, B.O.; formal analysis, B.O.; data curation, R.J. and A.A.; writing—original draft preparation, G.I. and B.O.; writing—review and editing, G.I., B.O., B.S., R.J., A.A., M.H.; supervision, G.I. and M.H. All authors have read and agreed to the published version of the manuscript.

Funding: This research received no external funding.

Conflicts of Interest: The authors declare no conflict of interest.

References

1. Kerlin, B.; Ayoob, R.; Smoyer, W.E. Epidemiology and pathophysiology of nephrotic syndrome-associated thromboembolic disease. *Clin. J. Am. Soc. Nephrol.* **2012**, *7*, 513–520. [CrossRef] [PubMed]
2. Glassock, R.J. Prophylactic anticoagulation in nephrotic syndrome: A clinical conundrum. *J. Am. Soc. Nephrol.* **2007**, *18*, 2221–2225. [CrossRef] [PubMed]
3. Singhal, R.; Brimble, K.S. Thromboembolic complications in the nephrotic syndrome: Pathophysiology and clinical management. *Thromb. Res.* **2006**, *118*, 397–407. [CrossRef] [PubMed]
4. Rostoker, G.; Durand-Zaleski, I.; Petit-Phar, M.; Maadi, A.B.; Jazaerli, N.; Radier, C.; Rahmouni, A.; Mathieu, D.; Vasile, N.; Rosso, J.; et al. Prevention of thrombotic complications of the nephrotic syndrome by low molecular weight heparin enoxaparin. *Nephron* **1995**, *69*, 20–28. [CrossRef] [PubMed]
5. KDIGO Working Group. KDIGO clinical practice guideline for glomerulonephritis. *Kidney Int. Suppl.* **2012**, *2*, 1–274.
6. Reich, L.M.; Bower, M.; Key, N.S. Role of the geneticist in testing and counseling for inherited thrombophilia. *Genet. Med.* **2003**, *5*, 133–143. [CrossRef] [PubMed]
7. Ismail, G.; Mircescu, G.; Ditoiu, A.V.; Tacu, B.D.; Jurubita, R.; Harza, M. Risk factors for predicting venous thromboembolism in patients with nephrotic syndrome: Focus on haemostasis-related parameters. *Int. Urol. Nephrol.* **2014**, *46*, 787–792. [CrossRef]
8. Barbour, S.J.; Greenwald, A.; Djurdjev, O.; Levin, A.; Hladunewich, M.; Nachman, P.H.; Hogan, S.L.; Cattran, D.C.; Reich, H.N. Disease-specific risk of venous thromboembolic events is increased in idiopathic glomerulonephritis. *Kidney Int.* **2012**, *81*, 190–195. [CrossRef]
9. Kumar, S.; Chapagain, A.; Nitsch, D.; Yaqoob, M.M. Proteinuria and hypoalbuminemia are risk factors for thromboembolic events in patients with idiopathic membranous nephropathy: An observational study. *BMC Nephrol.* **2012**, *13*, 107. [CrossRef]
10. Mahmoodi, B.K.; Ten Kate, M.K.; Waanders, F.; Veeger, N.J.G.M.; Brouwer, J.L.P.; Vogt, L.; Navis, G.; Van Der Meer, J. High absolute risks and predictors of venous and arterial thromboembolic events in patients with nephrotic syndrome: Results from a large retrospective cohort study. *Circulation* **2008**, *117*, 224–230. [CrossRef]
11. Beyan, C. Methylenetetrahydrofolate reductase gene polymorphisms in patients with nephrotic syndrome. *Clin. Nephrol.* **2013**, *80*, 311. [CrossRef] [PubMed]
12. Sahin, M.; Ozkurt, S.; Degirmenci, N.A.; Musmul, A.; Temiz, G.; Soydan, M. Assessment of genetic risk factors for thromboembolic complications in adults with idiopathic nephrotic syndrome. *Clin. Nephrol.* **2013**, *79*, 454–462. [CrossRef] [PubMed]
13. Fabri, D.; Belangero, V.M.S.; Annichino-Bizzacchi, J.M.; Arruda, V.R. Inherited risk factors for thrombophilia in children with nephrotic syndrome. *Eur. J. Pediatr.* **1998**, *157*, 939–942. [CrossRef] [PubMed]
14. Irish, B. The factor V Leiden mutation and risk of renal vein thrombosis in patients with nephrotic syndrome. *Nephrol. Dial. Transplant.* **1997**, *12*, 1680–1683. [CrossRef] [PubMed]
15. Price, D.T. Factor V Leiden Mutation and the Risks for Thromboembolic Disease: A Clinical Perspective. *Ann. Intern. Med.* **1997**, *127*, 895. [CrossRef] [PubMed]
16. Fay, W.P. Homocysteine and thrombosis: Guilt by association? *Blood* **2012**, *119*, 2977–2978. [CrossRef]
17. Dahlback, B. Advances in understanding pathogenic mechanisms of thrombophilic disorders. *Blood* **2008**, *112*, 19–27. [CrossRef]
18. Medjeral-Thomas, N.; Ziaj, S.; Condon, M.; Galliford, J.; Levy, J.; Cairns, T.; Griffith, M. Retrospective analysis of a novel regimen for the prevention of venous thromboembolism in nephrotic syndrome. *Clin. J. Am. Soc. Nephrol.* **2014**, *9*, 478–483. [CrossRef]
19. Llach, F. Hypercoagulability, renal vein thrombosis, and other thrombotic complications of nephrotic syndrome: Editorial review. *Kidney Int.* **1985**, *28*, 429–439. [CrossRef]
20. Rinaldo Bellomo, R.A. Membranous nephropathy and thromboembolism: Is prophylactic anticoagulation warranted? *Nephron* **1993**, *63*, 249–254. [CrossRef] [PubMed]
21. Wagoner, R.D.; Stanson, W.; Holley, K.E.; Winter, C.S. Renal vein thrombosis in idiopathic membranous glomerulopathy and nephrotic syndrome: Incidence and significance. *Kidney Int.* **1983**, *23*, 368–374. [CrossRef] [PubMed]

22. Velasquez Forero, F.; Garcia Prugue, N.; Ruiz Morales, N. Idiopathic Nephrotic Syndrome of the Adult with Asymptomatic Thrombosis of the Renal Vein. *Am. J. Nephrol.* **1988**, *8*, 457–462. [CrossRef] [PubMed]
23. Pincus, K.J.; Hynicka, L.M. Prophylaxis of thromboembolic events in patients with nephrotic syndrome. *Ann. Pharm.* **2013**, *47*, 725–734. [CrossRef] [PubMed]
24. Harza, M.; Ismail, G.; Mitroi, G.; Gherghiceanu, M.; Preda, A.; Mircescu, G.; Sinescu, I. Histological diagnosis and risk of renal vein thrombosis and other thrombotic complications in primitive nephrotic syndrome. *Rom. J. Morphol. Embryol.* **2013**, *54*, 555–560.
25. Balta, G.; Altay, C.; Gurgey, A. PAI-1 gene 4G/5G genotype: A risk factor for thrombosis in vessels of internal organs. *Am. J. Hematol.* **2002**, *71*, 89–93. [CrossRef]
26. Den Heijer, M.; Lewington, S.; Clarke, R. Homocysteine, MTHFR and risk of venous thrombosis: A meta-analysis of published epidemiological studies. *J. Thromb. Haemost.* **2005**, *3*, 292–299. [CrossRef]
27. Adams, R.L.C.; Bird, R.J. Coagulation cascade and therapeutics update: Relevance to nephrology. Part 1: Overview of coagulation, thrombophilias and history of anticoagulants. *Nephrology* **2009**, *14*, 462–470. [CrossRef]
28. Joffe, M.V.; Goldhaber, S.Z. Laboratory thrombophilias and venous thromboembolism. *Vasc. Med.* **2002**, *7*, 93–102. [CrossRef]
29. Ho, W.K.; Hankey, G.J.; Quinlan, D.J.; Eikelboom, J.W. Risk of Recurrent Venous Thromboembolism in Patients With Common Thrombophilia. *Arch. Intern. Med.* **2006**, *166*, 729. [CrossRef]
30. Brotman, D.J.; Necochea, A.J.; Wilson, L.M.; Crim, M.T.; Bass, E.B. Prothrombin G20210A in Adults With Venous Thromboembolism and in A Systematic Review. *JAMA* **2014**, *301*, 2472–2485.
31. Lijfering, W.M.; Middeldorp, S.; Veeger, N.J.G.M.; Hamulyák, K.; Prins, M.H.; Büller, H.R.; Van Der Meer, J. Risk of recurrent venous thrombosis in homozygous carriers and double heterozygous carriers of factor v leiden and prothrombin G20210A. *Circulation* **2010**, *121*, 1706–1712. [CrossRef] [PubMed]
32. Stevens, S.M.; Woller, S.C.; Bauer, K.; Kasthuri, R.; Cushman, M.; Streiff, M.; Lim, W.; Douketis, J.D. Guidance for the evaluation and treatment of hereditary and acquired thrombophilia. *J. Thromb. Thrombolysis* **2016**, *41*, 154–164. [CrossRef] [PubMed]
33. De Stefano, V.; Martinelli, I.; Mannucci, P.M.; Paciaroni, K.; Chiusolo, P.; Casorelli, I.; Rossi, E.; Leone, G. The risk of recurrent deep vein thrombosis among heterozygous carriers of both Factor V Leiden and the G20210A Prothrombin mutation. *N. Eng. J. Med.* **1999**, *341*, 801–806. [CrossRef] [PubMed]
34. González-Porras, J.R.; García-Sanz, R.; Alberca, I.; López, M.L.; Balanzategui, A.; Gutierrez, O.; Lozano, F.; San Miguel, J. Risk of recurrent venous thrombosis in patients with G20210A mutation in the prothrombin gene or factor V Leiden mutation. *Blood Coagul. Fibrinolysis* **2006**, *17*, 23–28. [CrossRef] [PubMed]
35. Palareti, G.; Legnani, C.; Cosmi, B.; Valdré, L.; Lunghi, B.; Bernardi, F.; Coccheri, S. Predictive value of D-dimer test for recurrent venous thromboembolism after anticoagulation withdrawal in subjects with a previous idiopathic event and in carriers of congenital thrombophilia. *Circulation* **2003**, *108*, 313–318. [CrossRef] [PubMed]

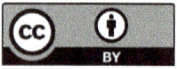

© 2020 by the authors. Licensee MDPI, Basel, Switzerland. This article is an open access article distributed under the terms and conditions of the Creative Commons Attribution (CC BY) license (http://creativecommons.org/licenses/by/4.0/).

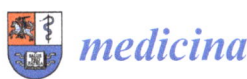

Article

Use of Glycated Hemoglobin (A1c) as a Biomarker for Vascular Risk in Type 2 Diabetes: Its Relationship with Matrix Metalloproteinases-2, -9 and the Metabolism of Collagen IV and Elastin

Krasimir Kostov [1],* and Alexander Blazhev [2]

1. Department of Pathophysiology, Medical University-Pleven, 1 Kliment Ohridski Str., 5800 Pleven, Bulgaria
2. Department of Biology, Medical University-Pleven, 1 Kliment Ohridski Str., 5800 Pleven, Bulgaria; yalishanda9@gmail.com
* Correspondence: dr.krasi_kostov@abv.bg; Tel.: +359-889-257-459

Received: 14 April 2020; Accepted: 5 May 2020; Published: 11 May 2020

Abstract: *Background and objectives*: HbA1c measurements may be useful not only in optimizing glycemic control but also as a tool for managing overall vascular risk in patients with diabetes. In the present study, we investigate the clinical significance of HbA1c as a biomarker for hyperglycemia-induced vascular damages in type 2 diabetes (T2D) based on the levels of matrix metalloproteinases-2, -9 (MMP-2, MMP-9), anti-collagen IV (ACIV), and anti-elastin (AE) antibodies (Abs) IgM, IgG, and IgA, and CIV-derived peptides (CIV-DP) reflecting collagen and elastin turnover in the vascular wall. The aim is to show the relationship of hyperglycemia with changes in the levels of vascular markers and the dynamics of this relationship at different degrees of glycemic control reported by HbA1c levels. *Materials and Methods*: To monitor elastin and collagen IV metabolism, we measured serum levels of these immunological markers in 59 patients with T2D and 20 healthy control subjects with an ELISA. *Results*: MMP-2, MMP-9, and the AEAbs IgA levels were significantly higher in diabetic patients than in control subjects, whereas those of the AEAbs IgM, ACIVAbs IgM, and CIV-DP were significantly lower. MMP-9 levels were significantly lower at HbA1c values >7.5%. *Conclusions*: A set of three tested markers (MMP-2, MMP-9, and AEAbs IgA) showed that vascular damages from preceding long-term hyperglycemia begin to dominate at HbA1c values ≥7.5%, which is the likely cut-point to predict increased vascular risk.

Keywords: type 2 diabetes; hemoglobin A1c; matrix metalloproteinases-2 and -9; anti-elastin antibodies; anti-collagen IV antibodies; diabetic retinopathy; diabetic nephropathy; macrovascular complications

1. Introduction

The prevalence of type 2 diabetes (T2D) is increasing worldwide, and it is expected to affect over 500 million adults worldwide by 2030 [1]. T2D is an important contributor to adverse cardiovascular complications, which are the leading causes of morbidity and mortality in Western countries [2].

Prevention of complications in T2D is closely linked to long-term control of hyperglycemia [3] since metabolic consequences extending beyond impaired glucose metabolism can affect almost every tissue and organ system of the body [4]. Despite the tendency in patients with good metabolic control to have a significantly reduced risk of developing complications, vascular disease can continue to develop and progress even under intensive treatment regimens due to the phenomenon known as "glycemic memory" [5]. Increased glucose levels can lead to metabolic derangements associated with vision loss, peripheral neuropathy, myocardial infarction, strokes, foot ulcers, and end-stage renal disease, which may cause permanent disability [6].

Despite the advancement of technologies to monitor blood glucose, for the vast majority of patients with diabetes, glycated hemoglobin (HbA1c) provides an excellent measure of glycemic control [7]. Nontraditional serum markers for short-term glucose control may enhance the ability to monitor hyperglycemia in people with diabetes. Fructosamine, glycated albumin, and 1,5-anhydroglucitol are of recent interest, especially in populations where the interpretation of HbA1c may be problematic such as in the setting of anemia, hemolysis, renal disease or pregnancy [8]. Most studies confirm a close linear relationship between HbA1c and mean blood glucose [9]. This suggests that HbA1c may be used not only as a diagnostic marker for the presence and severity of hyperglycemia during the preceding 4–12 weeks before the test but also over time as a "biomarker for a risk factor", i.e., hyperglycemia as a risk factor for diabetic retinopathy (DR), diabetic nephropathy (DN), and other vascular complications [4]. A 1% increase in absolute concentrations of HbA1c is associated with about 10–20% increase in cardiovascular disease risk [10]. The American Diabetes Association (ADA) now recommends the use of HbA1c to diagnose T2D with a cut-off value of ≥6.5%. Individuals with HbA1c levels of 5.7–6.4% are considered to be prediabetic. The ADA also recommends in patients with T2D, values of HbA1c less than 7% to prevent long-term complications associated with the disease [11,12].

As in the general population, in patients with diabetes, the treatment and prevention of cardiovascular disease require the use of specific biomarkers to predict risk. Most of these biomarkers are focused on already known pathophysiological pathways and mechanisms affecting the cardiovascular system. In the diabetic population the advanced glycation end products (AGEs), endothelin-1 (ET-1), matrix metalloproteinases (MMPs), high-sensitivity C-reactive protein (hsCRP), N-terminal fragment of brain natriuretic peptide (NT-proBNP), high-sensitivity troponin T (hsTnT), lipids, and albuminuria can be useful in predicting of cardiovascular disease [13,14]. In this regard, the markers for glucose-induced vascular damage, such as AGEs and urinary microalbumin levels, may be particularly useful in predicting the risk in individuals with diabetes [13].

Important factors in the development of vascular complications in T2D are the increased glycation, degradation, and/or accumulation of elastin and collagen in the vascular wall [15]. MMPs, which hydrolyze the protein components of the vascular extracellular matrix, are actively involved in this process. The subgroup of MMPs known as gelatinases, in particular gelatinase A (MMP-2) and gelatinase B (MMP-9), can degrade collagen (COL), denatured COL (gelatin), elastin (EL), laminin, fibronectin, and other substrates [16]. Dysregulation of gelatinase activity is associated with vascular inflammation, remodeling, and fibrosis and may contribute to the pathophysiology of diabetic complications [17]. In a previous study of patients with hypertension and T2D, we showed that elevated serum levels of MMP-2 and MMP-9 may reflect early structural changes in the vascular extracellular matrix [14]. Unlike the other MMPs, MMP-2 and MMP-9 differ in that they contain three type II fibronectin repeats that have a high binding affinity for collagen. These repeats direct the catalytic pocket of the gelatinases close to the collagen, thereby enhancing the rate of their hydrolysis [18]. The enhanced proteolytic activity of MMP-2 and MMP-9 is accompanied by the release of COL, EL and their derivatives (e.g., EL-derived peptides (EDPs), COL type IV (CIV)-derived peptides (CIV-DP)) in blood circulation, which is followed by the production of specific anti-elastin (AE) and anti-collagen (AC) antibodies (Abs) from IgM, IgG, and IgA classes (AEAbs IgM, AEAbs IgG, AEAbs IgA, ACAbs IgM, and ACAbs IgG) against their epitopes. These autoantibodies can serve as valuable control biomarkers for the turnover of protein components in the vascular extracellular matrix (ECM). Elevated levels of anti-CIV (ACIV) Abs IgG (ACIVAbs IgG) in hypertensive patients with T2D may indicate increased degradation of CIV [19], which is the most abundant structural component in the basement membrane (BM) of the small vessels [20]. Similarly, elevated levels of AEAbs IgA may indicate increased degradation of the elastic fibers in the vessel wall as a sign of microvascular [21] and/or macrovascular [22] disease in T2D.

In the present study, we investigate the clinical significance of HbA1c as a predictive biomarker for hyperglycemia-induced vascular damages in T2D, based on the statistical relationships between

HbA1c levels and corresponding levels of MMP-2, MMP-9, AEAbs (IgM, IgG, and IgA), ACIVAbs IgM, and the levels of CIV-DP, reflecting CIV and EL turnover in the vascular wall.

2. Materials and Methods

2.1. Study Population and Design

The study was approved by the University Research Ethics Committee and conducted in accordance with the Declaration of Helsinki (IRB approval no. 314-REC/Prot. 29). The study population consisted of 79 persons: 59 patients with T2D treated at the University Hospital Georgi Stranski, Pleven, and 20 healthy control subjects. Two groups were formed: Group I ($n = 20$): control group (Control); Group II ($n = 59$): patients with T2D. The clinical characteristics of the groups are shown in Table 1.

Table 1. Clinical characteristics of the groups in the study population.

Variables	Healthy Control Subjects ($n = 20$)	Patients with T2D ($n = 59$)
Men, n (%)	10 (50.0)	25 (42.0)
Women, n (%)	10 (50.0)	34 (58.0)
Age, years [1]	61.5 ± 2.9	60.7 ± 1.9
Duration of T2D [1]	N/A [2]	10.1 ± 1.0
HbA1c (%) [1]	N/A [2]	7.5 ± 0.2
BMI, kg/m^2 [1]	24.9 ± 0.5	28.4 ± 0.5 ***
TC, mmol/L [1]	4.2 ± 0.2	5.2 ± 0.2 *
LDL-C, mmol/L [1]	2.8 ± 0.2	3.0 ± 0.1
HDL-C, mmol/L [1]	1.2 ± 0.04	1.0 ± 0.03 ***
TG, mmol/L [1]	1.4 ± 0.1	2.7 ± 0.4
CRP, mg/L [1]	1.1 ± 0.2	8.4 ± 1.02 ***
Hypertension, n (%)	0 (0)	43 (73.0)
SBP, mmHg [1]	121.5 ± 1.9	149.2 ± 1.7 ***
DBP, mmHg [1]	78.2 ± 1.7	83.0 ± 1.5
Microangiopathy, n (%)	N/A [2]	50 (85.0)
Macroangiopathy, n (%)	N/A [2]	18 (31.0)
Neuropathy, n (%)	N/A [2]	8 (14.0)

* $p < 0.05$, *** $p < 0.001$; [1] Mean ± SEM; [2] N/A, not available; BMI: body mass index; TC: total cholesterol; LDL–C: low-density lipoprotein cholesterol; HDL–C: high-density lipoprotein cholesterol; TG: triglyceride; CRP: C-reactive protein; SBP: systolic blood pressure; DBP: diastolic blood pressure.

Selected control individuals were without diabetes mellitus, hypertension, or other vascular diseases, with a mean age of 61.5 ± 2.9 years. The mean age of patients with T2D was 60.7 ± 1.9 years. The patients were screened for microangiopathy using ophthalmoscopy and assessment of 24-h urine albumin excretion. Macroangiopathy was evaluated on the basis of clinical evidence for coronary artery disease, cerebrovascular disease, peripheral arterial disease, and/or history for acute arterial vascular events. Controls were screened for microangiopathy using ophthalmoscopy, and for macroangiopathy by physical examination, blood pressure measurement, electrocardiogram testing, measuring cholesterol levels, data on obesity and smoking, family history. The incidence of microangiopathy in the T2D group ($n = 50$) was 58%, and the incidence of macroangiopathy ($n = 18$) was 31%. Nine patients had both micro- and macrovascular diseases (Table 1).

According to the study design, our first aim was to compare the levels of MMP-2, MMP-9, AEAbs (IgM, IgG, and IgA), ACIVAbs IgM, and CIV-DP between patients and healthy controls. Our second aim was to compare within the patient group the levels of tested markers distributed below and above the different cut off values of HbA1c in the range between 6.0% and 8.0% (6.0%–6.5%–7.0%–7.5%–8.0%). All patients were divided into two subgroups according to these five cut-off values of HbA1c and we compared the levels of the markers between these subgroups (≤6.0% vs. >6.0%; ≤6.5% vs. >6.5%; ≤7.0% vs. >7.0%; ≤7.5% vs. >7.5%; ≤8.0% vs. >8.0%; see Table 2).

Table 2. Statistical significance between the levels of test markers in T2D subgroups at cut-off HbA1c values of 6.0%, 6.5%, 7.0%, 7.5%, and 8.0%.

HbA1c Subgroups	≤6.0% vs. >6.0%	≤6.5% vs. >6.5%	≤7.0% vs. >7.0%	≤7.5% vs. >7.5%	≤8.0% vs. >8.0%
MMP-2	NS	NS	NS	S *	NS
MMP-9	S **	S **	S *	S *	NS
AEAbs IgM	NS	NS	NS	NS	NS
AEAbs IgG	NS	NS	NS	NS	NS
AEAbs IgA	NS	NS	S *	S *	NS
ACIVAbs IgM	NS	NS	NS	NS	NS
CIV-DP	NS	NS	NS	NS	NS

* $p < 0.05$, ** $p < 0.01$, NS—not significant; S—significant; MMP-2: matrix metalloproteinase-2; MMP-9: matrix metalloproteinase-9; AEAbs: anti-elastin antibodies; ACIVAbs: anti-collagen IV antibodies; CIV-DP: CIV-derived peptides.

2.2. Immunological and Biochemical Assays

All laboratory determinations were performed after 12–14 h overnight fasting. To measured the levels of MMP-2, MMP-9, AEAbs, ACIVAbs, CIV-DP, and the other laboratory parameters, blood was drawn into serum tubes. Serum was obtained after centrifugation at 2500 rpm for 10 min. Until the immunological assay, the serums were stored at −70 °C.

2.2.1. Determination of MMP-2

To measure MMP-2 concentrations, an ELISA kit from R&D Systems (Cat. No. DMP2F0) (Minneapolis, MN, USA) was used. According to the manufacturer's instructions, 100 µL of assay diluent RD1-74 was added to each well-plate, then 50 µL tested sera, diluted 1:10 with calibrator diluent RD5-32 (20 µL serum + 180 µL calibrator diluent) or standards, was added at various concentrations to construct a calibration curve. After 2 h downtime at room temperature on a shaker, plates were washed three times with 400 µL wash buffer per well. After the last wash, 200 µL of the conjugate was added to each well and incubated for 2 h at room temperature on a shaker. The plate was washed again three times, and in each well, 200 µL substrate solution was added. This was incubated for 30 min at room temperature in the dark. The reaction was stopped by adding 50 µL of stop solution to each well. Within 30 min, the serum samples were assayed at 450 nm on an automatic micro-ELISA plate reader (Coulter Microplate Reader UV Max).

2.2.2. Determination of MMP-9

To measure MMP-9 concentrations, an ELISA kit from R&D Systems (Cat. No. DMP900) (Minneapolis, MN, USA) was used. According to the manufacturer's instructions, to each well-plate, 100 µL of assay diluent RD1-34 was added, then 100 µL tested sera, diluted 1:100 with calibrator diluent RD5-10 (10 µL serum + 990 µL calibrator diluent) or standards, was added at various concentrations to construct a calibration curve. After 2 h downtime at room temperature on a shaker, plates were washed three times with 400 µL wash buffer per well. After the last wash, 200 µL anti-MMP-9 antibody conjugated with peroxidase was added to each well and was incubated for 1 h at room temperature on a shaker. The plate was washed again three times, and in each well, 200 µL substrate solution was added. This was incubated for 30 min at room temperature in the dark. The reaction was stopped by adding 50 µL of stop solution to each well. Within 30 min, the serum samples were assayed at 450 nm on an automatic micro-ELISA plate reader (Coulter Microplate Reader UV Max).

2.2.3. Determination of AEAbs (IgM, IgG, and IgA)

To measure AEAbs IgM, AEAbs IgG, and AEAbs IgA concentrations, a sandwich ELISA was used. The assay was performed as follows: a microtiter 96-well polystyrene plate was coated with human aortic α-elastin, prepared as described by Baydanoff et al. [23] (1 µg of elastin in 100 µL of 0.05 M carbonate buffer, pH 9.6). Then the remaining "active" centers of the polystyrene wells were blocked by the plate incubation for 24 h with 1% solution of bovine serum albumin (BSA)

(Cat. No. A2153, Sigma-Aldrich, St. Louis, MO, USA) in phosphate-buffered saline (PBS), pH 7.4, containing 0.05% Tween 20. The next step was the addition of 100 μL of tested patient serum (diluted 1:10 with PBS) in each well of the microtiter plate, incubated for 1 h at 37 °C. After washing three times, incubation with anti-human immunoglobulin peroxidase conjugates to the heavy chain of IgM, IgG, and IgA, respectively (Sigma-Aldrich, St. Louis, MO, USA) followed. All immunoconjugates were diluted 1:10,000 with PBS containing 1% BSA and 0.05% Tween 20. Next, samples were incubated with substrate solution (ortho-phenylene diamine, 4 mg/mL in 10 mL 0.05 M citrate buffer, pH 5.0 with H_2O_2) for 1 h at room temperature in a dark chamber. The reaction was stopped by adding 50 μL of 4 M H_2SO_4 to each well, and the optical density was measured with a micro-ELISA plate reader (Coulter Microplate Reader UV Max) at a wavelength of 492 nm.

2.2.4. Determination of ACIVAbs IgM

To measure ACIVAbs IgM concentrations, a sandwich ELISA was used. The assay was performed as follows: a microtiter 96-well polystyrene plate was coated with 100 μL of 10 μg/mL of human CIV (Sigma-Aldrich, St. Louis, MO, USA) at room temperature for 3 h, followed by overnight incubation at 4 °C. The plate was washed with phosphate-buffered saline (PBS) containing 0.05% Tween 20 and 1% bovine serum albumin (BSA; Cat. No. A2153, Sigma-Aldrich, St. Louis, MO, USA). Then, a 100-μL serum sample (diluted 1:10) was placed in each well of a microtiter plate and incubated for 1 h at 37 °C. After washing three times, 100 μL of goat anti-human IgM Ab, Fc5μ, HRP conjugate (AP114P, Sigma-Aldrich, St. Louis, MO, USA) were added to each well for 1 h at 37 °C. All immunoconjugates were diluted 1:10,000 with PBS containing 1% BSA and 0.05% Tween 20. The plate was incubated for 1 h at 37 °C. Ortho-phenylenediamine (4 mg/mL in 0.05 M citrate buffer, pH 5.0 with H_2O_2) was used as a colorimetric substrate. The reaction was stopped by adding 50 μL of 4 M H_2SO_4 to each well, and the optical density was measured with a micro-ELISA plate reader (Coulter Microplate Reader UV Max) at a wavelength of 492 nm.

2.2.5. Determination of CIV-DP

To measure CIV-DP concentrations, a sandwich ELISA was used. The assay was performed as follows: each well of the microtiter plate was sensitized with 100 μL of 10 μg/mL of mouse monoclonal antibody to collagen IV (COL-94) (Cat. No. ab6311, Abcam, Cambridge, UK) at room temperature for 3 h, followed by overnight incubation at 4 °C. The plate was washed with phosphate-buffered saline (PBS) containing 0.05% Tween 20 and 0.1% bovine serum albumin (BSA) (Cat. No. A2153, Sigma-Aldrich, St. Louis, MO, USA). Then, a 100-μL serum sample (diluted 1:5) was placed in each well of a microtiter plate and incubated for 1 h at 37 °C. After washing three times, 100 μL of rabbit anti-human CIV polyclonal antibody (Cat. No. ab6586, Abcam, Cambridge, UK; diluted 1:2000) was allowed to react in each well at 37 °C for 1 h. The wells were washed with PBS + Tween 20, and peroxidase-conjugated goat anti-rabbit IgG H&L (HRP) (Cat. No. ab205718, Abcam, Cambridge, UK), diluted 10,000 fold, was then added to each well. The plate was incubated for 1 h at 37 °C. Ortho-phenylenediamine (0.4 mg/mL) was added to citrate buffer, and 100 μL of this solution was added to each well and allowed to react for 30 min. The reaction was stopped by adding 50 μL 4M H_2SO_4 to each well and the optical density was measured with a micro-ELISA plate reader (Coulter Microplate Reader UV Max) at a wavelength of 492 nm.

2.2.6. Biochemical Assays

The analysis was performed using an automatic biochemistry analyzer. HbA1c and CRP were measured by a turbidimetric immunoassay. Enzymatic methods were used to measure total cholesterol (TC), low-density lipoprotein cholesterol (LDL-C), high-density lipoprotein cholesterol (HDL-C), and triglyceride (TG).

2.3. Blood Pressure Measurements

Blood pressure (BP) was measured using a standard cuff mercury sphygmomanometer on the left arm in a sitting position, after 5–10 min rest. Normal BP was defined as SBP between 120 and 129 mmHg and/or DBP between 80 and 84 mmHg. Hypertension was defined as SBP ≥ 140 mmHg and/or DBP ≥ 90 mmHg, or if the patients have been diagnosed or had taken antihypertensive drugs at any time during the preceding six months.

2.4. Clinical Tests and Procedures

Each patient was subjected to the routine nephrologic (renal ultrasound, creatinine, blood urea nitrogen, urinary albumin excretion), ophthalmic (visual acuity test, ophthalmoscopy, tonometry) and neurologic (muscle reflexes, electromyography) examinations. Body mass index (BMI) was calculated using the standard metric BMI formula (Kg/m^2). BMI between 18.5 and 24.9 was considered normal, 25 to 29.9 was considered overweight, and equal to or higher than 30 was considered obese.

2.5. Statistical Analysis

All statistical analyses were performed using the SPSS 23.0 software (SPSS, Inc., Chicago, IL, USA). The data were expressed as mean ± standard error of the mean (SEM) or standard deviation (SD) (in the figures) and were calculated at a confidence level of 95%. The differences between the groups were assessed by Student's unpaired *t*-test. Correlation analysis was performed with Pearson's correlation test. Values of $p \leq 0.05$ were considered statistically significant.

3. Results

3.1. Comparison of the Tested Markers between the T2D and Control Groups

Patients with T2D showed statistically significantly higher serum levels of MMP-2 (30.68 ± 1.87 vs. 36.22 ± 1.50; $p = 0.026$), MMP-9 (25.84 ± 2.83 vs. 38.48 ± 2.69; $p = 0.002$), and AEAbs IgA (0.29 ± 0.03 vs. 0.55 ± 0.05; $p < 0.001$) than healthy controls (Figures 1A,B and 2A).

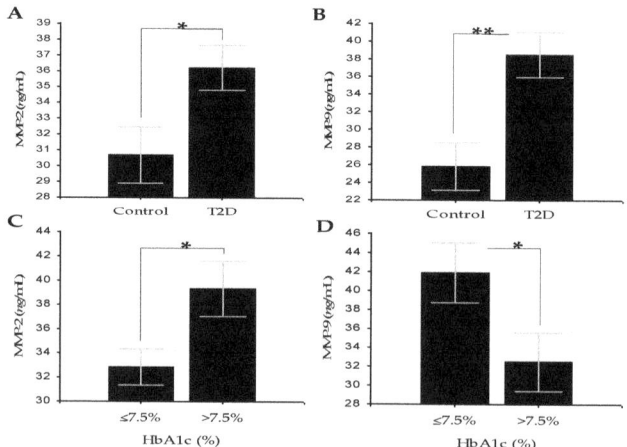

Figure 1. (**A**) Serum levels of MMP-2 in T2D group vs. control group. (**B**) Serum levels of MMP-9 in T2D group vs. control group. (**C**) Serum levels of MMP-2 in patients with HbA1c values ≤7.5% vs. patients with HbA1c values >7.5%. (**D**) Serum levels of MMP-9 in patients with HbA1c values ≤7.5% vs. patients with HbA1c values > 7.5%. Data are represented as mean ± SD. * $p \leq 0.05$, ** $p < 0.01$.

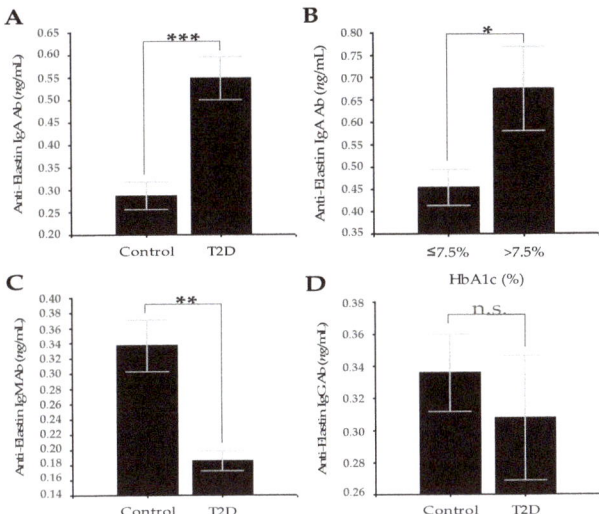

Figure 2. (**A**) Serum levels of AEAbs IgA in T2D group vs. control group (**B**) Serum levels of AEAbs IgA in patients with HbA1c values ≤7.5% vs. patients with HbA1c values >7.5%. (**C**) Serum levels of AEAbs IgM in the T2D group vs. control group. (**D**) Serum levels of AEAbs IgG in the T2D group vs. control group. Data are represented as mean ± SD. * $p < 0.05$, ** $p < 0.01$, and *** $p < 0.001$, n.s.—not significant.

Serum levels of AEAbs IgM were significantly lower in T2D group than in controls (0.34 ± 0.03 vs. 0.18 ± 0.01; $p = 0.001$; Figure 2C). The levels of AEAbs IgG were also lower in the T2D group than in controls, but the difference was not statistically significant (0.33 ± 0.02 vs. 0.31 ± 0.04; $p = 0.697$; Figure 2D). The levels of ACIVAbs IgM (0.18 ± 0.02 vs. 0.12 ± 0.01; $p = 0.016$) and CIV-DP (1.16 ± 0.05 vs. 0.74 ± 0.03; $p < 0.001$) in patients with T2D were significantly lower than in controls (Figure 3A,B).

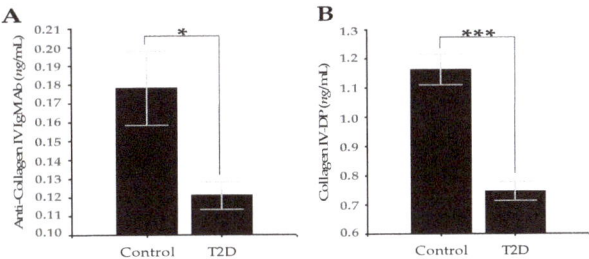

Figure 3. (**A**) Serum levels of ACIVAbs IgM in T2D group vs. control group (**B**) Serum levels of CIV-DP in T2D group vs. control group. Data are represented as mean ± SD. * $p < 0.05$, *** $p < 0.001$.

3.2. Comparison of the Tested Markers between T2D Subgroups at Cut-Off Values of HbA1c from 6.0 to 8.0%

Comparison of the tested markers levels at different HbAc cut-off values showed the most significant indication for vascular change at a cut-off HbA1c value of 7.5%. At this value, a set of three assessment markers for vascular risk (MMP-2, MMP-9, and AEAbs IgA) showed statistical significance (Table 2). In patients with poor glycemic control and increased vascular risk ($n = 25$), who have HbA1c values >7.5%, the levels of MMP-2 (32.85 ± 1.56 vs. 39.34 ± 2.39; $p = 0.022$) and AEAbs IgA (0.45 ± 0.04 vs. 0.67 ± 0.09; $p = 0.049$) were significantly increased compared to those with better control and HbA1c values ≤7.5% ($n = 34$; Figures 1C and 2B). In the same subgroups of patients, MMP-9, unlike MMP-2, showed significantly decreased levels at HbA1c values >7.5% compared with HbA1c values ≤7.5% (41.89 ± 3.31 vs. 32.51 ± 3.26; $p = 0.05$; Figure 1D).

At the cut-off HbA1c value of 7.0%, statistical significance showed a set of two markers (MMP-9 and AEAbs IgA). MMP-9 showed significantly decreased levels at HbA1c values >7.0% compared with HbA1c values ≤7.0% (43.12 ± 3.45 vs. 32.19 ± 3.05; $p = 0.023$). The levels of AEAbs IgA were significantly increased at HbA1c values >7.0% compared with HbA1c values ≤7.0% (0.44 ± 0.04 vs. 0.66 ± 0.09; $p = 0.031$; Table 2). Only one marker (MMP-9) showed significantly decreased levels at cut off HbA1c values of 6.0% (50.79 ± 5.64 vs. 34.15 ± 2.40; $p = 0.003$) and 6.5% (46.42 ± 4.32 vs. 33.36 ± 2.65; $p = 0.009$). None of the markers showed statistical significance at a cut-off value of HbA1c of 8.0% (Table 2). The relationship between the levels of test markers and HbA1 as a continuous variable is shown in Figure 4.

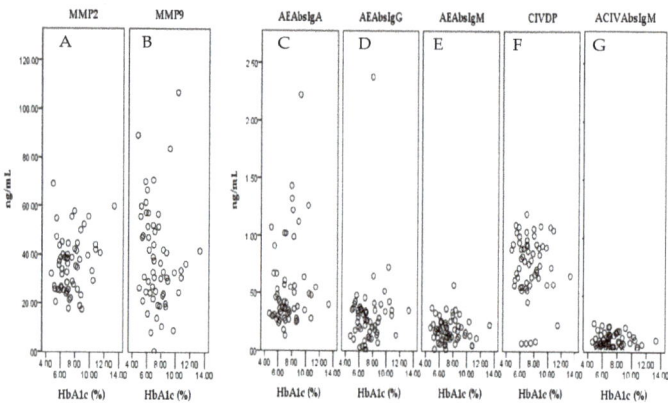

Figure 4. Scatterplots showing the relationship between the levels of (**A**) MMP-2, (**B**) MMP-9, (**C**) AEAbs IgA, (**D**) AEAbs IgG, (**E**) AEAbs IgM, (**F**) CIV-DP, (**G**) ACIVAbs IgM, and HbA1 as a continuous variable.

3.3. Correlations of Investigated Immunological Markers

There were significant correlations of the examined markers for vascular risk in the T2D group, which are presented in Table 3.

Table 3. Pearson's correlation coefficients and statistical significance between the variables in the T2D group.

Correlations	Correlation Coefficient	Statistical Significance
	r	p
MMP-2 vs. AEAbs IgG	0.273 *	0.036
MMP-2 vs. ACIVAbs IgM	0.343 **	0.008
AEAbs IgA vs. AEAbs IgM	0.327 *	0.012
AEAbs IgA vs. AEAbs IgG	0.500 ***	<0.001
AEAbs IgA vs. ACIVAbs IgM	0.365 **	0.005
AEAbs IgM vs. ACIVAbs IgM	0.679 ***	<0.001
AEAbs IgG vs. AEAbs IgM	0.308 *	0.017
AEAbs IgA vs. Systolic BP	−0.292 *	0.026
AEAbs IgA vs. Diastolic BP	−0.419 **	0.001
AEAbs IgM vs. Systolic BP	−0.306 *	0.019
AEAbs IgM vs. Diastolic BP	−0.263 *	0.045
AEAbs IgG vs. Systolic BP	−0.277 *	0.034
AEAbs IgG vs. Diastolic BP	−0.320 *	0.013
AEAbs IgA vs. CIV-DP	0.362 **	0.005
AEAbs IgA vs. BMI	−0.273 *	0.038

* $p < 0.05$, ** $p < 0.01$, *** $p < 0.001$; MMP-2: matrix metalloproteinase-2; AEAbs: anti-elastin antibodies; ACIVAbs: anti-collagen IV antibodies; CIV-DP: CIV-derived peptides; BP: blood pressure; BMI: body mass index.

4. Discussion

HbA1c is major tool for assessing glycemic control and has strong predictive value for diabetes complications [24]. Given the broad informativeness of the test, it is imperative to know how it can be optimally applied to the management and assessment of overall vascular risk (micro- and macrovascular) in patients with diabetes [25]. Systematic review and meta-analysis of multiple databases suggest that in people with diabetes, the target levels for HbA1c to minimize vascular complications should range from 6.0 to 8.0% [26]. The UK Prospective Diabetes Study (UKPDS) [27,28] and the Kumamoto Study [29] confirmed that intensive glycemic control significantly decreased rates of microvascular complications in patients with T2D [24]. The Diabetes Control and Complications Trial (DCCT) [30], a prospective randomized controlled trial of intensive (mean HbA1c about 7%) versus standard (mean HbA1c about 9%) glycemic control in patients with T1D, showed that better glycemic control is associated with 50–76% reductions in rates of development and progression of microvascular complications. Epidemiologic analyses of the DCCT and UKPDS also suggest that further lowering of A1C from 7 to 6% is associated with further reduction in the risk of microvascular complications, although the absolute risk reductions become much smaller [24]. The Analysis of the Action in Diabetes and Vascular disease: Preterax and Diamicron Modified Release Controlled Evaluation (ADVANCE) study has shown that microvascular event risk begins above an HbA1c of 6.5%. For macrovascular event risk, inflection of the curve was seen at around 7%, and the risk increased at higher HbA1c levels [31]. In a cohort of patients with T2D in the UK, Currie and colleagues report that the ideal HbA1c level is 7.5% and that the recommendations should target such a value. Their analyses demonstrate that an HbA1c of approximately 7.5% was associated with the lowest all-cause mortality and the lowest progression to large-vessel disease events. An increase or decrease from this mean HbA1c value was associated with a heightened risk of adverse outcomes [32]. The data in this study are consistent with our results, which give the highest indication of vascular change (set of three assessment markers—MMP-2, MMP-9, and AEAbs IgA) at a cut-off HbA1c value of 7.5% (Table 2). Therefore, vascular damage from preceding long-term hyperglycemia begins to dominate at an HbA1c value greater than 7.5%, which is the likely cut-off point to predict increased vascular risk.

Current consensus-based guidelines do not fix one exact cut-point of HbA1c, beyond which vascular risk increases. All recommend individualizing HbA1c targets on the basis of patient characteristics. The ADA recommends the reasonable target of HbA1c for many non-pregnant adults to be less than 7%. An HbA1c of <7.0% may be targeted in the majority of patients, acknowledging the individual needs [12]. When a patient has just been diagnosed and is free from significant cardiovascular disease, the aim should be a range from 6.0–6.5%. By contrast, in an elderly patient with long-standing and/or complicated disease, relaxing the target to 7.5–8.0% may be wiser, given that the vascular benefits in terms of life expectancy are less relevant [24]. The American Association of Clinical Endocrinologists and American College of Endocrinology (AACE/ACE) guidelines recommend a target of 6.5% (if it can be achieved safely). The National Institute for Health and Care Excellence (NICE) guideline specifies 6.5% or 7%, depending on the patient's treatment regimen. The Clinical Systems Improvement (ICSI) guideline recommends a target range less than 7% to less than 8% based on patient factors. According to recommendations of the American College of Physicians (ACP), for most patients with T2D, targets levels of HbA1c should be between 7.0% and 8.0% [6]. Our HbA1c cut-point of 7.5%, evaluated to predict higher vascular risk, falls in the middle of this recommended range.

When we compared the levels of MMP-2 and MMP-9 between the control group and the T2D group, we observed higher levels in patients with T2D (Figure 1A,B). As to our findings that MMP-2 and MMP-9 levels were significantly higher in T2D patients, similar findings have been reported by other researchers [33,34]. However, an impression in our study makes the observed opposite levels of the two gelatinases at HbA1c values greater than 7.5% (Figure 1C,D). In patients with poor glycemic control and increased vascular risk, who have HbA1c values >7.5%, MMP-2 levels were significantly increased compared to those with better control and HbA1c values ≤7.5% (Figure 1C). In the same subgroups of patients, MMP-9, unlike MMP-2, showed significantly decreased levels at HbA1c values >7.5% compared with HbA1c values ≤7.5% (Figure 1D). Similar results have been reported by Derosa and colleagues in children and adolescents with T1D. They reported that MMP-2 levels were significantly higher in patients with microangiopathic complications compared with control subjects and patients without complications. MMP-9 levels were significantly lower in patients with microangiopathic complications compared with control subjects and patients without complications. Based on these results, the authors postulated that MMP-2 may be a good index of the severity and stability of microangiopathy, and MMP-9 is a marker of macroangiopathy in diabetes [35]. We also found positive correlations between MMP-2 and AEAbs IgG and between MMP-2 and ACIVAbs IgM in the T2D group (Table 3). A possible explanation for this result is that MMP-2 may be involved in the process of elastin and collagen IV destruction and the development of vascular complications.

MMP-2 and MMP-9 play an important role in the development of microvascular and macrovascular complications in T2D patients. The recent results advocate that due to diabetes, the overexpression of MMP-2 and MMP-9 in the retina inhibits cell proliferation and differentiation and accelerates apoptosis, a phenomenon that precedes the development of histopathology characteristic of DR [36]. During the first stage of DR, increased retinal MMP-2 and MMP-9 enhance the permeability of the blood–retinal barrier via proteolytic degradation of tight junction protein occludin and disruption of the overall tight junction complex [37]. In addition, MMP-2 and MMP-9 facilitate apoptosis of retinal capillary cells and pericytes, which disrupts the normal vascular structure and leads to the formation of microaneurysms and hemorrhages [38]. During the advanced stage, MMP-2 and MMP-9 dissolve the vascular basement membrane and create the conditions for the formation of new vessels [39]. MMP-2 and MMP-9 are also implicated in the pathogenesis of diabetic macular edema and fibrovascular proliferation with tractional retinal detachment, which are the most common causes of vision loss in patients with DR [40–42]. The impact and contribution of MMP-2 and MMP-9 to the onset and progression of DN may be most critical in the earlier phases of the disease process, at a time in which enhanced matrix turnover, release of pro-fibrotic growth factors, and altered cell motility may damage the glomerular apparatus and tubular architecture [43]. In these phases of DN, MMP-9 can predict microalbuminuria several years before its appearance and can be prognostic marker for the renal involvement. In the late period of diabetes, decreased activity of MMP-2 and MMP-9 is observed with increased activity of tissue inhibitor of metalloproteinases-1 (TIMP-1). These leads to excessive deposition of type IV collagen and fibronectin in the BM and a decrease in effective filtration surface area [44]. In the advanced stage of chronic kidney disease, the activity of MMP-2 and MMP-9 is decreased and, in this late period, the fibrosis is difficult to reverse [45]. On the other hand, MMP-2 and MMP-9 are involved in the process of atherogenesis and development of arterial lesions in T2D [46,47]. They are synthesized in atheromatous plaques and are present at elevated levels in rupture-prone regions of arterial blood vessels. MMP-2 and MMP-9 were both correlated with plaque instability and there was a correlation between increased MMP-9 expression and cap rupture [48]. Plasma levels and zymographic activities of MMP-2 and MMP-9 are increased in T2D patients with peripheral arterial disease in comparison with healthy control subjects, and MMP-9 may be a useful marker for development of macrovascular complications in T2D [34].

EL fibers are essential structural elements of the vascular wall, especially of the arteries. They are considered the most resilient element of vascular ECM. The EL half-life is in the order of 40 years. [49]. Elastases are endopeptidases that cleave EL, resulting in the formation of EDPs. Elastases include serine- and cysteine- proteinases and four MMPs—MMP-2, MMP-9, MMP-7 (matrilysin), and MMP-12 (macrophage elastase) [50]. T2D is associated with an increase in the expression and activity of MMP-2 and MMP-9, and an increase generation of EDPs [51,52]. EDPs have immunogenic properties and favor the formation of specific AEAbs from IgM, IgG and IgA classes [53]. The presence of AEAbs can lead to the formation of circulating immune complexes and complement activation and K-cell-mediated antibody dependent cytotoxicity, which may further contribute to the destruction of EL in the arterial wall. This process can be maintained by specific T- and B-lymphocytes at sites of arterial damage [21,54,55]. When we compared the serum levels of AEAbs IgM, AEAbs IgG, and AEAbs

IgA in T2D patients with those of non-diabetic subjects, we observed significant increases in AEAbs IgA (Figure 2A), whereas the levels of AEAbs IgM and AEAbs IgG were decreased (Figure 2C,D). This feature of the humoral immune response, with the prevalence of higher serum levels of general or specific IgA Abs in diabetic patients, is a generalized phenomenon documented in a number of studies [56–59]. In one of these, the patients with T1D and T2D with micro- or macrovascular complications have had higher serum IgA concentrations than the corresponding groups of patients without complications. Furthermore, the patients with three kinds of microangiopathy had slightly higher IgA levels than patients with only one kind; those with nephropathy and hypertension had even higher levels. The macroangiopathy groups have shown the highest IgA levels among the T2D subgroups with complications, and the lowest among the T1D subgroups. These data suggest that monitoring IgA may provide early warning of the possible presence simultaneously of micro- or macrovascular complications in T2D [56]. Studies in T2D patients have also shown that poor glycemic control may be associated with an increase in serum IgA Abs [60]. Our results provide compelling evidence for this and show that the levels of AEAbs IgA are influenced by the degree of glycaemic control reflect by measurement of HbA1c (Figure 2B). In patients with poor glycemic control and increased vascular risk, who have HbA1c values >7.5%, AEAb IgA levels were significantly increased compared to those with better control and HbA1c values ≤7.5%. Similar to total IgA [56], an increase in AEAb IgA levels may indicate increased degradation of EL in the vascular wall and may be a specific marker for micro- or macrovascular damage in T2D [21,22]. These findings are also supported by the positive correlations that we found between AEAbs IgA and AEAbs IgM, AEAbs IgG, ACIVAbs IgM, and the CIV-DP. AEAbs also showed significant negative correlations with SBP, DBP, and BMI in the T2D group (Table 3).

CIV represents up to 50% of all BM proteins [61]. Unlike fibrillar COLs of type I, II, and III, CIV forms a network structure and it is found to be crucial for vascular BM assembly and stability [62]. MMP-2 and MMP-9 can cleave most of the major macromolecules of the ECM, including COL types IV, V, VII, and X. Processing of CIV gives rise to the release of fragments that are able to behave as epitopes since they can be bound by circulating Abs [63]. Autoantibodies (autoAbs) against CIV are present in various inflammatory and autoimmune diseases [64]. This is the case of recurrent Goodpasture's disease secondary to an autoreactive IgA Ab [63,65]. Moreover, autoAbs against CIV have been detected in children with T1D and vascular complications [66,67], as well as in hypertensive T2D patients with microangiopathy [19]. When we compared the serum levels of ACIVAbs IgM and CIV-DP, they were significantly lower in the patient group than in the control subjects (Figure 3A,B). A possible explanation for this result is that the levels and activity of MMP-9 in chronic hyperglycemia (HbA1c values >7.5%) are decreased, which leads to excessive deposition of CIV in the vascular BM and to its thickening [68]. Vascular BM thickening is the most characteristic structural abnormality of small blood vessels in DR and DN [69]. In addition, the highest HbA1c values exhibited the highest BM thickness in both the retinal and glomerular capillaries, which was observed in diabetic rats [70]. We also found positive correlations between ACIVAbs IgM and AEAbs IgM, between ACIVAbs IgM and AEAbs IgA, and between the CIV-DP and AEAbs IgA in the T2D group (Table 3).

Strengths of our study, unlike retrospective epidemiological studies, are that it reflects the direct relationship of hyperglycemia with vascular changes through the levels of appropriately selected biomarkers. Also, a design has been used in which the division of biomarkers into groups according to the degree of glycemic control (HbA1c levels) can provide valuable information on the vascular status of patients. A limitation of the study is the relatively small number studied persons, which requires these results to be confirmed in larger studies.

5. Conclusions

Considering the broad informativeness of the HbA1 test, it can be successfully applied to the management and assessment of overall vascular risk in patients with diabetes. Our results give the highest indication of vascular change (set of three assessment markers, MMP-2, MMP-9, and AEAbs IgA) at a cut-off HbA1c value of 7.5%. This indicates that vascular damage from preceding long-term hyperglycemia begins to dominate at HbA1c values ≥7.5%, which is the likely cut-off point to predict increased vascular risk.

Author Contributions: Conceptualization, software, formal analysis, writing—review and editing, visualization, K.K.; methodology, resources, A.B. All authors have read and agreed to the published version of the manuscript.

Funding: This study was accomplished with the financial support of the Medical University, Pleven.

Conflicts of Interest: The authors declare no conflict of interest.

References

1. Kostov, K. Effects of Magnesium Deficiency on Mechanisms of Insulin Resistance in Type 2 Diabetes: Focusing on the Processes of Insulin Secretion and Signaling. *Int. J. Mol. Sci.* **2019**, *20*, 1351. [CrossRef] [PubMed]
2. Nowak, C.; Carlsson, A.C.; Östgren, C.J.; Nyström, F.H.; Alam, M.; Feldreich, T.; Sundström, J.; Carrero, J.J.; Leppert, J.; Hedberg, P.; et al. Multiplex proteomics for prediction of major cardiovascular events in type 2 diabetes. *Diabetologia* **2018**, *61*, 1748–1757. [CrossRef] [PubMed]
3. Kohnert, K.D.; Heinke, P.; Zander, E.; Vogt, L.; Salzsieder, E. Glycemic Key Metrics and the Risk of Diabetes-Associated Complications. *Rom. J. Diabetes Nutr. Metab. Dis.* **2016**, *23*, 403–413. [CrossRef]
4. Lyons, T.J.; Basu, A. Biomarkers in diabetes: Hemoglobin A1c, vascular and tissue markers. *Transl. Res.* **2012**, *159*, 303–312. [CrossRef] [PubMed]
5. Keating, S.T.; Van Diepen, J.A.; Riksen, N.P.; El-Osta, A. Epigenetics in diabetic nephropathy, immunity and metabolism. *Diabetologia* **2018**, *61*, 6–20. [CrossRef] [PubMed]
6. Qaseem, A.; Wilt, T.J.; Kansagara, D.; Horwitch, C.; Barry, M.J.; Forciea, M.A. Hemoglobin A1c targets for glycemic control with pharmacologic therapy for nonpregnant adults with type 2 diabetes mellitus: A guidance statement update from the American College of Physicians. *Ann. Intern. Med.* **2018**, *168*, 569–576. [CrossRef]
7. Little, R.R.; Rohlfing, C.L.; Sacks, D.B. Status of hemoglobin A1c measurement and goals for improvement: From chaos to order for improving diabetes care. *Clin. Chem.* **2011**, *57*, 205–214. [CrossRef]
8. Juraschek, S.P.; Steffes, M.W.; Miller, E.R.; Selvin, E. Alternative markers of hyperglycemia and risk of diabetes. *Diabetes Care* **2012**, *35*, 2265–2270. [CrossRef]
9. Makris, K.; Spanou, L. Is there a relationship between mean blood glucose and glycated hemoglobin? *J. Diabetes Sci. Technol.* **2011**, *5*, 1572–1583. [CrossRef]
10. Khaw, K.T.; Wareham, N. Glycated hemoglobin as a marker of cardiovascular risk. *Curr. Opin. Lipidol.* **2006**, *17*, 637–643. [CrossRef]
11. American Diabetes Association. 2. Classification and Diagnosis of Diabetes: Standards of Medical Care in Diabetes—2020. *Diabetes Care* **2020**, *43*, S14–S31. [CrossRef] [PubMed]
12. American Diabetes Association. 6. Glycemic Targets: Standards of Medical Care in Diabetes—2020. *Diabetes Care* **2020**, *43*, S66–S76. [CrossRef] [PubMed]
13. Bachmann, K.N.; Wang, T.J. Biomarkers of cardiovascular disease: Contributions to risk prediction in individuals with diabetes. *Diabetologia* **2018**, *61*, 987–995. [CrossRef] [PubMed]
14. Kostov, K.; Blazhev, A.; Atanasova, M.; Dimitrova, A. Serum concentrations of endothelin-1 and matrix metalloproteinases-2,-9 in pre-hypertensive and hypertensive patients with type 2 diabetes. *Int. J. Mol. Sci.* **2016**, *17*, 1182. [CrossRef]
15. Singh, V.P.; Bali, A.; Singh, N.; Jaggi, A.S. Advanced glycation end products and diabetic complications. *Korean J. Physiol. Pharmacol.* **2014**, *18*, 1–14. [CrossRef]
16. Herouy, Y. The role of matrix metalloproteinases (MMPs) and their inhibitors in venous leg ulcer healing. *Phlebolymphology* **2004**, *44*, 231–243.
17. Thrailkill, K.M.; Bunn, R.C.; Moreau, C.S.; Cockrell, G.E.; Simpson, P.M.; Coleman, H.N.; Frindik, J.P.; Kemp, S.F.; Fowlkes, J.L. Matrix metalloproteinase-2 dysregulation in type 1 diabetes. *Diabetes Care* **2007**, *30*, 2321–2326. [CrossRef]
18. Kridel, S.J.; Chen, E.; Kotra, L.P.; Howard, E.W.; Mobashery, S.; Smith, J.W. Substrate hydrolysis by matrix metalloproteinase-9. *J. Biol. Chem.* **2001**, *276*, 20572–20578. [CrossRef]

19. Nikolov, A.G.; Nicoloff, G.; Tsinlikov, I.; Tsinlikova, I. Anti-collagen type IV antibodies and the development of microvascular complications in diabetic patients with arterial hypertension. *J. IMAB* **2012**, *18*, 315–322. [CrossRef]
20. Gatseva, A.; Sin, Y.Y.; Brezzo, G.; Van Agtmael, T. Basement membrane collagens and disease mechanisms. *Essays Biochem.* **2019**, *63*, 297–312.
21. Nikolov, A.; Nicoloff, G.; Tsinlikov, I.; Tsinlikova, I.; Blazhev, A.; Angelova, M.; Garev, A. Relationship between anti-elastin IgA and development of microvascular complications: A study in diabetic patients with arterial hypertension. *Diabetol. Croat.* **2013**, *41*, 103–111.
22. Nikolov, A.; Tsinlikov, I.; Tsinlikova, I.; Nicoloff, G.; Blazhev, A.; Garev, A. Levels of anti-elastin IgA antibodies are associated with high risk of atherosclerosis in diabetics with essential hypertension. *Atherosclerosis* **2017**, *263*, e124–e125. [CrossRef]
23. Baydanoff, S.; Nicoloff, G.; Alexiev, C. Age-related changes in the level of circulating elastin-derived peptides in serum from normal and atherosclerotic subjects. *Atherosclerosis* **1987**, *66*, 163–168. [CrossRef]
24. Care, D. 6. Glycemic Targets: Standards of Medical Care in Diabetes—2019. *Diabetes Care* **2019**, *42*, S61–S70.
25. Sandler, C.N.; McDonnell, M.E. The role of hemoglobin A1c in the assessment of diabetes and cardiovascular risk. *Cleve. Clin. J. Med.* **2016**, *83*, S4–S10. [CrossRef] [PubMed]
26. Cavero-Redondo, I.; Peleteiro, B.; Álvarez-Bueno, C.; Rodriguez-Artalejo, F.; Martínez-Vizcaíno, V. Glycated haemoglobin A1c as a risk factor of cardiovascular outcomes and all-cause mortality in diabetic and non-diabetic populations: A systematic review and meta-analysis. *BMJ Open* **2017**, *7*, e015949. [CrossRef]
27. UK Prospective Diabetes Study (UKPDS) Group. Effect of intensive blood-glucose control with metformin on complications in overweight patients with type 2 diabetes (UKPDS 34). *Lancet* **1998**, *352*, 854–865. [CrossRef]
28. UK Prospective Diabetes Study (UKPDS) Group. Intensive blood-glucose control with sulphonylureas or insulin compared with conventional treatment and risk of complications in patients with type 2 diabetes (UKPDS 33). *Lancet* **1998**, *352*, 837–853. [CrossRef]
29. Ohkubo, Y.; Kishikawa, H.; Araki, E.; Miyata, T.; Isami, S.; Motoyoshi, S.; Kojima, Y.; Furuyoshi, N.; Shichiri, M. Intensive insulin therapy prevents the progression of diabetic microvascular complications in Japanese patients with non-insulin-dependent diabetes mellitus: A randomized prospective 6-year study. *Diabetes Res. Clin. Pract.* **1995**, *28*, 103–117. [CrossRef]
30. Diabetes Control and Complications Trial Research Group. The effect of intensive treatment of diabetes on the development and progression of long-term complications in insulin-dependent diabetes mellitus. *N. Engl. J. Med.* **1993**, *329*, 977–986. [CrossRef]
31. Zoungas, S.; Chalmers, J.; Ninomiya, T.; Li, Q.; Cooper, M.E.; Colagiuri, S.; Fulcher, G.; de Galan, B.E.; Harrap, S.; Hamet, P.; et al. Association of HbA1c levels with vascular complications and death in patients with type 2 diabetes: Evidence of glycaemic thresholds. *Diabetologia* **2012**, *55*, 636–643. [CrossRef] [PubMed]
32. Currie, C.J.; Peters, J.R.; Tynan, A.; Evans, M.; Heine, R.J.; Bracco, O.L.; Zagar, T.; Poole, C.D. Survival as a function of HbA1c in people with type 2 diabetes: A retrospective cohort study. *Lancet* **2010**, *375*, 481–489. [CrossRef]
33. Derosa, G.; D'angelo, A.; Tinelli, C.; Devangelio, E.; Consoli, A.; Miccoli, R.; Penno, G.; Del Prato, S.; Paniga, S.; Cicero, A.F.G. Evaluation of metalloproteinase 2 and 9 levels and their inhibitors in diabetic and healthy subjects. *Diabetes Metab.* **2007**, *33*, 129–134. [CrossRef] [PubMed]
34. Signorelli, S.S.; Malaponte, G.; Libra, M.; Di Pino, L.; Celotta, G.; Bevelacqua, V.; Petrina, M.; Nicotra, G.S.; Indelicato, M.; Navolanic, P.M.; et al. Plasma levels and zymographic activities of matrix metalloproteinases 2 and 9 in type II diabetics with peripheral arterial disease. *Vasc. Med.* **2005**, *10*, 1–6. [CrossRef] [PubMed]
35. Derosa, G.; Avanzini, M.A.; Geroldi, D.; Fogari, R.; Lorini, R.; De Silvestri, A.; Tinelli, C.; d'Annunzio, G. Matrix metalloproteinase 2 may be a marker of microangiopathy in children and adolescents with type 1 diabetes. *Diabetes Care* **2004**, *27*, 273–275. [CrossRef] [PubMed]
36. Mohammad, G.; Siddiquei, M.M. Role of matrix metalloproteinase-2 and -9 in the development of diabetic retinopathy. *J. Ocul. Biol. Dis. Inform.* **2012**, *5*, 1–8. [CrossRef] [PubMed]
37. Giebel, S.J.; Menicucci, G.; McGuire, P.G.; Das, A. Matrix metalloproteinases in early diabetic retinopathy and their role in alteration of the blood–retinal barrier. *Lab. Investig.* **2005**, *85*, 597–607. [CrossRef]
38. Kowluru, R.A.; Zhong, Q.; Santos, J.M. Matrix metalloproteinases in diabetic retinopathy: Potential role of MMP-9. *Expert Opin. Investig. Drugs* **2012**, *21*, 797–805. [CrossRef]

39. Kłysik, A.B.; Naduk-Kik, J.; Hrabec, Z.; Goś, R.; Hrabec, E. Intraocular matrix metalloproteinase 2 and 9 in patients with diabetes mellitus with and without diabetic retinopathy. *Arch. Med. Sci.* **2010**, *6*, 375–381. [CrossRef]
40. Kwon, J.W.; Choi, J.A.; Jee, D. Matrix metalloproteinase-1 and matrix metalloproteinase-9 in the aqueous humor of diabetic macular edema patients. *PLoS ONE* **2016**, *11*, e0159720. [CrossRef]
41. Das, A.; McGuire, P.G.; Rangasamy, S. Diabetic macular edema: Pathophysiology and novel therapeutic targets. *Ophthalmology* **2015**, *122*, 1375–1394. [CrossRef] [PubMed]
42. Noda, K.; Ishida, S.; Inoue, M.; Obata, K.I.; Oguchi, Y.; Okada, Y.; Ikeda, E. Production and activation of matrix metalloproteinase-2 in proliferative diabetic retinopathy. *Investig. Ophthalmol. Vis. Sci.* **2003**, *44*, 2163–2170. [CrossRef] [PubMed]
43. Thrailkill, K.M.; Bunn, R.C.; Fowlkes, J.L. Matrix metalloproteinases: Their potential role in the pathogenesis of diabetic nephropathy. *Endocrine* **2009**, *35*, 1–10. [CrossRef] [PubMed]
44. Rogowicz, A.; Zozulińska, D.; Wierusz-Wysocka, B. The role of matrix metalloproteinases in the development of vascular complications of diabetes mellitus-clinical implications. *Pol. Arch. Med. Wewn.* **2007**, *117*, 43–48. [CrossRef] [PubMed]
45. Cheng, Z.; Limbu, M.; Wang, Z.; Liu, J.; Liu, L.; Zhang, X.; Chen, P.; Liu, B. MMP-2 and 9 in chronic kidney disease. *Int. J. Mol. Sci.* **2017**, *18*, 776. [CrossRef] [PubMed]
46. Newby, A.C. Metalloproteinases and vulnerable atherosclerotic plaques. *Trends Cardiovasc. Med.* **2007**, *17*, 253–258. [CrossRef]
47. Pasterkamp, G.; Schoneveld, A.H.; Hijnen, D.J.; De Kleijn, D.P.; Teepen, H.; Van Der Wal, A.C.; Borst, C. Atherosclerotic arterial remodeling and the localization of macrophages and matrix metalloproteases 1, 2 and 9 in the human coronary artery. *Atherosclerosis* **2000**, *150*, 245–253. [CrossRef]
48. Heo, S.H.; Cho, C.H.; Kim, H.O.; Jo, Y.H.; Yoon, K.S.; Lee, J.H.; Park, J.C.; Park, K.C.; Ahn, T.B.; Chung, K.C.; et al. Plaque rupture is a determinant of vascular events in carotid artery atherosclerotic disease: Involvement of matrix metalloproteinases 2 and 9. *J. Clin. Neurol.* **2011**, *7*, 69–76. [CrossRef]
49. Briones, A.M.; Arribas, S.M.; Salaices, M. Role of extracellular matrix in vascular remodeling of hypertension. *Curr. Opin. Nephrol. Hypertens.* **2010**, *19*, 187–194. [CrossRef]
50. Duca, L.; Blaise, S.; Romier, B.; Laffargue, M.; Gayral, S.; El Btaouri, H.; Kawecki, C.; Guillot, A.; Martiny, L.; Debelle, L.; et al. Matrix ageing and vascular impacts: Focus on elastin fragmentation. *Cardiovasc. Res.* **2016**, *110*, 298–308. [CrossRef]
51. Blaise, S.; Romier, B.; Kawecki, C.; Ghirardi, M.; Rabenoelina, F.; Baud, S.; Duca, L.; Maurice, P.; Heinz, A.; Schmelzer, C.E.; et al. Elastin-derived peptides are new regulators of insulin resistance development in mice. *Diabetes* **2013**, *62*, 3807–3816. [CrossRef] [PubMed]
52. Uemura, S.; Matsushita, H.; Li, W.; Glassford, A.J.; Asagami, T.; Lee, K.H.; Harrison, D.G.; Tsao, P.S. Diabetes mellitus enhances vascular matrix metalloproteinase activity: Role of oxidative stress. *Circ. Res.* **2001**, *88*, 1291–1298. [CrossRef] [PubMed]
53. Fülöp, J.T.; Wei, S.M.; Robert, L.; Jacob, M.P. Determination of elastin peptides in normal and arteriosclerotic human sera by ELISA. *Clin. Physiol. Biochem.* **1990**, *8*, 273–282. [PubMed]
54. Peterszegi, G.; Mandet, C.; Texier, S.; Robert, L.; Bruneval, P. Lymphocytes in human atherosclerotic plaque exhibit the elastin-laminin receptor: Potential role in atherogenesis. *Atherosclerosis* **1997**, *135*, 103–107. [CrossRef]
55. Péterszegi, G.; Texier, S.; Robert, L. Human helper and memory lymphocytes exhibit an inducible elastin-laminin receptor. *Int. Arch. Allergy Immunol.* **1997**, *114*, 218–223. [CrossRef]
56. Rodriguez-Segade, S.; Camina, M.F.; Carnero, A.; Lorenzo, M.J.; Alban, A.; Quinteiro, C.; Lojo, S. High serum IgA concentrations in patients with diabetes mellitus: Agewise distribution and relation to chronic complications. *Clin. Chem.* **1996**, *42*, 1064–1067. [CrossRef]
57. Ohmuro, H.; Tomino, Y.; Tsushima, Y.; Shimizu, M.; Kuramoto, T.; Koide, H. Elevation of serum IgA1 levels in patients with diabetic nephropathy. *Nephron* **1993**, *63*, 355. [CrossRef]
58. Vavuli, S.; Salonurmi, T.; Loukovaara, S.; Nissinen, A.E.; Savolainen, M.J.; Liinamaa, M.J. Elevated levels of plasma IgA autoantibodies against oxidized LDL found in proliferative diabetic retinopathy but not in nonproliferative retinopathy. *J. Diabetes Res.* **2016**, *2016*, 2614153. [CrossRef]

59. Guo, X.; Meng, G.; Liu, F.; Zhang, Q.; Liu, L.; Wu, H.; Du, H.; Shi, H.; Xia, Y.; Liu, X.; et al. Serum levels of immunoglobulins in an adult population and their relationship with type 2 diabetes. *Diabetes Res. Clin. Pract.* **2016**, *115*, 76–82. [CrossRef]
60. Awartani, F. Serum immunoglobulin levels in type 2 diabetes patients with chronic periodontitis. *J. Contemp. Dent. Pract.* **2010**, *11*, 1–8. [CrossRef]
61. Kalluri, R. Basement membranes: Structure, assembly and role in tumour angiogenesis. *Nat. Rev. Cancer* **2003**, *3*, 422–433. [CrossRef] [PubMed]
62. Hayden, M.R.; Sowers, J.R.; Tyagi, S.C. The central role of vascular extracellular matrix and basement membrane remodeling in metabolic syndrome and type 2 diabetes: The matrix preloaded. *Cardiovasc. Diabetol.* **2005**, *4*, 9. [CrossRef] [PubMed]
63. Monaco, S.; Sparano, V.; Gioia, M.; Sbardella, D.; Di Pierro, D.; Marini, S.; Coletta, M. Enzymatic processing of collagen IV by MMP-2 (gelatinase A) affects neutrophil migration and it is modulated by extracatalytic domains. *Protein Sci.* **2006**, *15*, 2805–2815. [CrossRef] [PubMed]
64. McLeod, O.; Dunér, P.; Samnegård, A.; Tornvall, P.; Nilsson, J.; Hamsten, A.; Bengtsson, E. Autoantibodies against basement membrane collagen type IV are associated with myocardial infarction. *Int. J. Cardiol. Heart Vasc.* **2015**, *6*, 42–47. [CrossRef]
65. Borza, D.B.; Chedid, M.F.; Colon, S.; Lager, D.J.; Leung, N.; Fervenza, F.C. Recurrent Goodpasture's disease secondary to a monoclonal IgA1-κ antibody autoreactive with the α1/α2 chains of type IV collagen. *Am. J. Kidney Dis.* **2005**, *45*, 397–406. [CrossRef]
66. Nicoloff, G.; Baydanoff, S.; Petrova, C.; Christova, P. Serum antibodies to collagen type IV and development of diabetic vascular complications in children with type 1 (insulin-dependent) diabetes mellitus: A longitudinal study. *Vascul. Pharmacol.* **2002**, *38*, 143–147. [CrossRef]
67. Nicoloff, G.; Baydanoff, S.; Stanimirova, N.; Petrova, C.; Christova, P. Detection of serum collagen type IV in children with type 1 (insulin-dependent) diabetes mellitus–a longitudinal study. *Pediatr. Diabetes* **2001**, *2*, 184–190. [CrossRef]
68. Ban, C.R.; Twigg, S.M. Fibrosis in diabetes complications: Pathogenic mechanisms and circulating and urinary markers. *Vasc. Health Risk Manag.* **2008**, *4*, 575–596.
69. Roy, S.; Ha, J.; Trudeau, K.; Beglova, E. Vascular basement membrane thickening in diabetic retinopathy. *Curr. Eye Res.* **2010**, *35*, 1045–1056. [CrossRef]
70. Cherian, S.; Roy, S.; Pinheiro, A.; Roy, S. Tight glycemic control regulates fibronectin expression and basement membrane thickening in retinal and glomerular capillaries of diabetic rats. *Investig. Ophthalmol. Vis. Sci.* **2009**, *50*, 943–949. [CrossRef]

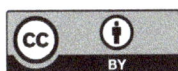

© 2020 by the authors. Licensee MDPI, Basel, Switzerland. This article is an open access article distributed under the terms and conditions of the Creative Commons Attribution (CC BY) license (http://creativecommons.org/licenses/by/4.0/).

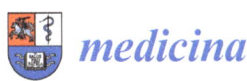

Article

Clinical Predictors of Preeclampsia in Pregnant Women with Chronic Kidney Disease

Bogdan Marian Sorohan [1,2], Andreea Andronesi [1,2], Gener Ismail [1,2,*], Roxana Jurubita [1,2], Bogdan Obrisca [1,2], Cătălin Baston [1,3] and Mihai Harza [1,3]

[1] Department of General Medicine, Carol Davila University of Medicine and Pharmacy, 050474 Bucharest, Romania; bogdan.sorohan@yahoo.com (B.M.S); andreea.andronesi@yahoo.com (A.A); roxana_jurubita@yahoo.com (R.J.); obriscabogdan@yahoo.com (B.O.); drcbaston@gmail.com (C.B.); mihai.harza@gmail.com (M.H.)
[2] Nephrology Department, Fundeni Clinical Institute, 022328 Bucharest, Romania
[3] Center of Uronephrology and Renal Transplantation, Fundeni Clinical Institute, 022328 Bucharest, Romania
* Correspondence: gener732000@yahoo.com

Received: 11 March 2020; Accepted: 24 April 2020; Published: 27 April 2020

Abstract: *Background and Objectives*: Pregnant women with chronic kidney disease (CKD) are at high risk of adverse maternal and fetal outcomes. Preeclampsia (PE) superimposed on CKD is estimated to occur in 21%–79% of pregnancies. Both conditions share common features such as proteinuria and hypertension, making differential diagnosis difficult. Objective: The aim of this study was to evaluate the incidence and the clinical-biological predictors of preeclampsia in pregnant women with CKD. *Material and Methods*: We retrospectively analyzed 34 pregnant women with pre-existing CKD admitted to our department between 2008 and 2017. *Results*: Among the 34 patients, 19 (55.8%) developed PE and the mean time of occurrence was 31.26 ± 2.68 weeks of gestation. The median value of 24-h proteinuria at referral was 0.87 g/day (interquartile range 0.42–1.50) and 47.1% of patients had proteinuria of ≥1 g/day. Patients with PE tended to be more hypertensive, with a more decreased renal function at referral and had significantly higher proteinuria (1.30 vs. 0.63 g/day, $p = 0.02$). Cox multivariate analysis revealed that proteinuria ≥1 g/day at referral and pre-existing hypertension were independently associated with PE (adjusted hazard ratio = 4.10, 95% confidence interval: 1.52–11.02, $p = 0.005$, adjusted hazard ratio = 2.62, 95% confidence interval: 1.01–6.77, $p = 0.04$, respectively). The cumulative risk of PE was significantly higher in pregnant women with proteinuria ≥1 g/day at referral (log-rank, $p = 0.003$). Proteinuria ≥ 1 g/day at referral and pre-exiting hypertension predicted PE development with accuracies of 73.5% and 64.7%, respectively. *Conclusions*: Pregnant patients with pre-existing CKD are at high risk of developing preeclampsia, while proteinuria ≥ 1 g/day at referral and pre-existing hypertension were independent predictors of superimposed preeclampsia.

Keywords: chronic kidney disease; preeclampsia; hypertension; proteinuria

1. Introduction

Pregnant women with chronic kidney disease (CKD) are at high risk of adverse maternal and fetal outcomes, such as preeclampsia, low birth weight and death, even in cases of mild CKD [1,2]. Moreover, pregnancy itself is a risk factor for CKD progression [3]. Preeclampsia is both a systemic and hypertensive disorder in pregnancy. Estimated to complicate 2–8% of all pregnancies, it is a leading cause of maternal and perinatal morbidity and mortality [4]. According to previous studies, preeclampsia superimposed on chronic hypertension and CKD are estimated to occur in 26% and 21–79% of pregnancies, respectively [5,6]. Preeclampsia superimposed on CKD is challenging for the clinician because both conditions share common features such as proteinuria and hypertension, making differential diagnosis difficult [7]. There is some evidence regarding biomarkers associated with preeclampsia in pregnant women with CKD, but further studies are needed in this regard [8]. The aim of this study was to evaluate the incidence and clinical and biological predictors of preeclampsia in pregnant women with CKD.

2. Materials and Methods

2.1. Study Population

We conducted a retrospective cohort study which included all pregnant women with pre-existing CKD that were referred to our department, between 2008 and 2017. Exclusion criteria were: Absence of CKD diagnosis, absence of pregnancy, referral to our department after 20 weeks' gestation and loss to follow-up. The final study population included 34 pregnant women with pre-existing CKD, out of 652 women of childbearing age monitored in our clinic between 2008–2017. All patients read and signed the informed consent form. The study was conducted in accordance with the Declaration of Helsinki, and the protocol was approved by the Ethics Committee of Fundeni Clinical Institute (No. 39622/ 12 December 2017).

2.2. Definitions

Preeclampsia was defined according to American College of Obstetricians and Gynecologists (ACOG) Task Force on Hypertension in Pregnancy (2013) and the revised statement (2014) of the International Society for the Study of Hypertension in Pregnancy (ISSHP) [9,10]. We considered the diagnosis of preeclampsia in CKD patients in every pregnant woman with pre-existing CKD who developed hypertension (≥140 mmHg systolic pressure or ≥90 mmHg diastolic pressure) after 20 weeks of gestation or a sudden exacerbation of preexisting hypertension or the need to improve antihypertensive therapy, plus the coexistence of one or more of the following new-onset conditions: proteinuria ≥ 300 mg/day or a significant sustained increase of preexisting proteinuria; liver involvement (elevated transaminases and/or severe right upper quadrant or epigastric pain); neurological complications (eclampsia, altered mental status, blindness, stroke, hyperreflexia when accompanied by clonus, severe headaches when accompanied by hyperreflexia, persistent visual scotomata); hematological complications (thrombocytopenia, disseminated intravascular coagulation, hemolysis); and fetal growth restriction. CKD was defined according to Kidney Disease Improving Global Outcomes (KDIGO) guidelines [11]. Referral was defined as the first visit of the patients to our clinic, between the beginning of pregnancy and week 20 of gestation.

2.3. Measurements

Clinical and biological parameters were collected from paper and electronic medical records. Renal function was evaluated based on serum creatinine and estimated with CKD-EPI formula. Proteinuria was measured from 24-h urine samples and reported in grams/day. Blood pressure was recorded by mercury sphygmomanometry and for the diagnosis of hypertension two determinations at least 4 h apart were taken into consideration.

2.4. Statistical Analysis

Values are reported as percentages for categorical data, mean ± SD for continuous parametric data, and median with interquartile range (IQR) for continuous nonparametric data. The chi-square, Student t-test, and Mann–Whitney U were used to evaluate the differences between groups. To analyze the clinical and biological determinants of superimposed preeclampsia, Cox regression analysis was performed, which included all the variables with $p \leq 0.10$ from the group comparison. The final variables in the model were then selected using a stepwise backward elimination process. Kaplan–Meier curves were used to determine the cumulative risk of preeclampsia and the risk difference was analyzed via the log-rank test. To test the predictive ability of the variables, we calculated the sensitivity, specificity, positive predictive value, negative predictive value, positive likelihood ratio, negative likelihood ratio, and accuracy. A p-value of <0.05 was considered statistically significant. Statistical analysis was performed with SPSS version 20 (SPSS Inc., Chicago, IL, USA) and STATA version 14 (StataCorp, College Station, TX, USA).

3. Results

3.1. Characteristics of the Study Group

Among the 34 pregnant patients with CKD, 19 (55.8%) developed preeclampsia, 26 (76.5%) had CKD stages 3-4, and the mean time of occurrence was at 31.26 ± 2.68 weeks of gestation. The mean maternal age was 24 ± 3.96 years and 3 (8.8%) patients were over 30 years old. The frequency of nulliparity in our group was 85.3%. The mean value of creatinine at referral was 1.6 ± 0.6 mg/dL. The median 24-h proteinuria at referral was 0.87 g/day (IQR 0.42–1.50) and 47.1% of patients had proteinuria of ≥1 g/day. The most frequent primary disease for CKD was glomerulonephritis (76.5%). Eight patients (23.5%) had a body mass index (BMI) of ≥25 kg/m^2 and half of the patients (50%) had pre-existing hypertension. None of our patients had a history of preeclampsia and there were no patients with CKD stage G5 (Table 1). Sixteen out of 19 (84.2%) patients developed PE < 34 weeks of gestation (early-onset PE) and in 3/19 (15.8%), PE occurred ≥ 34 weeks of gestation (late-onset PE).

Table 1. Characteristics of the study group.

Patients Characteristics	Overall (N = 34)	Preeclampsia (N = 19)	No Preeclampsia (N = 15)	p-value
Maternal age (mean, years)	24.26± 3.96	23.15±2.31	25.66±5.13	0.06
≥30 years (%)	3 (8.8%)	0 (%)	3 (20%)	0.02 [a]
Nulliparity (%)	29 (85.3%)	18 (94.7%)	11 (73.3%)	0.07
BMI (mean, kg/m^2)	21.91±3.36	22.28±3.26	21.45±3.54	0.48
≥25 kg/m^2 (%)	8 (23.5%)	4 (21.1%)	4 (26.7%)	0.70
Primary kidney disease (%)	26 (76.5%)	16 (84.2%)	10 (66.7%)	
Glomerulonephritis Tubulointerstitial disease (%)	5 (14.7%)	2 (10.5%)	3 (20%)	0.20
Diabetic kidney disease (%)	3 (8.8%)	1 (5.3%)	2 (13.3%)	
Pre-existing hypertension (%)	17 (50%)	12 (63.2%)	5 (33.3%)	0.08
Dyslipidemia (%)	9 (26.5%)	6 (31.6%)	3 (20%)	0.44
Hepatitis B virus infection (%)	3 (8.8%)	2(10.5%)	1(6.7%)	0.69
Hepatitis C virus infection (%)	3 (8.8%)	1 (5.3%)	2 (13.3%)	0.41
Urinary tract infections (%)	17 (50%)	11 (57.9%)	6 (40%)	0.30
Creatinine at referral (mean, mg/dL)	1.6 ±0.6	1.79±0.75	1.36±0.40	0.05
Creatinine at birth (mean, mg/dL)	1.6±0.8	1.93±0.98	1.20±0.33	0.01 [a]
eGFR at referral (mean, mL/min)	51.2± 22.8	46.16± 22.65	57.65±22	0.14
eGFR at birth (mean, mL/min)	51.5±21.8	42.62± 18	62.79± 21.4	0.005 [a]
CKD stage (%)				0.23
G1-G2	8 (23.5%)	3 (15.8%)	5 (33.3%)	
G3-G4	26(76.5%)	16 (84.2%)	10 (66.7%)	
Proteinuria at referral (median, g/24 h)	0.87 (0.42–1.50)	1.30 (0.67–1.50)	0.63 (0.30–0.85)	0.02 [a]
Proteinuria ≥ 1 g/day at referral (%)	16 (47.1%)	13 (68.7%)	3 (20%)	0.005 [a]
Fetal death (%)	1 (3.1%)	1 (5.3%)	0 (0%)	0.27
Low birth weight (%)	17 (50%)	16 (84.2%)	1 (6.7%)	<0.001 [a]

eGFR—estimated glomerular filtration rate; BMI—body mass index; CKD—chronic kidney disease; [a]—statistical significance.

3.2. Comparison between Women With and Without Preeclampsia

The characteristics of the women with superimposed preeclampsia on CKD and the differences between the two groups are summarized in Table 1. Patients with preeclampsia were more likely to be young (23.15 ± 2.31 vs. 25.66 ± 5.13, $p = 0.06$), hypertensive (63.2% vs. 33.3%, $p = 0.08$), dyslipidemic (31.6% vs. 20%, $p = 0.44$), and with decreased renal function at referral (46.16 ± 22.65 vs. 62.79 ± 21.4, $p = 0.005$) compared to those without preeclampsia. Furthermore, the preeclampsia group had significantly higher proteinuria (1.30 (IQR 0.67–1.50) vs. 0.63 (IQR 0.30–0.85) g/day, $p = 0.02$) and

13 of the 19 patients with preeclampsia had proteinuria ≥1 g/day at referral (68.7% vs. 20%, $p = 0.005$). Regarding fetal outcomes, fetal death occurred only in one pregnancy, the event taking place in the preeclampsia group (5.1%) and low birth weight was significantly higher in pregnant women with preeclampsia (84.2% vs. 6.7%, $p < 0.001$).

3.3. Predictors of Superimposed Preeclampsia

To assess variables associated with preeclampsia in CKD patients, Cox regression analysis with stepwise backward selection was performed (Table 2). Variables with $p < 0.10$ at the group comparison were included in the final model.

Table 2. Univariate and multivariate Cox regression analysis of predictors associated with superimposed preeclampsia on chronic kidney disease (CKD).

Variables	Cox Univariate Regression			Cox Multivariate Regression		
	HR	95% CI	p-value	HR	95% CI	p-value
Maternal age	0.88	0.75–1.03	0.12	-	-	-
Nulliparity	4	0.53–30.07	0.17	-	-	-
Creatinine at referral	1.57	0.87–2.73	0.13	-	-	-
Proteinuria ≥ 1 g/day at referral	3.91	3.74–9.98	0.008	4.10	1.52–11.02	0.005
Pre-existing hypertension	2.31	0.90–5.92	0.07	2.62	1.01–6.77	0.04

Cox multivariate regression with backward stepwise selection (variables introduced in the first step: maternal age, nulliparity, creatinine at referral, proteinuria ≥1 g/day at referral, pre-existing hypertension; variables that remained in the last step: proteinuria ≥1 g/day at referral, pre-existing hypertension); HR—hazard ratio; CI—confidence interval.

By univariate Cox analysis, proteinuria ≥ 1 g/day at referral was the only statistically significant variable as a risk factor for preeclampsia ($p = 0.008$), followed by pre-existing hypertension, which presented a tendency of significance ($p = 0.07$). In multivariate Cox analysis, proteinuria ≥1 g/day at referral and pre-existing hypertension after adjustment for age, nulliparity, and creatinine, were independent predictors of preeclampsia. The presence of proteinuria ≥1 g/day at referral and pre-existing hypertension increased the risk of preeclampsia 4.1 times (adjusted HR = 4.10, 95%CI: 1.52–11.02, $p = 0.005$) and 2.6 times (adjusted HR = 2.62, 95%CI: 1.01-6.77, $p = 0.04$), respectively.

In Figure 1A,B, the Kaplan–Meier curves show that the cumulative risk of preeclampsia at 35 and 38 weeks of gestation was significantly higher in pregnant women with proteinuria ≥1 g/day (68% and 81%, respectively) than in those with proteinuria <1 g/day at referral (27% and 34%, respectively) (log-rank, $p = 0.003$) and the cumulative risk of preeclampsia was also higher in pregnant women with pre-existing hypertension (67% and 70%, respectively) than is those without pre-existing hypertension (30% and 43%, respectively) (log-rank, $p = 0.05$).

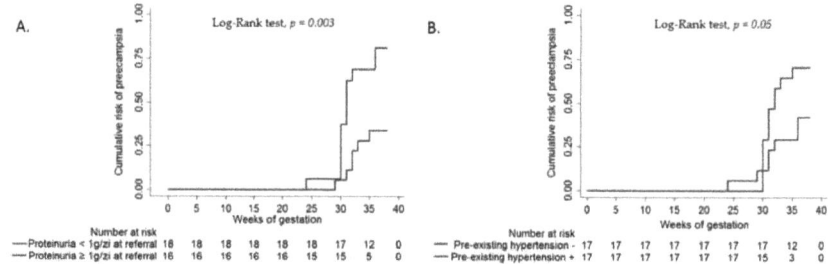

Figure 1. (**A**) Kaplan–Meier curves showing the cumulative risk of preeclampsia in pregnant women with proteinuria ≥1 g/day vs. <1 g/day at referral; (**B**) Kaplan–Meier curves showing the cumulative risk of preeclampsia in pregnant women with vs. without pre-existing hypertension.

We evaluated the predictive ability of the identified risk factors and found that proteinuria ≥1 g/day at referral and pre-existing hypertension could predict preeclampsia in pregnant women with CKD with an accuracy of 73.53% (95%CI: 55.6%–87.1%) and 64.71% (95%CI: 46.5%–80.3%), respectively (Table 3).

Table 3. Predictive analysis of risk factors for preeclampsia.

	Proteinuria ≥ 1 g/day at Referral		Pre-Existing Hypertension	
	Value	95% CI	Value	95% CI
Sensitivity (%)	68.42%	43.45%–87.42%	63.16%	38.36%–83.71%
Specificity (%)	80%	51.91%–95.67%	66.67%	38.38%–88.18%
+LHR	3.42	1.19%–9.85	1.89	0.86%–4.19
-LHR	0.39	0.19%–0.80	0.55	0.28%–1.10
PPV (%)	81.2%	60.09%–92.58%	70.59%	12.04%–84.15%
NPV (%)	66.67%	49.61%–80.25%	58.82%	41.77%–73.99%
Accuracy (%)	73.53%	55.64%–87.12%	64.71%	46.49%–80.25%

CI—confidence interval; LHR—likelihood ratio; PPV—positive predictive value; NPV—negative predictive value.

4. Discussion

Results from our study showed that pregnant women with CKD are at high risk of developing preeclampsia. Superimposed preeclampsia on CKD complicated 55.8% of the pregnancies in our study. This result is in agreement with other studies that reported values between 21% and 79% [6]. Moreover, the frequency of preeclampsia was increased in CKD stages 3–4. The increased incidence of preeclampsia compared to other studies could have been influenced by the diagnostic criteria we used, according to ACOG (2013) and the revised statement of ISSHP (2014), which exclude proteinuria as a mandatory condition for the diagnosis of preeclampsia [9,10]. The mechanisms by which CKD increases the risk of preeclampsia in not completely understood. Some mechanistic processes have been proposed, such as renin-angiotensin-aldosterone system (RAAS) dysregulation, endothelial dysfunction and complement dysregulation [12–14]. We reported no cases of postpartum preeclampsia within the first 6 months and no maternal deaths. However, one fetal death (5.3%) occurred in the preeclampsia group.

We evaluated possible clinical and biological predictors of superimposed preeclampsia in pregnant women with CKD and we found that the presence of proteinuria ≥1 g/day at referral and pre-existing hypertension increased the risk of superimposed preeclampsia 4.1 and 2.6 times, respectively. Other classic risk factors such as nulliparity, maternal age, BMI and the primary cause of CKD were not significantly associated with preeclampsia.

Proteinuria ≥1 g/day at referral was associated with a significantly increased cumulative risk of preeclampsia of 68% and 81% at 35 and 38 weeks respectively. Similar to our results, data from a prospective study, which included 504 pregnant women with CKD, showed that baseline proteinuria ≥1 g/day was an independent risk factor for pregnancy outcomes [15]. Also, data from a cohort study indicated that the proteinuria level at the beginning of pregnancy was strongly associated with subsequent preeclampsia in pregnant women with CKD [16]. A systemic review and meta-analysis which included 23 studies that evaluated the outcomes of pregnancy in CKD and CKD outcomes in pregnancy, demonstrated that proteinuria >0.5 g/day in pregnant women with CKD was a risk factor for superimposed preeclampsia [17]. Evaluation of proteinuria threshold at the time of referral in our study, until 20 weeks of gestation, is an expression of CKD and we proposed this clinical factor as a predictor and not as a diagnostic marker for superimposed preeclampsia.

According to our analysis, 63.2% of patients with preeclampsia had pre-existing hypertension. In agreement with our results, Braham et al reported that chronic hypertension increased the risk of superimposed preeclampsia 7.7 times in the US population and that the estimated incidence of disease was between 21% and 31.5% [5]. Another study by Webster et al. showed that the incidence of preeclampsia in women with chronic hypertension was 21% [18]. The higher percentage of preeclampsia in this subgroup could be explained by the fact that all these patients also had CKD and that a possible intrarenal renin-angiotensin-aldosterone system (RAAS) could be involved. It has been shown that in preeclamptic women, systemic RAAS components have lower circulating levels and there is an increased sensitivity to angiotensin II action, but little is known about the role of intrarenal RAAS [19,20]. Angiotensin II present in the renal tissue could be provided by angiotensinogen action, synthesized locally from tubular epithelial cells [21]. Furthermore, it has been demonstrated that angiotensin II promotes sFlt1 production in proximal tubular cells [22]. Yilmaz et al demonstrated that elevated intrarenal RAAS activity is involved in the development of preeclampsia, using elevated urinary angiotensinogen as a marker of local RAAS activation [23].

The diagnosis of superimposed preeclampsia on CKD is difficult to establish in clinical practice because of the common features shared by CKD and preeclampsia, thus making other parameters necessary for diagnosis. Promising results from previous studies showed that angiogenic (placenta growth factor (PIGF)) and antiangiogenic (soluble fms-like tyrosine kanise-1 (sFlt1)) factors and uteroplacental flows could be used as diagnostic tests for superimposed preeclampsia on CKD. However, they have not been implemented in clinical practice, making further study necessary [24–26]. More recently, plasma and urinary biomarkers derived from endothelial tissue (hyaluronan, intercellular adhesion molecule, vascular cell adhesion molecule, P-selectin, E-selectin), biomarkers of RASS and complement system activation have been studied in pregnant women with CKD. Kate Wiles et al. showed that increased plasma concentration of hyaluronan and vascular cell adhesion molecule had the potential to differentiate between pregnant women with superimposed preeclampsia on CKD and those without superimposed preeclampsia and that endothelial dysfunction had an important role in the pathophysiology of superimposed preeclampsia [13]. Relying on the latest evidence, the diagnostic utility of angiogenic, antiangiogenic and endothelial derived biomarkers in superimposed preeclampsia in CKD pregnant women is recognizable, but they are limited by availability and costs in clinical practice. Therefore, classical factors such as level of proteinuria at referral or pre-existing hypertension may still be useful in assessing the risk for superimposed preeclampsia on CKD [27] and could also contribute to the development of various prognostic tools alongside newly discovered biomarkers.

The strengths of our study are the use of adjusted models in the multivariate analysis and the diagnostic criteria used. However, its limitations such as the retrospective design, small size of the cohort study, and its single-center nature may limit its generalizability. Another limitation of our study that must be mentioned is regarding the selection bias. All patients included in the study had CKD and this could explain the higher incidence of PE than what was reported in other studies.

5. Conclusions

In conclusion, findings from our study indicate that pregnant women with pre-existing chronic kidney disease are at high risk of developing preeclampsia and that proteinuria ≥1 g/day at referral and pre-existing hypertension are independent predictors of superimposed preeclampsia. Consequently, maintaining proteinuria of <1 g/day in women with CKD who want to become pregnant could decrease the risk of preeclampsia. Moreover, women with pre-existing hypertension should be intensively monitored during pregnancy. However, to translate this conclusion into clinical practice is difficult considering the small size of our study population. Thus, larger studies are needed.

Author Contributions: Conceptualization, B.M.S, G.I., C.B and M.H.; Data curation, A.A., R.J. and B.O.; Formal analysis, B.M.S.; Investigation, A.A., R.J. and B.O; Methodology, B.M.S., G.I., C.B. and M.H.; Project administration, B.M.S.; Resources, A.A., R.J. and B.O.; Software, B.M.S.; Validation, A.A., R.J. and B.O.; Visualization, A.A.; Writing—original draft, B.M.S., G.I., C.B. and M.H.; Writing—review and editing, B.M.S., A.A., G.I., R.J., B.O., C.B. and M.H. All authors have read and agreed to the published version of the manuscript.

Funding: This research received no external funding.

Conflicts of Interest: The authors declare no conflict of interest.

References

1. Nevis, I.F.; Reitsma, A.; Dominic, A.; McDonald, S.; Thabane, L.; Akl, E.A.; Hladunewich, M.; Akbari, A.; Joseph, G.; Sia, W.; et al. Pregnancy outcomes in women with chronic kidney disease: A systematic review. *Clin. J. Am. Soc. Nephrol.* **2011**, *6*, 2587–2598. [CrossRef] [PubMed]
2. Piccoli, G.B.; Attini, R.; Vasario, E.; Conijn, A.; Biolcati, M.; D'Amico, F.; Consiglio, V.; Bontempo, S.; Todros, T. Pregnancy and chronic kidney disease: A challenge in all CKD stages. *Clin. J. Am. Soc. Nephrol.* **2010**, *5*, 844–855. [CrossRef] [PubMed]
3. Williams, D.; Davison, J. Chronic kidney disease in pregnancy. *BMJ* **2008**, *336*, 211–215. [CrossRef] [PubMed]
4. Steegers, E.A.; von Dadelszen, P.; Duvekot, J.J.; Pijnenborg, R. Pre-eclampsia. *Lancet* **2010**, *376*, 631–644. [CrossRef]
5. Bramham, K.; Parnell, B.; Nelson-Piercy, C.; Seed, P.T.; Poston, L.; Chappell, L.C. Chronic hypertension and pregnancy outcomes: Systematic review and meta-analysis. *BMJ* **2014**, *348*, g2301. [CrossRef] [PubMed]
6. Hirose, N.; Ohkuchi, A.; Usui, R.; Matsubara, S.; Suzuki, M. Risk of preeclampsia in women with CKD, dialysis or kidney transplantation. *Med. J. Obstet. Gynecol.* **2014**, *2*, 1028.
7. Piccoli, G.B.; Cabiddu, G.; Attini, R.; Vigotti, F.; Fassio, F.; Rolfo, A.; Giuffrida, D.; Pani, A.; Gaglioti, P.; Todros, T. Pregnancy in chronic kidney disease: Questions and answers in a changing panorama. *Best Pract. Res. Clin. Obstet. Gynaecol.* **2015**, *29*, 625–642. [CrossRef]
8. Rolfo, A.; Attini, R.; Nuzzo, A.M.; Piazzese, A.; Parisi, S.; Ferraresi, M.; Todros, T.; Piccoli, G.B. Chronic kidney disease may be differentially diagnosed from preeclampsia by serum biomarkers. *Kidney Int.* **2013**, *83*, 177–181. [CrossRef]
9. American College of Obstetricians and Gynecologists; Task Force on Hypertension in Pregnancy. Hypertension in pregnancy. Report of the American College of Obstetricians and Gynecologists' Task Force on Hypertension in Pregnancy. *Obstet. Gynecol.* **2013**, *122*, 1122–1131.
10. Tranquilli, A.L.; Dekker, G.; Magee, L.; Roberts, J.; Sibai, B.M.; Steyn, W.; Zeeman, G.G.; Brown, M.A. The classification, diagnosis and management of the hypertensive disorders of pregnancy: A revised statement from the ISSHP. *Pregnancy Hypertens.* **2014**, *4*, 97–104. [CrossRef]
11. Kidney Disease: Improving Global Outcomes (KDIGO) CKD Work Group. KDIGO clinical practice guideline for the evaluation and management of chronic kidney disease. *Kidney Int. Suppl.* **2013**, *3*, 1–150.
12. van der Graaf, A.M.; Toering, T.J.; Faas, M.M.; Lely, A.T. From preeclampsia to renal disease: A role of angiogenic factors and the renin-angiotensin aldosterone system? *Nephrol. Dial. Transplant.* **2012**, *27*, iii51–iii57. [CrossRef] [PubMed]
13. Wiles, K.; Bramham, K.; Seed, P.T.; Kurlak, L.O.; Mistry, H.D.; Nelson-Piercy, C.; Lightstone, L.; Chappell, L.C. Diagnostic Indicators of Superimposed Preeclampsia in Women With CKD. *Kidney Int. Rep.* **2019**, *4*, 842–853. [CrossRef] [PubMed]
14. Regal, J.F.; Burwick, R.M.; Fleming, S.D. The Complement System and Preeclampsia. *Curr. Hypertens. Rep.* **2017**, *19*, 87. [CrossRef] [PubMed]
15. Piccoli, G.B.; Cabiddu, G.; Attini, R.; Vigotti, F.N.; Maxia, S.; Lepori, N.; Tuveri, M.; Massidda, M.; Marchi, C.; Mura, S.; et al. Risk of adverse pregnancy outcomes in women with CKD. *J. Am. Soc. Nephrol.* **2015**, *26*, 2011–2022. [CrossRef] [PubMed]
16. Su, X.; Lv, J.; Liu, Y.; Wang, J.; Ma, X.; Shi, S.; Liu, L.; Zhang, H. Pregnancy and kidney outcomes in patients with IgA nephropathy: A cohort study. *Am. J. Kidney Dis.* **2017**, *70*, 262–269. [CrossRef] [PubMed]
17. Zhang, J.J.; Ma, X.X.; Hao, L.; Liu, L.J.; Lv, J.C.; Zhang, H. A systematic review and meta-analysis of outcomes of pregnancy in CKD and CKD outcomes in pregnancy. *Clin. J. Am. Soc. Nephrol.* **2015**, *10*, 1964–1978. [CrossRef]
18. Webster, P.; Webster, L.M.; Cook, H.T.; Horsfield, C.; Seed, P.T.; Vaz, R.; Santos, C.; Lydon, I.; Homsy, M.; Lightstone, L.; et al. A Multicenter Cohort Study of Histologic Findings and Long-Term Outcomes of Kidney Disease in Women Who Have Been Pregnant. *Clin. J. Am. Soc. Nephrol.* **2017**, *12*, 408–416. [CrossRef]
19. Langer, B.; Grima, M.; Coquard, C.; Bader, A.M.; Schlaeder, G.; Imbs, J.L. Plasma active renin, angiotensin I, and angiotensin II during pregnancy and in preeclampsia. *Obstet. Gynecol.* **1998**, *91*, 196–202. [CrossRef]
20. Stanhewicz, A.E.; Jandu, S.; Santhanam, L.; Alexander, L.M. Increased Angiotensin II Sensitivity Contributes to Microvascular Dysfunction in Women Who Have Had Preeclampsia. *Hypertension* **2017**, *70*, 382–389. [CrossRef]

21. Kobori, H.; Nangaku, M.; Navar, L.G.; Nishiyama, A. The intrarenal renin angiotensin system: From physiology to the pathobiology of hypertension and kidney disease. *Pharmacol. Rev.* **2007**, *59*, 251–287. [CrossRef] [PubMed]
22. Zhou, C.C.; Ahmad, S.; Mi, T.; Xia, L.; Abbasi, S.; Hewett, P.W.; Sun, C.; Ahmed, A.; Kellems, R.E.; Xia, Y. Angiotensin II induces soluble fms like tyrosine kinase-1 release via calcineurin signaling pathway in pregnancy. *Circ. Res.* **2007**, *100*, 88–95. [CrossRef] [PubMed]
23. Yilmaz, Z.; Yildirim, T.; Yilmaz, R.; Aybal-Kutlugun, A.; Altun, B.; Kucukozkan, T.; Erdem, Y. Association between urinary angiotensinogen, hypertension and proteinuria in pregnant women with preeclampsia. *J. Renin Angiotensin Aldosterone Syst.* **2015**, *16*, 514–520. [CrossRef] [PubMed]
24. Masuyama, H.; Nobumoto, E.; Okimoto, N.; Inoue, S.; Segawa, T.; Hiramatsu, Y. Superimposed preeclampsia in women with chronic kidney disease. *Gynecol. Obstet. Investig.* **2012**, *74*, 274–281. [CrossRef] [PubMed]
25. Rolfo, A.; Attini, R.; Tavassoli, E.; Neve, F.V.; Nigra, M.; Cicilano, M.; Nuzzo, A.M.; Giuffrida, D.; Biolcati, M.; Nichelatti, M.; et al. Is it possible to differentiate chronic kidney disease and preeclampsia by means of new and old biomarkers? A prospective study. *Dis. Markers.* **2015**, *127083*, 1–8. [CrossRef]
26. Bramham, K.; Seed, P.T.; Lightstone, L.; Nelson-Piercy, C.; Gill, C.; Webster, P.; Poston, L.; Chappell, L.C. Diagnostic and predictive biomarkers for pre-eclampsia in patients with established hypertension and chronic kidney disease. *Kidney Int.* **2016**, *89*, 874–885. [CrossRef]
27. Diaconu, C.C.; Nastasa, A.; Zaki, A.; Istratie, B.; Nazari, R.; Iancu, M.A.; Balaceanu, A. A comparative analysis of the hypertension treatment depending on comorbidities: Insights from clinical practice. *J. Hypertens.* **2016**, *34*, E320–E321. [CrossRef]

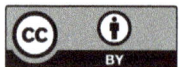

© 2020 by the authors. Licensee MDPI, Basel, Switzerland. This article is an open access article distributed under the terms and conditions of the Creative Commons Attribution (CC BY) license (http://creativecommons.org/licenses/by/4.0/).

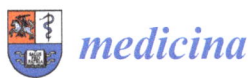

Case Report

Krukenberg Tumor in Association with Ureteral Stenosis Due to Peritoneal Carcinomatosis from Pulmonary Adenocarcinoma: A Case Report

Irina Balescu [1,2,*], Nona Bejinariu [3], Simona Slaniceanu [3], Mircea Gongu [4], Brandusa Masoud [5], Smarandita Lacau [5], George Tie [6], Maria Ciocirlan [7], Nicolae Bacalbasa [2,8] and Catalin Copaescu [1,9]

1. Department of Surgery, "Ponderas" Academic Hospital, 021188 Bucharest, Romania; catalin.copaescu@deltapromedical.ro
2. "Carol Davila" University of Medicine and Pharmacy, 020021 Bucharest, Romania; nicolae_bacalbasa@yahoo.ro
3. Department of Pathology, "Santomar Oncodiagnostic", 400664 Cluj Napoca, Romania; nona.bejinariu@gmail.ro (N.B.); simona.slaniceanu@gmail.ro (S.S.)
4. Department of Oncology, "Ponderas" Academic Hospital, 021188 Bucharest, Romania; mirceagongu@gmail.com
5. Department of Radiology, "Ponderas" Academic Hospital, 021188 Bucharest, Romania; brandusa.masoud@gmail.ro (B.M.); smarandita.lacau@gmail.ro (S.L.)
6. Department of Urology, "Ponderas" Academic Hospital, 021188 Bucharest, Romania; tiegeorge27@yahoo.com
7. Department of Gastroenterology, "Ponderas" Academic Hospital, 021188 Bucharest, Romania; maria.ciocirlan@gmail.ro
8. Center of Excellence in Translational Medicine, Fundeni Clinical Institute, 022328 Bucharest, Romania
9. "Grigore T Popa" University of Medicine and Pharmacy, 700115 Iasi, Romania
* Correspondence: irina.balescu@ponderas-ah.ro; Tel.: +40-724-077-709

Received: 10 March 2020; Accepted: 12 April 2020; Published: 17 April 2020

Abstract: Krukenberg tumors from pulmonary adenocarcinoma represent an extremely rare situation; only a few cases have been reported. The aim of this paper is to report an unusual such case in which almost complete dysphagia and ureteral stenosis occurred. The 62-year-old patient was initially investigated for dysphagia and weight loss. Computed tomography showed the presence of a thoracic mass compressing the esophagus in association with a few suspect pulmonary and peritoneal nodules, one of them invading the right ureter. A biopsy was performed laparoscopically on the peritoneal nodules. The right adnexa presented an atypical aspect; right adnexectomy was also found. The histopathological and immunohistochemical studies confirmed that the primitive origin was pulmonary adenocarcinoma. Although both peritoneal carcinomatosis and ovarian metastases from pulmonary adenocarcinoma represent a very uncommon situation, this pathology should not be excluded, especially in cases presenting suspect pulmonary lesions.

Keywords: pulmonary adenocarcinoma; Krukenberg tumors; ureteral stenosis

1. Introduction

Krukenberg tumors account for less than 2% of all ovarian carcinomas and represent ovarian metastases that usually originate from mucosecretory signet ring cell adenocarcinomas of the gastrointestinal tract. The most commonly encountered sites are the stomach and the colon [1–3]. In less common situations, Krukenberg tumors originate from other primaries such as the breast, small intestine, and appendix [3]. For lung cancer ovarian metastases, data are even scarcer, with only a few cases being reported so far [4–6]. Most often, these cases are represented by pulmonary adenocarcinomas (in up to 45% of cases), and the exact mechanism of development is not well understood [6]. The aim of this paper is to report the case of a patient diagnosed with Krukenberg tumor and peritoneal carcinomatosis invading the right ureter originating from pulmonary adenocarcinoma, in which the final diagnostic was established after performing a laparoscopic adnexectomy.

2. Case Report

A 62-year-old, nonsmoker woman with no significant pathological antecedents presented to our hospital for almost complete dysphagia. At the time of presentation, the patient was underweight, reporting an approximate weight loss of 15 kg during the last month. During this period, she also observed the apparition of dysphagia first for solids and later also for liquids, which worsened progressively. Biochemical tests demonstrated slow increase of cancer antigen CA 125 levels (74.2 U/mL—units per millilitre), whereas all the other tests (including tumoral markers, urinary and liver tests) were normal. The upper digestive endoscopy raised suspicion of an extrinsic compression of the medial third of the esophagus (at 26 cm from the dental arcade), which did not allow performing the maneuver with a 10 mm endoscope. The stenosis was hardly crossed by using a pediatric 5 mm endoscope, which showed the extension of the affected area on 5 cm. A gastrostomy feeding tube was placed during endoscopy. However, the esophageal lining was normal on the entire surface, again raising suspicion of extrinsic compression (Figure 1).

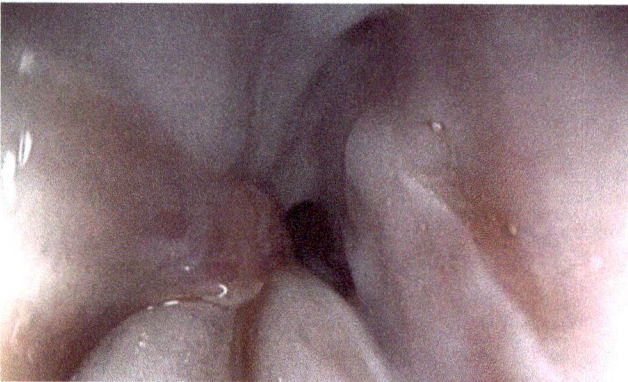

Figure 1. Upper digestive endoscopy revealed an extrinsic compression of the esophagus with normal esophageal lining.

In this context, an endoscopic ultrasound was attempted to retrieve a biopsy, but the maneuver was unsuccessful due to the extreme compression of the esophagus. The patient later underwent thoracic, abdominal, and pelvic computed tomography that demonstrated the presence of suspect pulmonary nodules in association with a mass compressing the esophagus and invading the pleura, the pericardium, the esophageal wall, and the aortic wall (Figures 2 and 3), as well as a tumoral nodule in close proximity to the uterine cervix invading the right ureter and creating an ureteral stenosis. The cardiologic evaluation demonstrated the presence of a mild pericardial effusion, with no other significant modifications of the cardiac function.

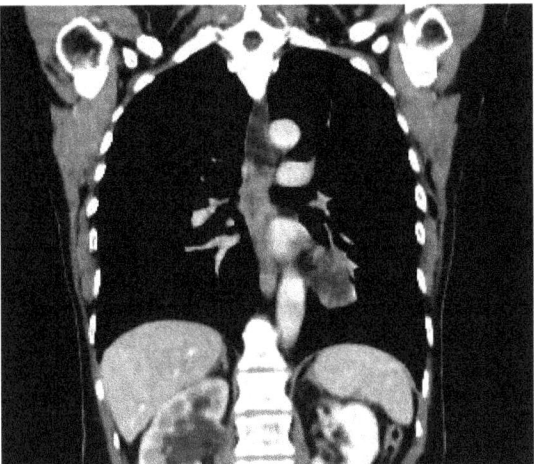

Figure 2. Computed tomography revealing extrinsic compression of the medial third of the esophagus.

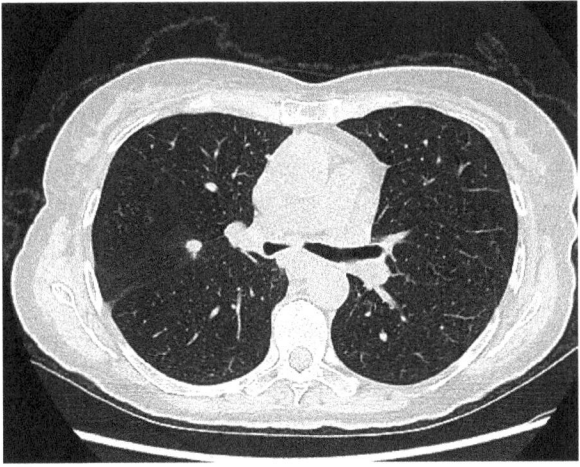

Figure 3. Computed tomography revealing extrinsic compression of the medial third of the esophagus in association with suspect pulmonary nodules.

The imagistic studies were further completed by pelvic magnetic resonance, which raised the suspicion of peritoneal nodules at the pelvic level and confirmed the presence of the tumoral nodule in close proximity to the uterine cervix invading the right ureter and with no apparent connection to the uterine cervix (Figures 4 and 5). In the meantime, other few-millimeter nodules of peritoneal carcinomatosis were found in the pelvic area with no other suspect aspects. The gynecological examination confirmed the presence of a tumoral mass of 3/1.5 cm invading the right ureter, developed in close proximity to the uterine cervix but with no apparent appurtenance to the gynecological tract. No other pathological images were encountered, and the Papanicolaou test failed to demonstrate any modification.

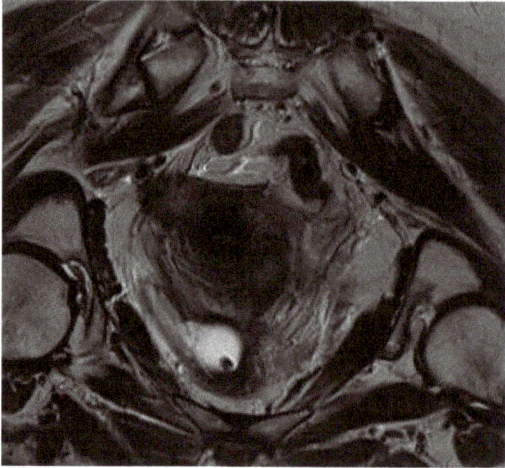

Figure 4. Pelvic magnetic resonance imaging (MRI) revealing the presence of a large tumoral nodule compressing the right ureter.

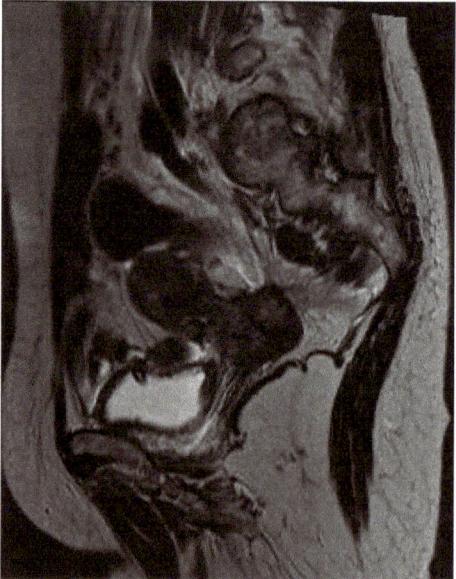

Figure 5. Pelvic MRI revealing the presence of a large tumoral nodule compressing the right ureter.

Due to an important ureteral stenosis being found, the patient also underwent Cook catheter placement on the right side. At the time of the catheter placement, a cisto-ureteroscopy was performed, which demonstrated an extrinsic compression of the right ureter, with the ureteral and urinary bladder mucosa being normal (Figures 6–8).

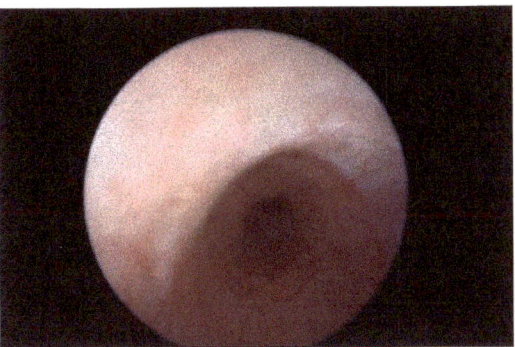

Figure 6. Right ureteroscopy presenting right ureteral stenosis probably due to external compression, a normal aspect of the ureteral lining.

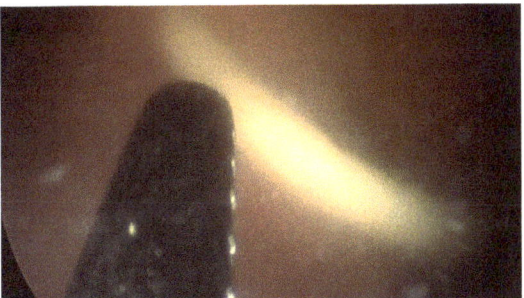

Figure 7. Intravesical positioning of the right Cook catheter.

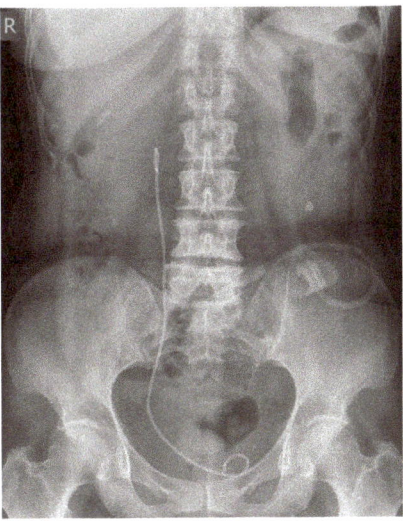

Figure 8. Abdominal X-ray revealing the correct position of the Cook catheter.

A diagnostic laparoscopy was performed on the patient, which demonstrated the presence of a few peritoneal nodules at the level of the pelvic area, retrieved in association with the nodule invading the right ureter. However, the right ovary was also found to have a pathological aspect, so it was retrieved by performing a right adnexectomy (Figures 9–11).

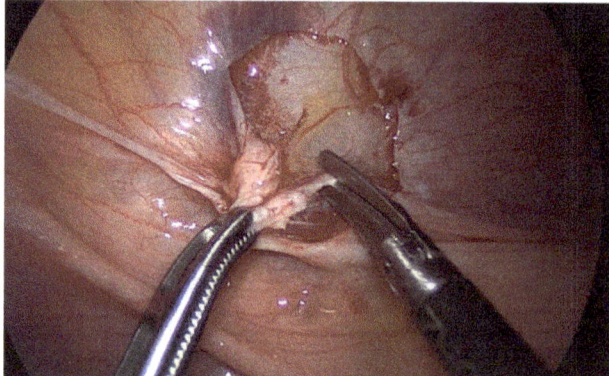

Figure 9. Laparoscopic biopsy of a peritoneal nodule on the anterior surface of the left broad uterine ligament.

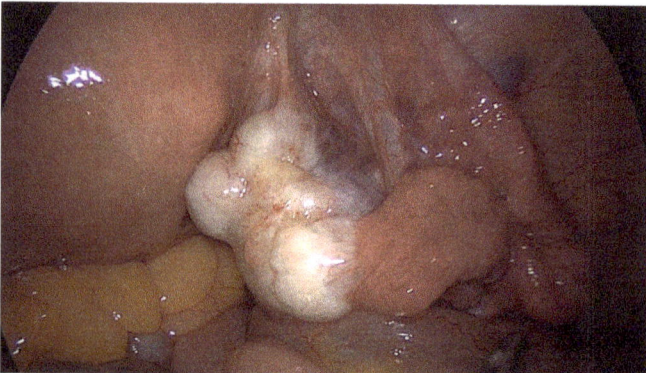

Figure 10. Laparoscopic exploration revealed tumoral transformation of the right adnexa, so a right adnexectomy was performed.

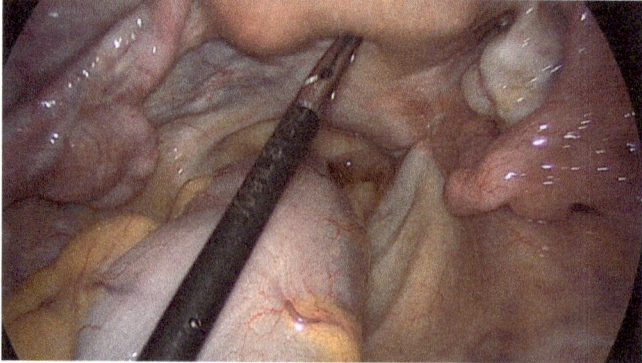

Figure 11. Laparoscopic exploration revealing the nodule of peritoneal carcinomatosis invading the right ureter.

The final histopathological studies of the specimens demonstrated the presence of a well-differentiated adenocarcinoma, with the ovarian parenchyma presenting tumoral invasion on up to 90% of the volume (Figure 12a–d). The immunohistochemical studies established the final diagnostic of pulmonary adenocarcinoma (diffuse and intense positivity for cytokeratin 7 (CK7) and thyroid transcription factor-1 (TTF-1); positivity for carcinoembryonic antigen (CEA); poor positivity for estrogen receptors (ERs); negativity for GATA3 transcription factor, paired-box gene 8 (PAX8), Wilms' tumor 1 (WT1) factor, homeobox protein (CDX2), p16-cyclin-dependent kinase inhibitor 2A, and S-100 proteins; Figure 13a–f). In this context, the genital, breast, gastric, colonic, esophageal, and pancreatic malignancies were excluded, with the final aspect pulmonary adenocarcinoma. Epidermal growth factor receptor (EGFR), anaplastic lymphoma kinase (ALK), and programmed cell death ligand 1 (PD-L1) tests were performed demonstrating the presence of mutations, so the patient was later confined to the medical oncology clinic for biological treatment.

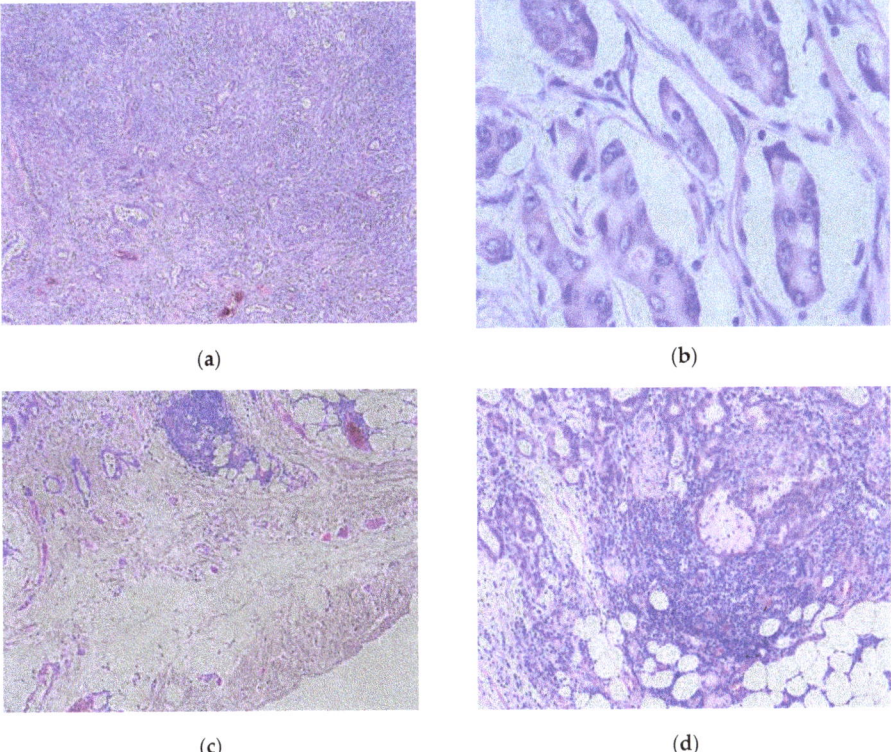

Figure 12. Histopathological study. (a) Hematoxylin and eosin (H&E) staining of the ovarian parenchyma revealing tumoral infiltration in more than 90% of the parenchyma (5×); (b) H&E staining of the ovarian parenchyma revealing tumoral infiltration in more than 90% of the parenchyma (40×); (c) H&E staining of the peritoneum revealing the presence of tumoral deposits (5×); (d) H&E staining of the peritoneum revealing perineural invasion (10×).

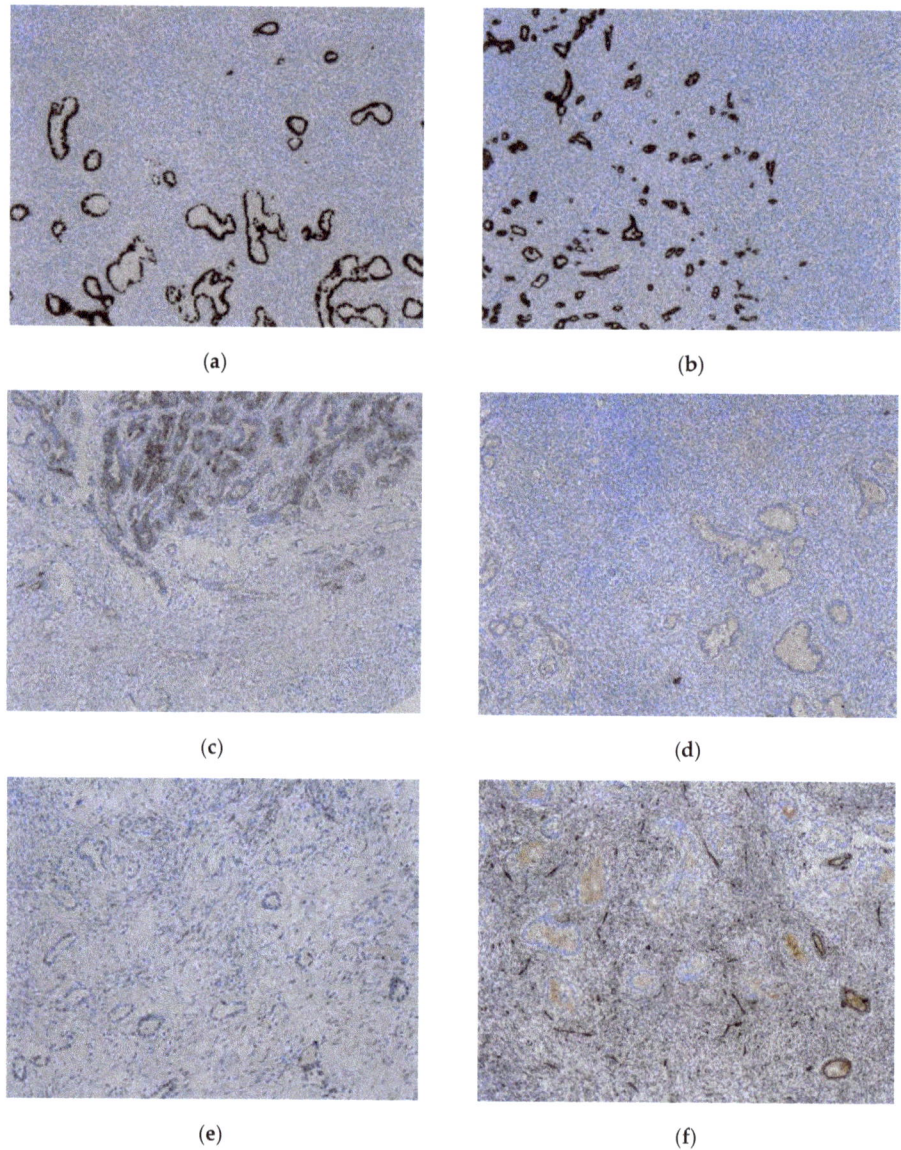

Figure 13. Immunohistochemical study revealing diffuse positivity. (**a**) TTF-1 staining; (**b**) CK7 staining; (**c**) CEA staining; (**d**) PAX8 staining; (**e**) ER staining; (**f**) WT1 staining.

3. Discussion

Krukenberg tumors were initially described by Friedrich Ernst Krukenberg in 1896, when he revealed the first five such cases [7]. Since then, this histopathological finding has been treated as a separate entity, and further studies demonstrated that the most common origins of the primaries that might lead to the development of such tumors are represented by gastric cancer (up to 76% of cases), followed by colorectal cancer (up to 11% of cases). Other possible origins include the breast, biliary system, pancreas, urinary tract, and gynecological tract [2,3]. Most often, Krukenberg tumors are found bilaterally, and in up to half of cases, they are associated with the presence of ascites [8]. As for Krukenberg tumors with lung cancer origins, it is estimated that less than 4% of all lung cancers lead to the development of ovarian metastases, with up to half of them being represented by small cell carcinomas [4]. To establish that an ovarian tumor has a metastatic origin from a primary lung carcinoma, detection of TTF-1 at the level of the ovarian lesion plays a central role [4]. In our case, the identification of this marker at the level of the specimen of adnexectomy enabled us to suspect the pulmonary origin of the metastatic islets that had been found at the level of the ovarian tissue. The final diagnostic in our case was established based on immunohistochemical studies, which were strongly suggestive for pulmonary adenocarcinoma. The lesions proved to have positive staining for TTF1, CK7, and CEA. In a recent study conducted on a group of 665 specimens of resected pulmonary cancer and 425 resected metastases, Vidarsdottir et al. routinely studied the presence of CK7, CK20, CDX2, CK5, p40, p63, TTF-1, napsin A, GATA3, and PAX8, and demonstrated that primary adenocarcinoma of the lung presented strong positive expression for TTF1 in 90% of cases and for napsin A in 84%, whereas only less than 10% of cases were positive for p63, CDX2, CK20, and GATA3. Additionally, 68% of cases with pulmonary adenocarcinoma presented positive staining for CK7, TTF-1, and napsin A and were negative for the other studied parameters [9]. The authors demonstrated that the presence of TTF1 and CK7 could also be used to differentiate pulmonary adenocarcinoma by squamous cell carcinoma. In the latter histopathological subtype, the positivity of TTF-1 and CK7 was demonstrated in only 3% and 44% of cases, respectively [9].

The therapeutic strategies in such cases are mainly decided according to the primary tumor; however, due to the metastatic character of Krukenberg lesions, the presence of ovarian metastases is usually considered as a sign of a systemic disease, which transforms the patient into a candidate for palliative systemic treatment. This pathological finding is usually associated with poor rates of long-term survival [5]. However, in our case, a right adnexectomy was performed as part of the diagnostic strategy and not with curative intent. The patient also showed a large mediastinal mass and peritoneal carcinomatosis nodules invading the ureter as a sign of systemic disease.

Another particularity of our case is the presence of peritoneal carcinomatosis with a pulmonary adenocarcinoma origin. One nodule of peritoneal carcinomatosis developed in close proximity with the right ureter, where almost complete stenosis had developed. Based on autopsy studies, peritoneal carcinomatosis from pulmonary adenocarcinoma can be encountered in up to 16% of cases; however, clinical manifestation of such lesions are rarely encountered, with obstructive symptomatology being the most common [10,11]. Although this symptomatology is to be expected at the level of the gastrointestinal tract due to the presence of mesenteric nodules, in rare cases, other abdominal structures might be involved. In the case we presented here, obstruction of the right ureter caused a grade III uretero-hydronephrosis. In our case, during laparoscopy, no other nodules of peritoneal carcinomatosis were found, except for few-millimeter lesions at the level of the pelvic area, especially on the uterine serosa and its ligaments.

The rarity of peritoneal carcinomatosis from lung cancer was also demonstrated by the study conducted by Satoh et al., which included 1041 cases with pulmonary cancer over a period of 26 years. Among these cases, only eight patients developed clinically evident peritoneal carcinomatosis [12]; however, regarding histopathological subtypes of pulmonary cancer that present the highest risk of developing peritoneal metastases, adenocarcinoma seems to play the most important role. In another more recent study conducted on the issue of peritoneal carcinomatosis from non-small cell lung carcinoma, Nassereddine et al. included 12 patients diagnosed with peritoneal carcinomatosis from non-small cell lung carcinoma, with 11 cases diagnosed with pulmonary adenocarcinoma. The authors underlined that all cases presented other metastases at the time of the initial diagnosis. The most commonly encountered sites for the metastatic disease were represented by pleura, bone, adrenal glands, liver, and colon. These authors also reported the presence of ovarian metastases, but the incidence of this finding was not reported. In this case series, the most commonly encountered positivity of the immunostaining was the one for PD-L1 (in 37.5% of cases), a finding that was also encountered in the case we reported [13].

The prognosis for these cases seems to be extremely poor, with the overall survival time usually only a few months from the time peritoneal carcinomatosis is diagnosed. Regardless, attention should be paid to identifying the cases that present with EGFR mutation (consisting of exon 19 deletion), which seem to be associated with a more favorable outcome [14]. In such cases tyrosine kinase inhibitors might be administrated, and a significant benefit of survival (of more than 1 year) is expected [15,16]. In the aforementioned case, the presence of EGFR mutation allowed us to introduce this biological treatment with good chances of prolonging the patient's survival. In addition, a differential diagnostic of the primary tumor with pleural mesothelioma should be ruled out; immunohistochemical studies are the cornerstone process by which to establish this differential diagnosis [17].

4. Conclusions

Association between peritoneal carcinomatosis creating urinary tract obstruction and Krukenberg tumor is an extremely rare eventuality in patients with pulmonary adenocarcinoma. The case we reported presents a series of particularities: the symptomatology at the time of presentation, almost complete dysphagia due to a thoracic mass compressing the esophagus, the modality in which the final diagnostic was established, and laparoscopic adnexectomy in association with peritoneal nodules biopsy, which revealed positive immunohistochemical staining for TTF-1, CK7, and CEA. The demonstration of EGFR, PD-L1, and ALK mutations offered a chance for improved survival for our patient, who thereby became a candidate for immunotherapy.

Author Contributions: I.B. performed surgery; N.B. and S.S. performed histopathological and immunohistochemical studies; M.G. advised about oncologic testing; B.M. and S.L. performed the imaging studies; G.T. performed urological procedure; M.C. performed endoscopic evaluation; N.B. performed literature data review; C.C. finally reviewed the manuscript. All authors have read and agreed to the published version of the manuscript.

Funding: This research received no external funding.

Conflicts of Interest: The authors have no conflicts of interest to declare regarding this study.

References

1. Aziz, M.; Kasi, A. *Cancer, Krukenberg Tumor*; StatPearls Publishing: Treasure Island, FL, USA, 2018.
2. Man, M.; Cazacu, M.; Oniu, T. Krukenberg tumors of gastric origin versus krukenberg tumors of colorectal origin. *Chirurgia* **2007**, *102*, 407–410. [PubMed]
3. McGill, F.; Ritter, D.B.; Rickard, C.; Kaleya, R.N.; Wadler, S.; Greston, W.M. Management of krukenberg tumors: An 11-year experience and review of the literature. *Prim. Care Update. Ob Gyns* **1998**, *5*, 157–1588. [CrossRef]
4. Losito, N.S.; Scaffa, C.; Cantile, M.; Botti, G.; Costanzo, R.; Manna, A.; Franco, R.; Greggi, S. Lung cancer diagnosis on ovary mass: A case report. *J. Ovarian. Res.* **2013**, *6*, 34. [CrossRef] [PubMed]
5. Sota Yoldi, L.A.; Vigil, V.L.; Martin, D.C.; Antunes, P.B. Krukenberg tumor secondary to lung adenocarcinoma. *Arch. Bronconeumol.* **2019**, *55*, 380–381. [CrossRef] [PubMed]
6. Irving, J.A.; Young, R.H. Lung carcinoma metastatic to the ovary: A clinicopathologic study of 32 cases emphasizing their morphologic spectrum and problems in differential diagnosis. *Am. J. Surg. Pathol.* **2005**, *29*, 997–1006. [PubMed]
7. Young, R.H. From krukenberg to today: The Ever present problems posed by metastatic tumors in the ovary: Part, I. Historical perspective, general principles, mucinous tumors including the krukenberg tumor. *Adv. Anat. Pathol.* **2006**, *13*, 205–227. [CrossRef] [PubMed]
8. Tan, K.L.; Tan, W.S.; Lim, J.F.; Eu, K.W. Krukenberg tumors of colorectal origin: A dismal outcome—Experience of a tertiary center. *Int. J. Colorectal Dis.* **2010**, *25*, 233–238. [CrossRef] [PubMed]
9. Vidarsdottir, H.; Tran, L.; Nodin, B.; Jirstrom, K.; Planck, M.; Jonsson, P.; Mattsson, J.S.M.; Botling, J.; Micke, P.; Brunnstrom, H. Immunohistochemical profiles in primary lung cancers and epithelial pulmonary metastases. *Hum. Pathol.* **2019**, *84*, 221–230. [CrossRef] [PubMed]

10. Sereno, M.; Rodriguez-Esteban, I.; Gomez-Raposo, C.; Merino, M.; Lopez-Gomez, M.; Zambrana, F.; Casado, E. Lung cancer and peritoneal carcinomatosis. *Oncol. Lett.* **2013**, *6*, 705–708. [CrossRef] [PubMed]
11. McNeill, P.M.; Wagman, L.D.; Neifeld, J.P. Small bowel metastases from primary carcinoma of the lung. *Cancer* **1987**, *59*, 1486–1489. [CrossRef]
12. Satoh, H.; Ishikawa, H.; Yamashita, Y.T.; Kurishima, K.; Ohtsuka, M.; Sekizawa, K. Peritoneal carcinomatosis in lung cancer patients. *Oncol. Rep.* **2001**, *8*, 1305–1307. [CrossRef] [PubMed]
13. Nassereddine, H.; Sannier, A.; Brosseau, S.; Rodier, J.M.; Khalil, A.; Msika, S.; Danel, C.; Couvelard, A.; Theou-Anton, N.; Cazes, A. Clinicopathological and molecular study of peritoneal carcinomatosis associated with non-small cell lung carcinoma. *Pathol. Oncol. Res.* **2019**. [CrossRef] [PubMed]
14. Meneses Grasa, Z.; Coll Salinas, A.; Macías Cerrolaza, J.A.; Aguayo Albasini, J.L.; Campillo Soto, A.; Guillén Paredes, M.P. Intestinal obstruction by metastasis in mesentery from squamous cell lung carcinoma. *Rev. Esp. Enferm. Dig.* **2009**, *101*, 817–818. (In Spanish) [CrossRef] [PubMed]
15. Su, H.T.; Tsai, C.M.; Perng, R.P. Peritoneal Carcinomatosis in Lung Cancer. *Respirology* **2008**, *13*, 465–467. [CrossRef] [PubMed]
16. Grigoroiu, M.; Tagett, R.; Draghici, S.; Dima, S.; Nastase, A.; Florea, R.; Sorop, A.; Ilie, V.; Bacalbasa, N.; Tica, V.; et al. Gene-Expression Profiling in Non-Small Cell Lung Cancer with Invasion of Mediastinal Lymph Nodes for Prognosis Evaluation. *Cancer Genom. Proteom.* **2015**, *12*, 231–242.
17. Kushitani, K.; Takeshima, Y.; Amatya, V.J.; Furonaka, O.; Sakatani, A.; Inai, K. Immunohistochemical marker panels for distinguishing between epithelioid mesothelioma and lung adenocarcinoma. *Pathol. Int.* **2007**, *57*, 190–199. [CrossRef] [PubMed]

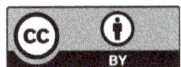

© 2020 by the authors. Licensee MDPI, Basel, Switzerland. This article is an open access article distributed under the terms and conditions of the Creative Commons Attribution (CC BY) license (http://creativecommons.org/licenses/by/4.0/).

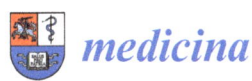

Article

Pleural Solitary Fibrous Tumors—A Retrospective Study on 45 Patients

Cornel Savu [1,2,*], Alexandru Melinte [1], Radu Posea [1], Niculae Galie [1,2], Irina Balescu [3], Camelia Diaconu [4,5], Dragos Cretoiu [6,7], Simona Dima [8], Alexandru Filipescu [9,10], Cristian Balalau [11,12] and Nicolae Bacalbasa [8,9,13]

1. Department of Thoracic Surgery, "Marius Nasta" Institute of Pneumonology, 050152 Bucharest, Romania; alexandru.melinte@gmail.ro (A.M.); radu.posea@gmail.ro (R.P.); niculae.galie@gmail.ro (N.G.)
2. Department of Thoracic Surgery, "Carol Davila" University of Medicine and Pharmacy, 020021 Bucharest, Romania
3. Department of Surgery, "Ponderas" Academic Hospital, 021188 Bucharest, Romania; irina_balescu206@yahoo.com
4. Department of Internal Medicine, "Floreasca" Clinical Emergency Hospital, 105402 Bucharest, Romania; drcameliadiaconu@gmail.com
5. Department of Internal Medicine, "Carol Davila" University of Medicine and Pharmacy, 020021 Bucharest, Romania
6. "Alessandrescu-Rusescu" National Institute of Mother and Child Health, Fetal Medicine Excellence Research Center, 020395 Bucharest, Romania; dragos.cretoiu@gmail.ro
7. Department of Cell and Molecular Biology and Histology, "Carol Davila" University of Medicine and Pharmacy, 020021 Bucharest, Romania
8. Center of Excellence in Translational Medicine, Fundeni Clinic Institute, 022328 Bucharest, Romania; simona.dima@gmail.ro (S.D.); nicolae_bacalbasa@yahoo.ro (N.B.)
9. Department of Obstetrics and Gynecology, "Carol Davila" University of Medicine and Pharmacy, 020021 Bucharest, Romania; alexandru.filipescu@gmail.ro
10. Department of Obstetrics and Gynecology, "Elias" Emergency Hospital, 105402 Bucharest, Romania
11. Department of Surgery, "Carol Davila" University of Medicine and Pharmacy, 020021 Bucharest, Romania; cristian.balalau@gmail.ro
12. Department of Surgery, "Pantelimon" Clinical Hospital, 021661 Bucharest, Romania
13. Department of Obstetrics and Gynecology, "I Cantacuzino" Clinical Hospital, 030167 Bucharest, Romania
* Correspondence: drsavu25@yahoo.com

Received: 4 March 2020; Accepted: 14 April 2020; Published: 16 April 2020

Abstract: *Introduction*: The purpose of this paper is to study the type, the clinical presentation, and the best diagnostic methods for pleural solitary fibrous tumors (PSFTs), as well as to evaluate which is the most appropriate treatment, especially as PSFTs represent a rare occurrence in the thoracic pathology. *Material and Method*: A retrospective study was conducted on a group of 45 patients submitted to surgery between January 2015 and December 2019. In most cases, the diagnosis was established through imaging studies—thoracic computed tomography (CT) scan with or without contrast—but also using magnetic resonance imaging (MRI) or positron emission tomography (PET) scans when data from CT scans were scarce. All patients were submitted to surgery with curative intent. *Results*: Most patients included in this study were asymptomatic, with this pathology being more common in patients over 60 years of age, and more common in women. The occurrence of malignant PSFT in our study was 17.77% (8 cases). All cases were submitted to surgery with curative intent, with a single case developing further recurrence. In order to achieve complete resection en bloc resection of the tumor with the chest wall, resection was performed in two cases, while lower lobectomy, pneumectomy, and hemidiaphragm resection, respectively, were needed in each case. Postoperative mortality was null. *Conclusion*: Thoracic CT scan remains the most important imagistic investigation in diagnosing. MRI is superior to thoracic CT, especially in cases that involved the larger blood vessels within the thorax, spinal column, or diaphragm. Complete surgical resection is the gold standard in treatment of PSFT, and the prognosis in benign cases is very good.

Keywords: PSFT; resection; surgery

1. Introduction

Pleural solitary fibrous tumors (PSFTs) are rare tumors, and their evolution is considered unpredictable. The incidence of this disease is considered to be lower than 5% of the total number of pleural tumors [1]. The first case of PSFT was described from a histological view by Wagner in 1870 [2], however, the first pleural tumor was presented by Lieutaud in 1767 [3,4]. In 1931, Klemperer and Rabin published a histopathological description and divided the tumors in two categories: diffuse and localised [5]. Stout and Murray (1942) were the first to identify the mesenchymal origin of pleural tumors, which was later confirmed by electronic microscopy and immunohistochemistry [6]. Over time, these tumors have had different names: localised mesothelioma, benign mesothelioma, fibrous mesothelioma, pleural fibroma, benign pleural fibroma, pleural fibromyxoma, localised fibrous tumor, and so on [7].

Over the last 20 years, the term mesothelioma was replaced by solitary fibrous pleural tumor. These tumors were first described as being within the pleura, but it was later observed that it can also have an extra pleural localisation. There were also cases described of fibrous solitary tumors in various locations: liver, pelvis, peritoneum, meningeal, adrenal gland, intrapulmonary, urinary bladder, pericardium, and almost every organ system [8,9].

PSFTs are found within the pleura in 57.7% of cases, with the rest (42.3%) being localized extrapleural [8,10]. The World Health Organization (2015) reviewed the classification of pleural tumors from a pathological view and placed them in three categories: mesothelial tumors, mesenchymal tumors, and lympho-proliferative disorder. Both benign and malignant solitary fibrous tumors are part of the mesenchymal tumor group, along with desmoid tumors and calcified fibrous tumors.

2. Materials and Methods

This paper represents a retrospective study on a series of 45 patients diagnosed with PSFT who were submitted to surgery in our thoracic surgery clinic from the Institute of Pneumology, Bucharest over a period of five years (2015–2019). After obtaining the approval of the Ethical Committee no 12/9 February 2020, data of these patients were retrospectively reviewed. The analyzed parameters were represented by age, sex, clinical presentation, blood test results, imaging aspects, histopathological examination of the tumor after surgery, type of surgical resection, complementary treatment, and postoperative evolution. For a better classification of our series, we used the tumor size criteria (larger or smaller than 10 cm), with the De Perrot staging of pleural fibrous tumors (Table 1).

Table 1. Pleural solitary fibrous tumor (PSFT) staging De Perrot.

Stage 0	Pedunculated Tumor Without Signs of Malignity
Stage I	Sessile or "inverted" tumor without signs of malignity
Stage II	Pedunculated tumor with histological signs of malignity
Stage III	Sessile or "inverted" tumor with histological signs of malignity
Stage IV	Multiple synchronous metastatic tumors

Differentiation between malignant and benign PSFT was done using the criteria established by England et al. [11]: presence of tumoral necrosis; presence of atypical nuclei, cellular pleomorphism, and hypercellularity; presence ≥4 mitosis/10 HPF (high power field). Immunohistochemistry tests were performed for both types of PSFTs.

Imaging studies consisted of chest X-ray, thoracic computed tomography (CT) scan, magnetic resonance imaging (MRI), and positron emission tomography (PET) scan. Both CT guided biopsy as well as direct tumor biopsy were used for histological diagnosis. Bronchoscopy was used in larger tumors with compression of the lung with a visible impact on the bronchial tree. Other routine tests performed were electrocardiography (EKG), lung function tests, blood gas levels, and transthoracic echography associated with a cardiology exam. Patients were also classified according to their smoking status as well as according to their exposure to asbestos or ionizing radiation.

Follow-up was done with the following protocol: standard chest X-ray at three and six months postoperative, thoracic CT scan every six months in the first two years and once a year for the next five years. Most patients from our series are still in the postoperative follow-up program, as we have set a 15 year monitoring period.

3. Results

From our 45 patient series, 35 were women (77.7%) and were 10 men (22.2%) with a ratio of 1 male/3.5 female (1:3.5). The age of our patients was between 32 and 84 years with an average of 61.84 years. The representation of age groups was as follows: 1 case between 30 and 40 years old (woman) (2.22%), 5 cases between 40 and 50 years old (women) (11.1%), 6 cases between 50 and 60 years old (5 women, 1 male) (13.3%), 19 cases between 60 and 70 years old (14 women and 5 male) (42.22%), 11 cases between 70 and 80 years old (7 women and 4 male) (24.44%), and 3 cases over 80 years old (2 women and 1 male) (6.66%).

According to the size of the tumors, in the case of PSFT, the largest was 34/24/15 cm and weighed 3800 g, and the smallest was 2.5/1.7/1.5 cm with a weight of 64 g. In our series, 60% of the tumors were under 10 cm (27 cases), and 40% over 10 cm (18 cases) (Figure 1).

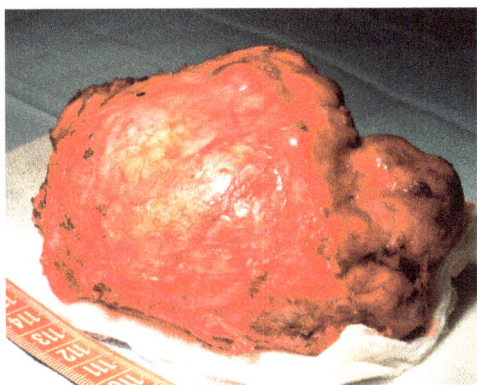

Figure 1. Surgical specimen.

Regarding the risk factors in our series, 15 cases (33.33%) were smokers, 2 cases were exposed to asbestos (4.44%), 1 case had a genetic factor (2.22%) (mother with pleural mesothelioma), 1 case had exposure to ionising radiation (2.22%), and 1 case had exposure to benzene (2.22%). In conclusion, 20 cases (44.44%) had exposure to risk factors.

From a clinical view, 24 cases (53.33%) were asymptomatic and 21 cases (46.66%) had a diversity of clinical manifestations (Table 2).

We can observe that most symptomatic presentations (14 cases—31.11%) were with chest pain, dyspnea, or cough. The rest of the symptoms found are associated with paraneoplastic syndrome: Doege–Potter syndrome, Pierre–Marie–Bamberger syndrome, arthralgia, articular oedema, or weight loss. Moreover, a correlation between the tumor size and symptoms was noted. Most asymptomatic patients had tumors <10 cm (23 cases—51.11%), with only one case presenting with chest pain (2.22%), with $p < 0.01$. From the symptomatic patients (21 cases—44.44%), 20 of them had tumors >10 cm with only one case (2.22%) under 10 cm. Regarding tumor localisation, 20 cases (44.44%) were in the right hemithorax and 25 cases (55.55%) in the left hemithorax. As a point of origin of the tumor, 21 cases

(46.66%) where in the parietal pleura and 22 cases (48.88%) in the visceral pleural, with one case (2.22%) in the mediastinal pleural and one case (2.22%) in the left hemidiafragm.

Table 2. Clinical presentation in PSFT.

Symptoms	Number of Cases
Hypertrophic osteoarthropathy Pierre–Marie–Bamberger syndrome	2 (4.44%)
Hypoglycemia Doege–Potter Syndrome	2 (4.44%)
Thoracic pain	5 (11.11%)
Cough	6 (13.33%)
Dyspnea	3 (6.66%)
Facial and upper body oedema Superior vena cava syndrome	1 (2.22%)
Arthralgia and articular oedema	1 (2.22%)
Weight loss	1 (2.22%)

Using de Perrot staging and England pathology criteria, there were 19 cases in stage 0, 18 cases in stage I, 1 case in stage II, 7 cases in stage III, and no cases for stage IV. Benign tumors (82.22%) were discovered in stages 0 and I, while malignant tumors (17.77%) were diagnosed in stages II and III (Table 3).

Table 3. Malignant PSFT—correlation between symptoms, tumor size, and staging (De Perrot).

Symptoms	Size	Stage
Symptoms of Doege–Potter	34 cm	III
Doege–Potter syndrome	21 cm	III
Pierre–Marie–Bamberger syndrome	23 cm	III
Pierre–Marie–Bamberger syndrome	25 cm	III
Superior vena cava syndrome	15 cm	III
Arthralgia and articular oedema	18 cm	III
Weight loss	9 cm	II
Dyspnea	24 cm	III

Immunohistochemistry studies were used in 15 cases (33.33%) for both histological types. These tests were positive for cluster of differentiation 34 (CD34), B cell lymphoma (bcl-2), Vimentin, cluster of differentiation 99 (CD99), and signal transducer and activator of transcription 6 (STAT 6) in eight cases of malignant PSFT (17.77%), and were negative in seven cases (15.55%) of benign PSFT. Imaging diagnosis was based on simple chest X-ray, which was performed for all 45 patients. In 39 cases (86.66%), nodular or pleural masses were identified, two cases (4.44%) presented a normal aspect, while the remaining four cases (8.88%) were thought to have pulmonary or mediastinal masses. Further on, CT scan was performed in 35 cases (77.77%), of which 15 patients (42.85%) were diagnosed with pleural fibrous tumors, pleural mesothelioma was suspected (14.28%) in 5 cases, while a clear diagnosis could not be set in 8 cases (22.85%) (Figure 2). In another four cases (11.42%), a mediastinal tumor was suspected, while in three cases (8.57%), benign pulmonary tumors were suspected.

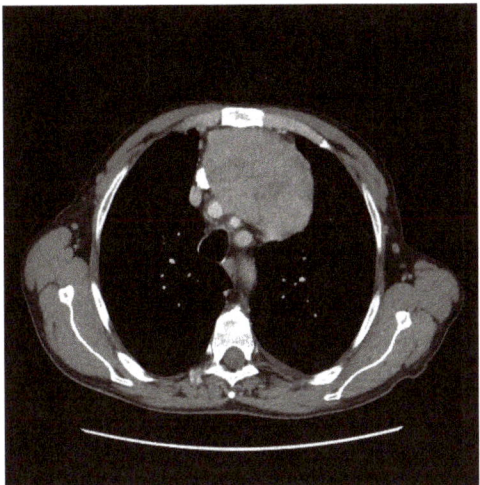

Figure 2. Computed tomography (CT) aspect.

In six cases (17.14%), further investigations were performed, consisting of biopsy through thoracotomy in three cases (8.57%) and CT guided biopsy in another three cases (8.57%). In four cases (8.88%), along with thoracic CT scan, an MRI was performed in order to establish a diagnosis. In total, nine patients received an MRI (20%), in cases in which we suspected spinal involvement (two cases—4.44%), mediastinal blood vessels involvement (six cases—13.33%), or diaphragmatic invasion (one case—2.22%). Only one case in which a malignant thoracic tumor was suspected was submitted to a PET scan.

Comparing patients investigated through thoracic CT scan (35 cases) with those who received an MRI (nine cases), we noticed a higher diagnostic accuracy in cases in which MRI was used. Diagnosis was established by CT scan in 42.85% of cases (15 patients), while MRI established a clear diagnosis in all nine patients (100%). This further proves the greater accuracy of MRI studies when compared with thoracic CT scan in cases in which spinal column, blood vessels, or diaphragmatic invasion is suspected.

Treatment of PSFT consisted of surgery in all 45 cases, with only one case (2.22%) having a recurrence that required another surgical procedure in association with chemotherapy and radiotherapy.

En bloc surgical resection with 2 cm margins surrounding the tumor was performed in 38 cases (84.4%). The tumor was resected en bloc with chest wall resection (involving the first three ribs) in one case (2.22%), lower left lobectomy in one case (2.22%), left pneumonectomy in one case (2.22%), partial resection of the left hemidiaphragm in one case (2.22%), and posterior chest wall resection (involving the third, fourth, and fifth ribs) in one case (2.22%).

The correlation between the type of PSFT and the type of performed surgical procedure is presented in Table 4. Open surgery was performed in most cases (40 cases—88.8%) and video assisted thoracic surgery (VATS) surgery only in five cases (11.11%).

Most cases reported no postoperative complications. However, there were eight cases (17.77%) that required an extended postoperative stay, the most commonly encountered postoperative complications consisting of bleeding in two cases (4.44%), upper gastrointestinal bleeding owing to a gastric ulceration in one case (2.22%), cardiac arrhythmias in one case (2.22%), surgical wound infection in one case (2.22%), and paralysis of the left hemidiaphragm in one case (2.22%). The overall mortality was null.

Table 4. Surgery performed according to the histopahological form of PSFT.

Malignant Tumors	Benign PSFT
Tumoral resection (2.22%)	Tumoral resection 37 cases (82.22%)
Tumoral resection en bloc with left pneumonectomy (2.22%)	
Tumoral resection en bloc with left chest wall resection involving the first three ribs (2.22%)	
Tumoral resection en bloc with lower left lobectomy (2.22%)	
Tumoral resection en bloc with upper right lobectomy (2.22%)	
Tumoral resection en bloc with right chest wall resection involving the third, fourth, and fifth ribs (2.22%)	
Tumoral resection en bloc with left pneumonectomy (2.22%)	
Tumoral resection en bloc with partial diaphragm resection (2.22%)	

Follow-up was structured in two intervals: an initial period for the first five years, during which 36 patients were introduced (80% of cases), with the other nine cases (20%) having yet to come in. The second period for follow-up will be until 15 years postoperative. Follow-up PET-CT scan was performed for only one patient with malignant PSFT, who after five years presented with local recurrence. PET-CT was not usually performed in order to differentiate between malignant or benign PSFT.

Two-year follow-up from surgery reviewed 34 cases (75.55%) and five-year follow-up reviewed 7 patients (15.55%). Of those reviewed after two years, 6 patients had malignant PSFT (with malignant histologic characteristics) (75%) and 28 patients had benign PSFT (benign histological characters) (62.22%). At the five-year follow-up, we only have five cases of benign PSFT and two cases of malignant PSFT. We mention that the five-year follow-up on all 45 patients is not yet completed.

4. Discussion

PSFTs are not as common as other types of pleural tumors, such as diffuse malignant pleural mesothelioma. They account for less than 5% of cases of pleural tumors and are more frequently encountered in men, during the sixth or seventh decade of their life [12]. Other authors consider it more common in women, with a proportion of 1:1.35 [11]. In our observation, we encountered a higher preponderance of women compared with men (77.7% of cases), with the proportion of women to men being 3.5:1.

Even though this affection may occur at any age, the sixth decade of life indicates a higher prevalence, as mentioned in the literature [13,14]. In our study group, we encountered an average age of 61.84, with the majority of cases being situated in the 60–70 age group (19 cases, or 42.22%) and in the 70–80 age group (11 cases, or 24.44%), similar to the data from the literature.

In the literature, there is no suggestive mentioning of the factors that may lead to PSFT development, excepting one published case, which mentioned the genetic character of this disease [15]. In addition, exposure to asbestos, tobacco, or other nitrogen oxide gases was not linked to PSFT. In our series, even though there were patients with previous exposure to smoking, asbestos, ionizing radiation, or benzene (19 cases—42.22%), a correlation could not have been established between exposure and PSFT development.

Some authors consider that up to 87% of cases diagnosed with PSFT have their origin in the visceral pleura and only 13% of them in the parietal pleura [16]. However, in our cases, a heterogenic localization was found, with an even 22 cases (48.88%) in the visceral pleura and 21 cases (46.66%) in the parietal pleura. As for the cellular origin of PSFT, the opinions are very diverse, leading to the numerous names of this disease. At present, the origin is accepted to be a mesenchymal one, at the level of the mesenchymal cells of the pleura. Nonetheless, there were cases of fibrous solitaire tumors with extrapleural localization at the level of the urinary bladder [17], retroperitoneum [18], salivary gland, meninges, thyroid, paranasal sinuses, or even with intrapulmonary location.

PSFT is a benign tumor in most cases, but in some cases, it can have malignant characters. The proportion of benign PSFT and malign PSFT is 7:1 [19]. The incidence of malign PSFT is considered as 12% of the entire cases of solitary fibrous tumors [20]. In our study, the majority of cases were benign (82.22%), and only eight cases were malign PSFT (17.77%), which is a higher number than those presented in the literature (Figure 3).

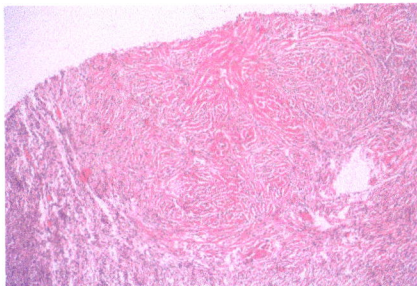 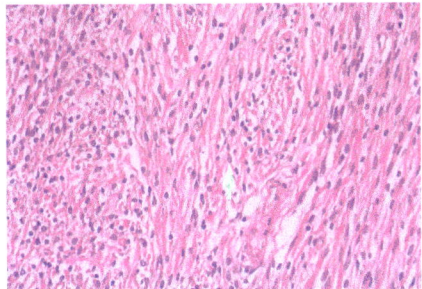

Figure 3. Histopathological aspects.

Some others consider that the incidence of malign PSFT is much higher, with the percentile reaching 43% of the cases [21]. Even though, it is accepted that approximately 78–88% of the cases represent benign PSFT and only 12% to 22% represent malignant cases [22]. In this context, there were some major criteria of malignancy put in place: mitotic index higher than 4/10 HPF, intratumoral necrosis or haemorrhage, pleomorphic cells, and the presence of metastasis; a minor criterion is represented by a size larger than 10 cm [13].

The histopathological diagnosis is usually accompanied by immunohistochemistry studies. The cases of malign PSFT are usually positive for CD35, CD99, bcl-2, or vimentin [23]. In our case, immunohistochemistry was used in 15 cases (33%), representing a disadvantage in getting a rigorous, definitive diagnosis. In addition, for a complete diagnosis, the Ki-67 antigen, associated with cellular proliferation, should be used (MIB-1-monoclonal antibody) for a better histological differentiation of the two cases of PSFT. Ki-67 is a nuclear protein, used as a marker of cellular proliferation, and MIB-1- monoclonal antibody for proliferation, linked with Ki-67. A Ki67 level <1% is suggestive for the lack of malignancy [1]. A more biological aggressiveness of PSFT is characterised by higher values of Ki-67 and p53 and variable CD-34 levels [7].

The recent oncological studies have shown, in the cases of PSFT, a fusion of NAB2–STAT6 gene, which is a result of intrachromosomal inversion 12q13.3., characteristic for this type of disease. This type of fusion leads to the development of STAT6 antibody, an immunohistochemical marker for this type of tumor [24]. Moreover, the mitotic number equal to higher than 4/10 HPF, TERD promoter, and mutation TP53 were correlated with the biological aggressiveness of the tumor [25]. NAB2–R593W fusion plays a major role in malign PSFT. Meanwhile, FLT1–R593W and KDR–V2971I somatic mutations are proof of the existence of a malignant angiogenetic phenotype [10].

There are correlation studies between sanguine inflammatory parameters and types of PSFT, which is the reason that fibrinogen, C reactive protein, and the neutrophil to lymphocyte ratio >5 were measured. An increase in these parameters was observed, especially in tumors larger than 10 cm, and especially in advanced stages from De Perrot classification as markers of malignity [26].

PSFTs are in most cases asymptomatic, but with their growth, they can lead to compression of the nearby organs (lungs, heart, large vessels, and thoracic wall), associated with a diversity of clinical symptoms [9,27,28]. In our case, the proportion of symptomatic and asymptomatic patients was almost equal, with 21 of them (46.66%) being symptomatic and 24 of them (53.33%) being asymptomatic. It should also be mentioned that, in most cases, the symptomatology was associated with the presence of larger tumors, with the size of over 10 cm—in our study, we have noticed that the symptomatology in patients with tumors larger than 10 cm was present in 44.44% of the cases, and in only one patient (2.22%), with a tumor smaller than 10 cm (who presented chest pain due to thoracic wall compression). The most frequent paraneoplastic syndromes mentioned in the literature are Doege–Potter syndrome (hypoglycaemic syndrome), hypertrophic pulmonary osteoarthopathy (Pierre–Marie–Bamberger syndrome), or the growth of the levels of beta human chorionic gonadotropin (BHCG) [29]. Refractory hypoglycaemia in PSFT context was first described in 1930, independently, by Doege and Potter, with no particularities in men or women incidences being observed [30–32]. Actually, hypoglycaemia associated with PSFT is considered a non-islet cell tumor hypoglycaemia (NICTH). NICTH is associated with solitary fibroma, hemangiopericytoma, or myxofibrosarcoma [33].

NITCH is encountered in approximately 4–5% of PSFT cases [34], and can be present in solitary pleural fibroma as well as in pelvic ones [35,36]. In our study group, out of 45 cases, Doege–Potter syndrome was present in two patients with malignant PSFT (4.44%). It is worth mentioning that NICHT can be associated with PSFT, regardless of the localization, but is more frequently associated with the malignant form (60.3%), representing an important prognostic factor [23,34]. In our study, out of the malignant forms of PSFT (eight cases), Doege–Potter was encountered in 25% of cases (six cases). Some studies have shown that PSFTs associated with hypoglycaemia represent 68% of the cases of pediculate tumors [19]. In our study group, we remarked that PSFTs were sessile or inverted tumors with histological sign of malignity. The main reasons for NICTH are the following: high level glucose usage by the tumor cells; insulin receptors proliferation; high levels of insulin like growth factor (IGF)-II, owing to tumor secretion; as well as a decrease in peptide C insulin, gonadotropin hormone (GH), and IGF-I. To sum up, the most important aspect of this pathology is the high level of IGF-II, as well as a significant change in IGF-II/IGF-I proportions (>10), and can confirm the NICTH diagnosis [37,38].

NICTH syndrome disappears with the tumor resection, a few days after the surgical procedure (3–4 days) [35]. In the cases of tumors that cannot be surgically removed, presenting with hypoglycaemia, some authors suggest alternative treatments such as a combination of two agents (Temozolomide and Bevacizumab), or radio embolization with yttrium 90 (Y^{90})-labelled glass microsphere [36,37]. Some other authors consider that, even if the tumor was completely removed, an adjuvant oncologic treatment is still needed [39]. Moreover, for an intraoperative control of glycaemia, it is recommended to use an artificial pancreas, which is capable to continually monitor glycaemia, and permanently adjust glucose and insulin intake [40].

Another paraneoplastic syndrome associated with PSFT is hypertrophic pulmonary osteoarthopathy, or Pierre–Marie–Bamberger syndrome [41]. In our study, the incidence was 4.44% (two cases) of malign PSFT. Causes of clubbing of the fingers and toes and of hypertrophic pulmonary osteoarthopathy are as follows: an abnormal production of hepatocyte growth factor (HGF) or a high level of hyaluronic acid, secreted by the fibrous tumor [16]. Digital clubbing can be measured using Schamroth sign, indicating the severity of the digital modification. However, they disappear with the complete tumor removal in two to six months from intervention [42]. We have acknowledged this with our two cases that presented Pierre–Marie–Bamberger syndrome—digital clubbing disappeared in about 2–5 months post-operative. Superior vena cava syndrome associated with PSFT is rarely described, even though it is frequently associated with bronchopulmonary cancer or lymphoproliferative disorders [43]. It is more frequently associated with malign PSFT [44]. In our cases, this syndrome was encountered in only one patient (2.22%) and was associated with malign PSFT, which leads to the apparition of arm and cephalic extremity oedema owing to the compression of superior vena cava and of the right atrium.

From a radiological view, the most frequent diagnosis is achieved through a simple thoracic radiography, in posterior–anterior incidence, which can determine the diagnosis of thoracic disease, as we have used in our research. Most commonly, the diagnosis is then confirmed using computed tomography of the thorax. For a complete diagnosis, with a definitive demarcation between malign

PSFT and benign PSFT, a multislice computed tomography is used. This method can create a multidimensional reconstruction, revealing the exact localization and size (less or more than 10 cm), tumor density, and vascularization, as well as the existence of pleural effusion, which can be a criteria of malignancy of PSFT [45]. Usually, in thoracic CT scans, in PSFT cases, there are some criteria that should be studied: the connection between the tumor and the mediastinal pleura (acute or obtuse angle formed with the adjacent pleura), tumor characteristics (lobulated, smooth with clear edges), shape of the tumor, homogenous or heterogeneous aspects, and associated characteristics. These are represented by the presence or absence of lymphadenopathy and pleural metastasis, or of the cleavage plane between the tumor and mediastinal structure, the "geographic pattern" of a rich vascularization of the tumor, and the necrosis or calcifications. All these aspects of the CT scan can reveal the differences between malign and benign PSFT [46,47].

In contrast, some authors consider these aspects to not be definitive for a proper demarcation between malignant and benign PSFT, underlining the fact that there are no clear differences that could be revealed by CT scan [48]. Nonetheless, computed tomography was used as a first-line investigation in our case, being the elective investigation in 35 of the cases (77.77%). The accuracy of the diagnosis was 42.85% (15 cases). Later, in 20% of the cases (nine cases), the investigation was then followed up with thoracic MRI. It had the patenting to supply with quantitative and qualitative data, as well as anatomical and functional ones without using radiation from the administeration of nephrotoxic contrast dye, making it excellent to be used in differential diagnosis of malign or benign pleural diseases [49]. In addition, it is useful in determining the existence of mediastinal invasion (larger vessels, main bronchi, and trachea), of the spinal cord or of the diaphragm, conferring precious information for the surgical treatment. The postoperative histopathological diagnosis enriches the accuracy of the CT diagnosis, as was emphasized in three cases (6.66%) using cutting needle biopsy with CT guidance [49]. In three other cases (6.66%) of large tumors, adjacent to the thoracic wall and approachable by standard radiology guiding, we also used direct needle biopsy. We consider these types of procedures (fine needle biopsy of the tumor) as not mandatory, as they do not influence the necessity of surgical removal. Still, they are useful in cases in which the tumor cannot be excised or metastases are present.

The elective treatment in PSFT is surgical resection. In malignant cases, an en bloc extensive and complex resection is proposed (thoracic wall, pulmonary lobe, lung, diaphragm, and so on), using oncological margins. The survival rate in malignant PSFT is considered by some authors to be 68% [9]. Malignant PSFTs metastasize using the hematogenous path to the liver, central nervous system, spleen, bones, kidneys, and adrenal glands [9]. In our study, out of eight cases of malignant PSFT, just one case had a recurrence two years after the first surgical intervention, and needed another intervention associated with adjuvant oncological treatment.

According to some authors, even benign PSFT can be unpredictable (10–15% of cases), especially if the size of the tumor is larger than 10 cm and has infiltrated the pleural margins [7]. This is the reason why in the case of our patients, tumor resection was done with oncological margins of 2 cm and in association with histopathological examination from pleural margins (37 cases, 82.22%). Some other authors stated that cancer recurrence in benign PSFT is between 11.2% and 20%, with a prolonged follow-up being required for this reason [27,50]. Some other authors expressed that, in the case of recurrence of benign PSFT, surgical treatment is the main option, eith oncologic treatment remaining as the sole option for inoperable tumors or in the presence of metastatic disease [20,51].

Even though surgical treatment is essential, some other authors consider that in the cases of malignant PSFT, adjuvant oncologic treatment should be associated [9]. From our eight patients with malignant PSFT, we have considered the surgical treatment to be the key treatment of this pathology. In our opinion, adjuvant oncologic treatment is reserved for recurrent cases (one case, 2.22% from our study). The prognosis of patients with PSFT is good, with the majority of cases being benign (88%), and only 12% showing a malignant behaviour [14]. Some other authors consider the recurrence to be 16% in the cases of malignant PSFT and only 2% in the benign cases [21]. In our study, we have observed that malignant recurrence represents 12.5% of the cases (n = 1). This represented the recurrence at about two years after the first surgery, and now, it is one-year cancer free since the moment of reintervention and the end of adjuvant oncologic treatment. For benign PSFT, there was no disease recurrence. It is also worth mentioning that the follow-up of the 45 patients is not completed yet. There were 34 patients who were re-evaluated two years after surgery (75.55%), with seven of them being also re-evaluated at the five-year follow-up (15.55%). As the follow-up period is not yet finished for the whole study group, it is premature to conclude, as we have proposed a 15-year follow-up period.

Tapias proposes an evaluation score and late follow-up of the patients, based on a series of pathologic signs: the origin of the tumor in parietal pleura, sesil morphology of the tumor, size larger than 10 cm, hypercellularity, high necrosis, and mitotic activity. On the basis of this score, a recurrence free survival interval of 100% was determined, if the score is less than three points [31].

Tumor recurrence is the main risk factor that can lead to death, appearing mostly in malign PSFT, even with en bloc resection of the multimodal treatment and even with close follow-up [21].

5. Conclusions

In conclusion, PSFTs are rare pleural tumors, most of which are benign; moreover, most of them are associated with a good prognostic, with the rates of malignant lesions being under 20% of cases. Most often, they are asymptomatic, with no signs and symptoms for a long period of time, and being usually discovered at a routine chest X-ray. In our study, PSFT was most commonly found in women over 40 years of age. Most of the cases were in patients over the age of 60 years. Thoracic CT scan is the main radiological instrument used for diagnosing this disease. MRI is complementary and, in some cases, superior to a CT scan. As for the therapeutic strategy, en bloc surgical resection with negative oncological margins is the gold standard in the treatment of PSFT. Chemotherapy and radiotherapy should be used in recurrent disease or inoperable stages.

Author Contributions: C.S., A.M., R.P. and N.G. performed surgical procedures; I.B., N.B. and C.D. performed literature search and review; D.C., A.F., C.B. and S.D. performed data analysis; C.S. and N.G. finally reviewed the manuscript. All authors have read and agreed to the published version of the manuscript.

Funding: This research received no external funding.

Acknowledgments: This work was supported by the project entitled "Multidisciplinary Consortium for Supporting the Research Skills in Diagnosing, Treating, and Identifying Predictive Factors of Malignant Gynecologic Disorders", project number PN-III-P1-1.2-PCCDI2017-0833.

Conflicts of Interest: The authors have no conflicts of interest to declare regarding this study.

References

1. Yagyu, H.; Hara, Y.; Murohashi, K.; Ishikawa, Y.; Isaka, T.; Woo, T.; Kaneko, T. Giant Solitary Fibrous Tumor of Pleura Presenting Both Benign and Malignant Features. *Am. J. Case Rep.* **2019**, *20*, 1755–1759. [CrossRef] [PubMed]
2. Wagner, E. Das tuberkelahnliche Lymphadenom (Der cytogene oder reticulirte Tuberkel). *Arch. Heilk. (Leipzig)* **1870**, *11*, 497.
3. Kucuksu, N.; Thomas, W.; Ezdinli, E.Z. Chemotherapy of Malignant Diffuse Mesothelioma. *Cancer* **1976**, *37*, 1265–1274. [CrossRef]
4. Ehrenhaft, J.L.; Sensenig, D.M.; Lawrence, M.S. Mesotheliomas of the Pleura. *J. Thorac. Cardiovasc. Surg.* **1960**, *40*, 393–409. [CrossRef]
5. Klemperer, P.; Coleman, B.R. Primary Neoplasms of the Pleura. A Report of Five Cases. *Am. J. Ind. Med.* **1992**, *22*, 1–31. [CrossRef] [PubMed]
6. Stout, A.P.; Himadi, G.M. Solitary (Localized) Mesothelioma of the Pleura. *Ann. Surg.* **1951**, *133*, 50–64. [CrossRef] [PubMed]

7. Attanoos, R.L.; Pugh, M.R. The Diagnosis of Pleural Tumors Other Than Mesothelioma. *Arch. Pathol. Lab. Med.* **2018**, *142*, 902–913. [CrossRef]
8. Yonli, D.S.; Chakroun, M.; Mokadem, S.; Saadi, A.; Rammeh, S.; Chebil, M. Adrenal Solitary Fibrous Tumor: A Case Report. *Urol. Case Rep.* **2019**, *27*, 100919. [CrossRef]
9. Ronchi, A.; Cozzolino, I.; Zito, M.F.; Accardo, M.; Montella, M.; Panarese, I.; Roccuzzo, G.; Toni, G.; Franco, R.; De Chiara, A. Extrapleural Solitary Fibrous Tumor: A Distinct Entity From Pleural Solitary Fibrous Tumor. An Update on Clinical, Molecular and Diagnostic Features. *Ann. Diagn. Pathol.* **2018**, *34*, 142–150. [CrossRef]
10. Song, Z.; Yang, F.; Zhang, Y.; Fan, P.; Liu, G.; Li, C.; Ding, W.; Zhang, Y.; Xu, X.; Ye, Y. Surgical Therapy and Next-Generation Sequencing-Based Genetic Alteration Analysis of Malignant Solitary Fibrous Tumor of the Pleura. *Onco Targets Ther.* **2018**, *11*, 5227–5238. [CrossRef]
11. England, D.M.; Hochholzer, L.; McCarthy, M.J. Localized Benign and Malignant Fibrous Tumors of the Pleura. A Clinicopathologic Review of 223 Cases. *Am. J. Surg. Pathol.* **1989**, *13*, 640–658. [CrossRef] [PubMed]
12. Mendez-Sanchez, H.; Mendez-Vivas, W.; Vargas-Mendoza, G.K.; Vazquez-Lopez, S.; Williams-Jacquez, A.D.; Cortes-Telles, A. Solitary Fibrous Tumors of the Pleura: A Clinical-Pathological Characterization Emphasizing Changes in Lung Function. *Adv. Respir. Med.* **2019**, *87*, 247–251. [CrossRef] [PubMed]
13. Briselli, M.; Mark, E.J.; Dickersin, G.R. Solitary Fibrous Tumors of the Pleura: Eight New Cases and Review of 360 Cases in the Literature. *Cancer* **1981**, *47*, 2678–2689. [CrossRef]
14. Jha, V.; Gil, J.; Teirstein, A.S. Familial Solitary Fibrous Tumor of the Pleura: A Case Report. *Chest* **2005**, *127*, 1852–1854. [CrossRef] [PubMed]
15. Cardillo, G.; Facciolo, F.; Cavazzana, A.O.; Capece, G.; Gasparri, R.; Martelli, M. Localized (Solitary) Fibrous Tumors of the Pleura: An Analysis of 55 Patients. *Ann. Thorac. Surg.* **2000**, *70*, 1808–1812. [CrossRef]
16. Urbina-Lima, A.D.; Roman-Martin, A.A.; Crespo-Santos, A.; Martinez-Rodriguez, A.; Cienfuegos-Belmonte, I.R.; Olmo-Ruiz, M.; Esteban-Artiaga, R.; Molina-Suarez, J.L. Solitary Fibrous Tumor of the Urinary Bladder Associated with Hypoglycemia: An Unusual Case of Doege-Potter Syndrome. *Urol. Int.* **2019**, *103*, 120–124. [CrossRef] [PubMed]
17. Prado, F.; Dos Ramos, J.P.; Larranaga, N.; Espil, G.; Kozima, S. Solitary Fibrous Tumor and Doege-Potter Syndrome. *Medicina (B Aires)* **2018**, *78*, 47–49.
18. Yanik, F.; Karamustafaoglu, Y.A.; Yoruk, Y. Surgical Outcomes and Clinical Courses of Solitary Fibrous Tumors of Pleura. *Niger. J. Clin. Pract.* **2019**, *22*, 1412–1416. [CrossRef]
19. Tapias, L.F.; Mercier, O.; Ghigna, M.R.; Lahon, B.; Lee, H.; Mathisen, D.J.; Dartevelle, P.; Lanuti, M. Validation of a Scoring System to Predict Recurrence of Resected Solitary Fibrous Tumors of the Pleura. *Chest* **2015**, *147*, 216–223. [CrossRef]
20. Lahon, B.; Mercier, O.; Fadel, E.; Ghigna, M.R.; Petkova, B.; Mussot, S.; Fabre, D.; Le Chevalier, T.; Dartevelle, P. Solitary Fibrous Tumor of the Pleura: Outcomes of 157 Complete Resections in a Single Center. *Ann. Thorac. Surg.* **2012**, *94*, 394–400. [CrossRef]
21. de Perrot, M.; Fischer, S.; Brundler, M.A.; Sekine, Y.; Keshavjee, S. Solitary Fibrous Tumors of the Pleura. *Ann. Thorac. Surg.* **2002**, *74*, 285–293. [CrossRef]
22. Ventura, L.; Gnetti, L.; Braggio, C.; Carbognati, P.; Rusca, M.; Silini, E.M.; Ampolini, L. Solitary Fibrous Tumor of the Pleura Associated with Severe Hypoglycemia: The Doege-Potter syndrome. *J. Thorac. Oncol.* **2017**, *12*, S1019–S1020. [CrossRef]
23. Galateau-Salle, F.; Churg, A.; Roggli, V.; Travis, W.D. The 2015 World Health Organization Classification of Tumors of the Pleura: Advances since the 2004 Classification. *J. Thorac. Oncol.* **2016**, *11*, 142–154. [CrossRef] [PubMed]
24. Huang, S.C.; Huang, H.Y. Solitary Fibrous Tumor: An Evolving and Unifying Entity with Unsettled Issues. *Histol. Histopathol.* **2019**, *34*, 313–334.
25. Ghanim, B.; Hess, S.; Bertoglio, P.; Celik, A.; Bas, A.; Oberndorfer, F.; Melfi, F.; Mussi, A.; Klepetko, W.; Pirker, C.; et al. Intrathoracic Solitary Fibrous Tumor—An International Multicenter Study on Clinical Outcome and Novel Circulating Biomarkers. *Sci. Rep.* **2017**, *7*, 12557. [CrossRef]
26. Cao, Y.Y.; Fan, N.; Xing, F.; Xu, L.Y.; Qu, Y.J.; Liao, M.Y. Computed Tomography-Guided Cutting Needle Pleural Biopsy: Accuracy and Complications. *Exp. Ther. Med.* **2015**, *9*, 262–266. [CrossRef]

27. Mavarez, J.D.A.; Montes, M.A.V.; Seoane, M.R.R.; Shao, M.L. Hypoglycemia as an Atypical Presentation of a Pleural Tumor. *Arch. Bronconeumol.* **2019**, *55*, 652–654. [CrossRef]
28. Karki, A.; Yang, J.; Chauhan, S. Paraneoplastic Syndrome Associate with Solitary Fibrous Tumor of Pleura. *Lung India* **2018**, *35*, 245–247. [CrossRef]
29. Meng, W.; Zhu, H.H.; Li, H.; Wang, G.; Wei, D.; Feng, X. Solitary Fibrous Tumors of the Pleura With Doege-Potter Syndrome: A Case Report and Three-Decade Review of the Literature. *BMC Res. Notes* **2014**, *7*, 515. [CrossRef]
30. Gomez, F.D.; Robin, L.; Jakubowicz, D.; Sillou, S.; Lab, J.P.; Balian, C. Solitary Fibrous Tumor of the Retroperitoneum With Urinary Symptoms Revealing a Doege-Potter's Syndrome. *Prog. Urol.* **2019**, *29*, 136–137. [CrossRef]
31. Tapias, L.F.; Lanuti, M. Solitary fibrous tumors of the pleura: Review of literature with up-to-date observations. *Lung Cancer Manag.* **2015**, *4*, 169–179. [CrossRef]
32. Jannin, A.; Espiard, S.; Benomar, K.; Do, C.C.; Mycinski, B.; Porte, H.; D'Herbomez, M.; Penel, N.; Vantyghem, M.C. Non-Islet-Cell Tumour Hypoglycaemia (NICTH): About a Series of 6 Cases. *Ann. Endocrinol. (Paris)* **2019**, *80*, 21–25. [CrossRef] [PubMed]
33. Aridi, T.; Tawil, A.; Hashem, M.; Khoury, J.; Raad, R.A.; Youssef, P. Unique Presentation and Management Approach of Pleural Solitary Fibrous Tumor. *Case Rep. Surg.* **2019**, *2019*, 9706825. [CrossRef] [PubMed]
34. Wada, Y.; Okano, K.; Ando, Y.; Uemura, J.; Suto, H.; Asano, E.; Kishino, T.; Oshima, M.; Kumamoto, K.; Usuki, H.; et al. A Solitary Fibrous Tumor in the Pelvic Cavity of a Patient with Doege-Potter Syndrome: A Case Report. *Surg. Case Rep.* **2019**, *5*, 60. [CrossRef] [PubMed]
35. Kim, D.W.; Na, K.J.; Yun, J.S.; Song, S.Y. Doege-Potter Syndrome: A Report of a Histologically Benign but Clinically Malignant Case. *J. Cardiothorac. Surg.* **2017**, *12*, 64. [CrossRef]
36. Han, G.; Zhang, Z.; Shen, X.; Wang, K.; Zhao, Y.; He, J.; Gao, Y.; Shan, X.; Xin, G.; Li, C.; et al. Doege-Potter Syndrome: A Review of the Literature Including a New Case Report. *Medicine (Baltimore)* **2017**, *96*, e7417. [CrossRef]
37. Villemain, A.; Menard, O.; Mandry, D.; Siat, J.; Vignaud, J.M.; Martinet, Y.; Tiotiu, A. Paraneoplastic Hypoglycemia: The Hopes of Pathophysiological Documentation. *Rev. Pneumol. Clin.* **2017**, *73*, 140–145. [CrossRef]
38. Kuhn-Velten, U.; Hohmann, C.; Strauss, T.; Heizmann, O.; Kloppel, G. Solitary Fibrous Tumor: A Rare Cause of Recurrent Severe Hypoglycemia. *Dtsch. Med. Wochenschr.* **2018**, *143*, 824–829.
39. Rena, O.; Filosso, P.L.; Papalia, E.; Molinatti, M.; Di Marzio, P.; Maggi, G.; Oliaro, A. Solitary Fibrous Tumour of the Pleura: Surgical Treatment. *Eur. J. Cardiothorac. Surg.* **2001**, *19*, 185–189. [CrossRef]
40. Pirvu, A.; Angelescu, D.; Savu, C. Localized Fibrous Tumor of the Pleura an Unusual Cause of Severe Hypoglycaemia. Case Report. *Rev. Med. Chir. Soc. Med. Nat. Iasi* **2016**, *120*, 628–630.
41. Bailly, C.; Bichali, A.M.; Douane, F.; Ansquer, C.; Drui, D. Metastatic Solitary Fibrous Tumor with Doege-Potter Syndrome: Hypoglycemia Treated by 90Y Radioembolization. *Clin. Nucl. Med.* **2018**, *43*, e93–e95. [CrossRef] [PubMed]
42. Ogunsakin, A.A.; Hilsenbeck, H.L.; Portnoy, D.C.; Nyenwe, E.A. Recurrent Severe Hypoinsulinemic Hypoglycemia Responsive to Temozolomide and Bevacizumab in a Patient With Doege-Potter Syndrome. *Am. J. Med. Sci.* **2018**, *356*, 181–184. [CrossRef] [PubMed]
43. Sugimoto, M.; Tokitou, R.; Kadosaki, M.; Takeuchi, M. Intraoperative Glycemic Control Using an Artificial Endocrine Pancreas in a Patient with a Recurrent Pleural Solitary Fibrous Tumor Producing Insulin-Like Growth Factor 2: A Case Report. *JA Clin. Rep.* **2019**, *5*, 6. [CrossRef] [PubMed]
44. Bossart, S.; Rammlmair, A.; Haneke, E. Reversible Schamroth Sign after Pleural Tumor Resection. *Skin Appendage Disord.* **2019**, *5*, 327–328. [CrossRef] [PubMed]
45. Galie, N.; Vasile, R.; Savu, C.; Petreanu, C.; Grigorie, V.; Tabacu, E. Superior Vena Cava Syndrome—Surgical Solution—Case Report. *Chirurgia (Bucur.)* **2010**, *105*, 835–838. [PubMed]
46. Shiono, S.; Abiko, M.; Tamura, G.; Sato, T. Malignant Solitary Fibrous Tumor with Superior Vena Cava Syndrome. *Gen. Thorac. Cardiovasc. Surg.* **2009**, *57*, 321–323. [CrossRef]
47. You, X.; Sun, X.; Yang, C.; Fang, Y. CT Diagnosis and Differentiation of Benign and Malignant Varieties of Solitary Fibrous Tumor of the Pleura. *Medicine (Baltimore)* **2017**, *96*, e9058. [CrossRef]

48. Cardinale, L.; Dalpiaz, G.; Pulzato, I.; Ardissone, F. Computed Tomography of Solitary Fibrous Tumor of the Pleura Abutting the Mediastinum: A Diagnostic Challenge. *Lung India* **2018**, *35*, 121–126.
49. Aluja, J.F.; Gutierrez, F.; Bhalla, S. Pleural Tumours and Tumour-Like Lesions. *Clin. Radiol.* **2018**, *73*, 1014–1024. [CrossRef]
50. Abu, A.W. Solitary Fibrous Tumours of the Pleura. *Eur. J. Cardiothorac. Surg.* **2012**, *41*, 587–597. [CrossRef]
51. Gupta, A.; Souza, C.A.; Sekhon, H.S.; Gomes, M.M.; Hare, S.S.; Agarwal, P.P.; Kanne, J.P.; Seely, J.M. Solitary Fibrous Tumour of Pleura: CT Differentiation of Benign and Malignant Types. *Clin. Radiol.* **2017**, *72*, 796. [CrossRef] [PubMed]

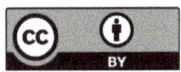

© 2020 by the authors. Licensee MDPI, Basel, Switzerland. This article is an open access article distributed under the terms and conditions of the Creative Commons Attribution (CC BY) license (http://creativecommons.org/licenses/by/4.0/).

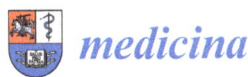

Case Report

Synchronous Cervical Adenocarcinoma and Ovarian Serous Adenocarcinoma—A Case Report and Literature Review

Nicolae Bacalbasa [1,2,3,†], Irina Cecilia Balescu [4,5,*], Camelia Diaconu [6,7,†], Simona Dima [3], Laura Iliescu [7,8,†], Mihaela Vilcu [9,10], Alexandru Filipescu [1,11,†], Ioana Halmaciu [12], Dragos Cretoiu [13,14] and Iulian Brezean [9,10]

1. Department of Obstetrics and Gynecology, "Carol Davila" University of Medicine and Pharmacy, 020021 Bucharest, Romania; nicolae_bacalbasa@yahoo.ro (N.B.); alexandru.filipescu@gmail.ro (A.F.)
2. Department of Obstetrics and Gynecology, "I. Cantacuzino" Clinical Hospital, 030167 Bucharest, Romania
3. Department of Visceral Surgery, Center of Excellence in Translational Medicine "Fundeni" Clinical Institute, 022328 Bucharest, Romania; simona.dima@gmail.ro
4. Department of Surgery, "Ponderas" Academic Hospital, 021188 Bucharest, Romania
5. Department of Surgery, "Carol Davila" University of Medicine and Pharmacy, 020021 Bucharest, Romania
6. Department of Internal Medicine, "Floreasca" Clinical Emergency Hospital, 105402, Bucharest, Romania; drcameliadiaconu@gmail.com
7. Department of Internal Medicine, "Carol Davila" University of Medicine and Pharmacy, 020021 Bucharest, Romania; laura.iliescu@gmail.ro
8. Department of Internal Medicine, "Fundeni" Clinical Institute, 022328 Bucharest, Romania
9. Department of Visceral Surgery, "Carol Davila" University of Medicine and Pharmacy, 020021 Bucharest, Romania; mihaela.vilcu@gmail.ro (M.V.); iulian.brezean@gmail.ro (I.B.)
10. Department of Visceral Surgery, "I. Cantacuzino" Clinical Hospital, 030167 Bucharest, Romania
11. Department of Obstetrics and Gynecology, "Elias" Emergency Hospital, 105402 Bucharest, Romania
12. Department of Anatomy, "George Emil Palade" University of Medicine, Pharmacy, Science and Technology, 540139 Târgu Mureș, Romania; ioana.halmaciu@gmail.ro
13. "Alessandrescu-Rusescu" National Institute of Mother and Child Health, Fetal Medicine Excellence Research Center, 020395 Bucharest, Romania; dragos.cretoiu@gmail.ro
14. Department of Cell and Molecular Biology and Histology, "Carol Davila" University of Medicine and Pharmacy, 020021 Bucharest, Romania
* Correspondence: irina.balescu@ponderas-ah.ro; Tel.: +40-724077709
† These authors contributed equally to this work.

Received: 9 February 2020; Accepted: 24 March 2020; Published: 29 March 2020

Abstract: *Background/Aim:* Synchronous gynecological malignancies are rarely encountered, and most often these cases are represented by synchronous ovarian and endometrial cancer. The aim of this paper is to present the case of a 53-year-old patient who was diagnosed with synchronous cervical and ovarian cancer. *Case presentation:* The patient had been initially investigated for vaginal bleeding and was submitted to a biopsy confirming the presence of a cervical adenocarcinoma. Once the diagnostic of malignancy was confirmed, the patient was submitted to a computed tomography which revealed the presence of large abdominal tumoral nodules of peritoneal carcinomatosis and was submitted to palliative chemotherapy with poor response. Eighteen months later she developed intestinal obstruction and was submitted to surgery. At that moment, synchronous ovarian and cervical tumors were diagnosed. Total radical hysterectomy with bilateral adnexectomy, pelvic and para-aortic lymph node dissection, omentectomy, and pelvic peritonectomy was performed; in the meantime, the histopathological studies confirmed the presence of two synchronous malignancies. *Conclusion:* Although synchronous lesions are rarely encountered, this eventuality should not be omitted. In such cases, surgery should be taken in consideration and the intent of radicality should regard both lesions.

Keywords: synchronous malignancies; cervical adenocarcinoma; serous ovarian adenocarcinoma

1. Introduction

Synchronous gynecological malignancies can rarely be encountered in patients with gynecological tract tumors, the most commonly encountered lesions being represented by ovarian and endometrial cancer [1–3]. As for the association of cervical and ovarian cancer, this situation has been rarely reported, the most common association being of human papillomavirus (HPV)-induced cervical cancer and mucinous ovarian adenocarcinoma; only few cases have been reported so far [4–6]. The aim of the paper is to present the case of a patient who was initially diagnosed with advanced stage mucinous adenocarcinoma of the uterine cervix and presumed peritoneal carcinomatosis who was diagnosed at the time of surgery with synchronous cervical and ovarian carcinoma.

2. Case Presentation

The study was approved by the local ethics committee (11/27.01.2020) and the patient signed an informed consent form. The 53-year-old postmenopausal woman with no significant family oncological background was initially investigated for postmenopausal vaginal bleeding, diffuse pelvic pain, and weight loss. At that moment, vaginal examination revealed the presence of a cervical tumor which was biopsied.

The histopathological studies revealed the presence of a moderately differentiated cervical adenocarcinoma, so the patient was submitted to a pelvic magnetic resonance imaging and to a thoracic and abdominal computed tomography, which revealed the presence of large abdominal masses of peritoneal carcinomatosis. In the meantime, biological parameters did not reveal any significant modifications—the serum levels of cancer antigen 125 (CA125), human epididymis 4 (HE4), and carcinoembryonic antigen (CEA) reported minimal modification (CA125 = 76 U/mL, HE4 = 43 U/mL, CEA = 25 ng/mL). Therefore, the diagnostic for that moment was of cervical adenocarcinoma with peritoneal metastases; hence, the patient was submitted to platinum-based chemotherapy with palliative intent; however, at six months follow-up the imagistic studies revealed no significant response, and the patient became refractory to this treatment and decided to interrupt the oncological treatment. Therefore, due to the lack of compliance partially induced by the poor response to treatment, the patient was lost from follow up for more than a year.

However, eighteen months later she came back due to the presence of diffuse abdominal pain and intestinal obstructive syndrome. The patient was submitted to surgery in order to treat the intestinal obstruction; at the time of surgery bilateral ovarian tumors were identified in association with peritoneal nodules of carcinomatosis and with the already known cervical tumor. The intraoperative frozen section demonstrated the presence of a serous ovarian adenocarcinoma and confirmed the fact that the peritoneal lesions had an ovarian origin; therefore, she was submitted to surgery with curative intent; in this respect, a total radical hysterectomy with bilateral adnexectomy, pelvic and para-aortic lymph node dissection, omentectomy, and pelvic peritonectomy were performed (Figures 1 and 2).

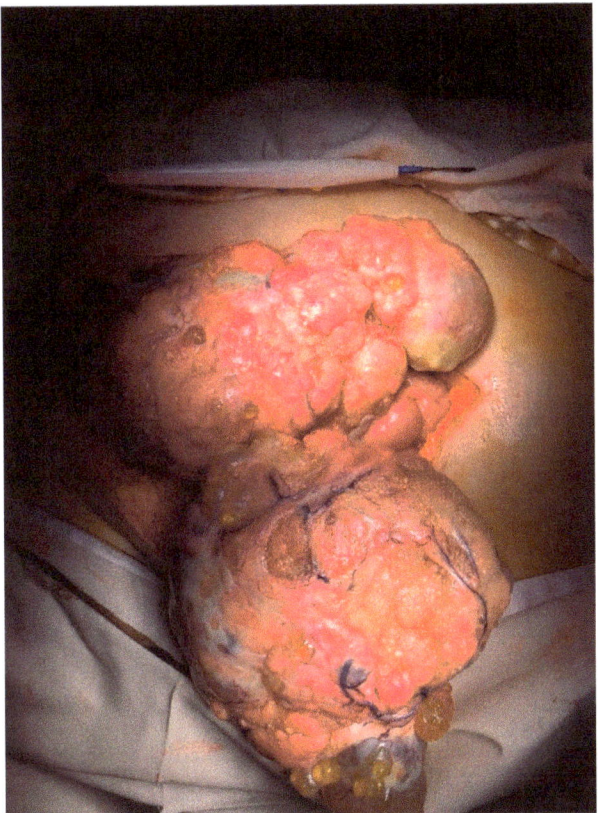

Figure 1. Initial intraoperative aspect—large nodules of peritoneal carcinomatosis.

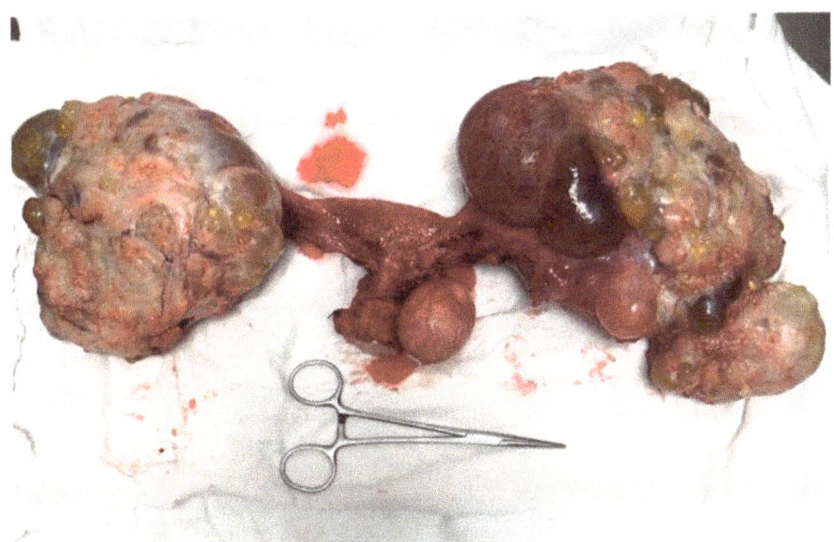

Figure 2. The final aspect—the specimen of total radical hysterectomy with bilateral adnexectomy and excision of the nodules of peritoneal carcinomatosis.

The final histopathological findings confirmed the presence of a moderately differentiated mucinous cervical adenocarcinoma, in association with well differentiated ovarian serous adenocarcinoma with peritoneal involvement; in the meantime, three of the 21 pelvic lymph nodes presented tumoral involvement. The final staging was of stage IIIC ovarian adenocarcinoma (cancer has spread to the peritoneum and the cancer in the peritoneum is larger than 2 centimeters and/or cancer has spread to lymph nodes in the abdomen) and stage IIA cervical cancer (cancer has spread to the uterus and/or fallopian tubes (the long slender tubes through which eggs pass from the ovaries to the uterus); according to the World Health Organization (WHO) 2014 classification, the ovarian lesion was classified as a low grade serous carcinoma, while the cervical lesion was classified as a not otherwise specified mucinous carcinoma [7]. Postoperatively she was confined to the oncology service in order to be submitted to adjuvant consolidation chemotherapy. In the meantime, after establishing the final histopathological diagnostic, BRCA1/2 (BReast CAncer genes 1 and 2) testing was performed; however, none of these mutations were encountered.

3. Discussion

Synchronous gynecological malignancies have been encountered in up to 2% of women diagnosed with any kind of gynecological cancers; however, the most commonly encountered association consists of ovarian and endometrial cancer [3–6]. As for the association between ovarian and cervical cancer, isolated cases have been reported so far: Therefore, in a study conducted by Turkish authors on a period of 20 years, there were only five patients diagnosed with synchronous ovarian and cervical cancer [8]. In a more recent study conducted by Young et al. on 20 patients with synchronous gynecological malignancies, a single patient was diagnosed with synchronous ovarian and cervical carcinoma [6].

In such cases the most important question which is raised is if the two lesions are real synchronous, distinct malignancies, or if one of them is the metastasis of the other tumor. This fact can be clearly ruled out in cases in which the tumors exhibit different subtypes, as well as in cases in which areas of normal parenchyma can be evidenced between the two lesions. Therefore, in our case, the presence of two different histopathological subtypes (serous ovarian adenocarcinoma and mucinous cervical adenocarcinoma) sustained the hypothesis of synchronous lesions in an indubitable manner.

Uterine cervix adenocarcinoma represents the second most common histopathological subtype of cervical cancer after squamous cell carcinoma, ranging for up to 20% of cases with cervical cancer. However, in the last decades, the incidence of cervical adenocarcinoma increased, especially due to the fact that screening tests are less effective for this histopathological subtype [9–11]. The low efficacy of detection of this histopathological subtype during routine evaluation is rather related to the endocervical development of these tumors; therefore, an important number of cases are diagnosed at a more advanced stage of the disease, when local extension or distant metastases transform the patient into a candidate for palliative treatment [12,13]. Moreover, this histopathological subtype has been initially considered as being associated with a poorer outcome when compared to squamous cell carcinoma [14]. However, more recent and larger studies came to demonstrate that association of targeted therapies such as monoclonal antibodies, angiogenic kinases by tyrosine kinase inhibitors, immune checkpoint programmed cell death 1, and T-lymphocyte-associated molecule-4 inhibitors might significantly improve the outcomes of these patients, especially when used in the setting of advanced or recurrent disease [15]. In the meantime, in cases diagnosed with cervical adenocarcinoma, the risk of lymph node metastases development is rather related to the presence of stromal invasion and lymph vascular invasion than to the dimensions of the tumor [13,14]. Another important feature of this histopathological subtype is represented by the capacity to develop distant metastases at the level of the ovaries and lymph nodes, when compared to squamous cell carcinoma [16–19]. However, in our case, the fact that the ovarian tumors proved to have a serous component, while the cervical adenocarcinoma proved to be a mucinous tumor, enabled us to consider that the two malignancies were synchronous and not metastatic lesions. Moreover, the degree of differentiation of the ovarian tumor probably explained the absence of a negative impact of the long period of time in which the patient did not undergo any treatment; in the meantime, the patient's decision to interrupt the treatment against the medical recommendation and her poor compliance with the initial treatment can be explained by the fact that under this treatment only minor improvement of the general status was observed.

As for the type of treatment of cervical adenocarcinoma, it is usually similar to the one for squamous cell cervical cancer [20–22]. However, association of monoclonal antibodies in the setting of advanced stage or recurrent disease provided a significant improvement of the long-term outcomes of these cases [15]. These data were also sustained by the study conducted between 2004 and 2014 at the Royal Marsden Hospital, which demonstrated that second line therapy in the setting of advanced and recurrent cervical cancer is associated with poor rates of response; moreover, the authors underlined the necessity of exploring the effectiveness of novel targeted agents and immunotherapy in such cases. Data related in this study are particularly important due to the fact that different and aggressive biological subtypes such as clear cell, adenocarcinoma, and even neuroendocrine uterine cervix carcinomas have been included [23]. As for the cases diagnosed in early stages of the disease, fertility sparing surgery should not be taken into consideration, due to the more aggressive biological behavior of this histopathological subtype.

Mucinous adenocarcinomas of the uterine cervix are an even scarcer biological subtype, being considered as a particular subgroup since 2014; one of the largest studies which came to investigate the prognostic factors in patients with mucinous adenocarcinoma of uterine cervix has been recently published in the *Journal of Gynecology Obstetrics and Human Reproduction* and included 82 cases diagnosed with cervical adenocarcinomas, 21 of them being diagnosed with the mucinous subtype [24]. Among these cases, the mean age was of 42 years, while the most commonly encountered symptoms were represented by vaginal bleeding, followed by mucinous discharge; moreover, only 72% of cases presented a modified smear test. As for the type of performed treatment, it consisted of total radical hysterectomy with bilateral adnexectomy and sentinel node biopsy in cases diagnosed in early stages of disease and complete lymph node dissection in more advanced stages; in the meantime, surgery was followed by adjuvant oncological treatment. After a mean follow-up of 30 months, 13 cases were alive and free of disease, one was alive with disease, three were dead of disease, one was dead due to other causes, and the remaining three cases were lost from follow-up [24]. These data come to suggest that although this histopathological subtype is significantly scarcer, it benefits from the same type of oncological and surgical treatment when compared to squamous cell carcinoma. As for the case we presented, it was treated in a similar manner once the hypothesis of peritoneal carcinomatosis with cervical origin was excluded; therefore, the patient benefitted from a radical hysterectomy with extended pelvic and para-aortic lymph node dissection.

However, the correct and complete diagnostic in our case was delayed with almost two years, especially due to the fact that the ovarian malignancy was not associated with increased levels of CA125 and HE4, being a non-secretory tumor; this aspect in association with the poor compliance of the patient with the proposed treatment led to a delay of the treatment with curative intent.

When it comes to the utility of CA125 in ovarian cancer diagnostic, attention should be focused on the fact that only half of patients are in early stages of the disease and up to 90% of cases diagnosed in advanced stages present increased levels, the remaining 10% of cases presenting normal or minimal increase, of the serum levels of CA125 [25]. In the meantime, in order to maximize the rates of detection of ovarian cancer even in cases in which serum levels of CA125 could not give a diagnostic clue, HE4 has been proposed; therefore, it is estimated that two thirds of patients diagnosed with early or advanced stage of the disease will exhibit increased levels of HE4. Moreover, certain studies have shown that one third of patients with normal levels of CA125 and ovarian cancer will exhibit increased levels of HE4; however, in our case, neither CA125 nor HE4 did report any suggestive modification for the diagnostic of ovarian cancer. In this respect, the treatment was initially tailored according to the suspicion of diagnostic of cervical adenocarcinoma and peritoneal carcinomatosis with cervical origin. Other serum markers which might increase the rates of preoperative diagnostic of ovarian cancer in postmenopausal women are represented by alpha fetoprotein and β-human chorionic gonadotrophin; however, these parameters seem to be beneficial, especially in cases diagnosed with particular histopathological subtypes, such as germ cell ovarian tumors [26]. In this respect, novel tumor markers and scores are still needed in order to provide a better preoperative identification of such pathologies.

4. Conclusions

Although rarely seen, synchronous cervical and ovarian cancer might be encountered and might benefit from surgery with curative intent. However, in the case we reported, the presence of a non-secretory ovarian adenocarcinoma, even in the presence of large nodules of peritoneal carcinomatosis in association with the indubitable diagnostic of cervical adenocarcinoma, led to a confusing initial diagnostic. Moreover, the fluctuant evolution of this patient was also caused by the initial poor compliance of the patient with treatment and follow-up. However, the final diagnostic was established at the time of surgery for obstructive syndrome, which revealed the presence of two different lesions and which offered the chance to the patient to be submitted to surgery with curative intent, radical procedures being performed for both ovarian and cervical malignant lesions.

Author Contributions: N.B., M.V., I.B. and A.F. performed the surgical procedure; I.C.B. reviewed literature data; I.C.B., L.I., C.D., I.H. and D.C. prepared the draft of the manuscript; I.B. was advisor of the surgical oncology procedures; I.B. reviewed the final version of the manuscript. All Authors read and approved the final version of the manuscript.

Funding: This research received no external funding.

Acknowledgments: This work was supported by the project entitled "Multidisciplinary Consortium for Supporting the Research Skills in Diagnosing, Treating and Identifying Predictive Factors of Malignant Gynecologic Disorders", project number PN-III-P1-1.2-PCCDI2017-0833.

Conflicts of Interest: The Authors have no conflict of interest to declare regarding this study.

References

1. Williams, M.G.; Bandera, E.V.; Demissie, K.; Rodriguez-Rodriguez, L. Synchronous Primary Ovarian and Endometrial Cancers: A Population-Based Assessment of Survival. *Obstet. Gynecol.* **2009**, *113*, 783–789. [CrossRef]
2. Lee, T.S.; Jung, J.Y.; Kim, J.W.; Park, N.H.; Song, Y.S.; Kang, S.B.; Lee, H.P. Feasibility of Ovarian Preservation in Patients with Early Stage Endometrial Carcinoma. *Gynecol. Oncol.* **2007**, *104*, 52–57. [CrossRef] [PubMed]
3. Bacalbasa, N.; Stoica, C.; Popa, I.; Mirea, G.; Balescu, I. Endometrial Carcinoma Associated with Ovarian Granulosa Cell Tumors—A Case Report. *Anticancer Res.* **2015**, *35*, 5547–5550. [PubMed]
4. Ronnett, B.M.; Yemelyanova, A.V.; Vang, R.; Gilks, C.B.; Miller, D.; Gravitt, P.E.; Kurman, R.J. Endocervical Adenocarcinomas with Ovarian Metastases: Analysis of 29 Cases with Emphasis on Minimally Invasive Cervical Tumors and the Ability of the Metastases to Simulate Primary Ovarian Neoplasms. *Am. J. Surg. Pathol.* **2008**, *32*, 1835–1853. [CrossRef] [PubMed]
5. Vinokurova, S.; Wentzensen, N.; Einenkel, J.; Klaes, R.; Ziegert, C.; Melsheimer, P.; Sartor, H.; Horn, L.C.; Hockel, M.; von Knebel, D.M. Clonal History of Papillomavirus-Induced Dysplasia in the Female Lower Genital Tract. *J. Natl. Cancer Inst.* **2005**, *97*, 1816–1821. [CrossRef]
6. Tong, S.Y.; Lee, Y.S.; Park, J.S.; Bae, S.N.; Lee, J.M.; Namkoong, S.E. Clinical Analysis of Synchronous Primary Neoplasms of the Female Reproductive Tract. *Eur. J. Obstet. Gynecol. Reprod. Biol.* **2008**, *136*, 78–82. [CrossRef] [PubMed]
7. Lax, S.F.; Horn, L.C.; Loning, T. Categorization of Uterine Cervix Tumors: What's New in the 2014 WHO Classification. *Pathologe* **2016**, *37*, 573–584. [CrossRef]
8. Ayhan, A.; Yalcin, O.T.; Tuncer, Z.S.; Gurgan, T.; Kucukali, T. Synchronous Primary Malignancies of the Female Genital Tract. *Eur. J. Obstet. Gynecol. Reprod. Biol.* **1992**, *45*, 63–66. [CrossRef]
9. Bray, F.; Carstensen, B.; Moller, H.; Zappa, M.; Zakelj, M.P.; Lawrence, G.; Hakama, M.; Weiderpass, E. Incidence Trends of Adenocarcinoma of the Cervix in 13 European Countries. *Cancer Epidemiol. Biomark. Prev.* **2005**, *14*, 2191–2199. [CrossRef]

10. Wang, S.S.; Sherman, M.E.; Hildesheim, A.; Lacey, J.V., Jr.; Devesa, S. Cervical Adenocarcinoma and Squamous Cell Carcinoma Incidence Trends Among White Women and Black Women in the United States for 1976–2000. *Cancer* **2004**, *100*, 1035–1044. [CrossRef]
11. Castellsague, X.; Diaz, M.; de Sanjose, S.; Munoz, N.; Herrero, R.; Franceschi, S.; Peeling, R.W.; Ashley, R.; Smith, J.S.; Snijders, P.J.; et al. Worldwide Human Papillomavirus Etiology of Cervical Adenocarcinoma and Its Cofactors: Implications for Screening and Prevention. *J. Natl. Cancer Inst.* **2006**, *98*, 303–315. [CrossRef] [PubMed]
12. Sherman, M.E.; Wang, S.S.; Carreon, J.; Devesa, S.S. Mortality Trends for Cervical Squamous and Adenocarcinoma in the United States: Relation to Incidence and Survival. *Cancer* **2005**, *103*, 1258–1264. [CrossRef] [PubMed]
13. Sasieni, P.; Castanon, A.; Cuzick, J. Screening and Adenocarcinoma of the Cervix. *Int. J. Cancer* **2009**, *125*, 525–529. [CrossRef] [PubMed]
14. Ryu, S.Y.; Kim, M.H.; Nam, B.H.; Lee, T.S.; Song, E.S.; Park, C.Y.; Kim, J.W.; Kim, Y.B.; Ryu, H.S.; Park, S.Y.; et al. Intermediate-Risk Grouping of Cervical Cancer Patients Treated with Radical Hysterectomy: A Korean Gynecologic Oncology Group Study. *Br. J. Cancer* **2014**, *110*, 278–285. [CrossRef] [PubMed]
15. Boussios, S.; Seraj, E.; Zarkavelis, G.; Petrakis, D.; Kollas, A.; Kafantari, A.; Assi, A.; Tatsi, K.; Pavlidis, N.; Pentheroudakis, G. Management of Patients with Recurrent/Advanced Cervical Cancer beyond First Line Platinum Regimens: Where Do We Stand? A Literature Review. *Crit. Rev. Oncol. Hematol.* **2016**, *108*, 164–174. [CrossRef] [PubMed]
16. Gadducci, A.; Guerrieri, M.E.; Cosio, S. Adenocarcinoma of the Uterine Cervix: Pathologic Features, Treatment Options, Clinical Outcome and Prognostic Variables. *Crit. Rev. Oncol. Hematol.* **2019**, *135*, 103–114. [CrossRef]
17. Eifel, P.J.; Morris, M.; Oswald, M.J.; Wharton, J.T.; Delclos, L. Adenocarcinoma of the Uterine Cervix Prognosis and Patterns of Failure in 367 Cases. *Cancer* **1990**, *65*, 2507–2514. [CrossRef]
18. Eifel, P.J.; Burke, T.W.; Morris, M.; Smith, T.L. Adenocarcinoma as an Independent Risk Factor for Disease Recurrence in Patients with Stage IB Cervical Carcinoma. *Gynecol. Oncol.* **1995**, *59*, 38–44. [CrossRef]
19. Irie, T.; Kigawa, J.; Minagawa, Y.; Itamochi, H.; Sato, S.; Akeshima, R.; Terakawa, N. Prognosis and Clinicopathological Characteristics of Ib-IIb Adenocarcinoma of the Uterine Cervix in Patients Who Have Had Radical Hysterectomy. *Eur. J. Surg. Oncol.* **2000**, *26*, 464–467. [CrossRef]
20. Gien, L.T.; Beauchemin, M.C.; Thomas, G. Adenocarcinoma: A Unique Cervical Cancer. *Gynecol. Oncol.* **2010**, *116*, 140–146. [CrossRef]
21. Baalbergen, A.; Veenstra, Y.; Stalpers, L.L.; Ansink, A.C. Primary Surgery versus Primary Radiation Therapy with or without Chemotherapy for Early Adenocarcinoma of the Uterine Cervix. *Cochrane Database Syst. Rev.* **2010**, CD006248. [CrossRef]
22. Park, J.Y.; Kim, D.Y.; Kim, J.H.; Kim, Y.M.; Kim, Y.T.; Nam, J.H. Outcomes After Radical Hysterectomy in Patients with Early-Stage Adenocarcinoma of Uterine Cervix. *Br. J. Cancer* **2010**, *102*, 1692–1698. [CrossRef] [PubMed]
23. McLachlan, J.; Boussios, S.; Okines, A.; Glaessgen, D.; Bodlar, S.; Kalaitzaki, R.; Taylor, A.; Lalondrelle, S.; Gore, M.; Kaye, S.; et al. The Impact of Systemic Therapy beyond First-Line Treatment for Advanced Cervical Cancer. *Clin. Oncol. (R. Coll. Radiol.)* **2017**, *29*, 153–160. [CrossRef] [PubMed]
24. Bonin, L.; Devouassoux-Shisheboran, M.; Golfier, F. Clinicopathological Characteristics of Patients with Mucinous Adenocarcinoma of the Uterine Cervix: A Retrospective Study of 21 Cases. *J. Gynecol. Obstet. Hum. Reprod.* **2019**, *48*, 319–327. [CrossRef] [PubMed]
25. Kobayashi, E.; Ueda, Y.; Matsuzaki, S.; Yokoyama, T.; Kimura, T.; Yoshino, K.; Fujita, M.; Kimura, T.; Enomoto, T. Biomarkers for Screening, Diagnosis, and Monitoring of Ovarian Cancer. *Cancer Epidemiol. Biomark. Prev.* **2012**, *21*, 1902–1912. [CrossRef] [PubMed]
26. Boussios, S.; Attygalle, A.; Hazell, S.; Moschetta, M.; McLachlan, J.; Okines, A.; Banerjee, S. Malignant Ovarian Germ Cell Tumors in Postmenopausal Patients: The Royal Marsden Experience and Literature Review. *Anticancer Res.* **2015**, *35*, 6713–6722.

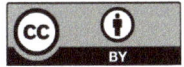

© 2020 by the authors. Licensee MDPI, Basel, Switzerland. This article is an open access article distributed under the terms and conditions of the Creative Commons Attribution (CC BY) license (http://creativecommons.org/licenses/by/4.0/).

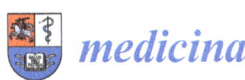

Article

The Risk of Para-Aortic Lymph Node Metastases in Apparent Early Stage Ovarian Cancer

Nicolae Bacalbasa [1,2,3,†], Irina Balescu [1,4,*], Mihaela Vilcu [1,5], Simona Dima [3], Camelia Diaconu [1,6,†], Laura Iliescu [1,7,†], Alexandru Filipescu [1,8,†], Mihai Dimitriu [1,9] and Iulian Brezean [1,6]

1. "Carol Davila" University of Medicine and Pharmacy, 020021 Bucharest, Romania; nicolae_bacalbasa@yahoo.ro (N.B.); mihaela.vilcu@gmail.com (M.V.); drcameliadiaconu@gmail.com (C.D.); laura.iliescu@gmail.ro (L.I.); alexandru.filipescu@gmail.ro (A.F.); mihai.dimitriu@gmail.com (M.D.); iulian.brezean@gmail.ro (I.B.)
2. Department of Obstetrics and Gynecology, "I. Cantacuzino" Clinical Hospital, 030167 Bucharest, Romania
3. Department of Visceral Surgery, Center of Excellence in Translational Medicine, "Fundeni" Clinical Institute, 022328 Bucharest, Romania; simonadima@gmail.ro
4. Department of Surgery, "Ponderas" Academic Hospital, 021188 Bucharest, Romania
5. Department of Visceral Surgery, "I. Cantacuzino" Clinical Hospital, 030167 Bucharest, Romania
6. Department of Internal Medicine, Clinical Emergency Hospital of Bucharest, 105402 Bucharest, Romania
7. Department of Internal Medicine, "Fundeni" Clinical Institute, 022328 Bucharest, Romania
8. Department of Obstetrics and Gynecology, "Elias" Emergency University Hospital, 011461 Bucharest, Romania
9. Department of Obstetrics and Gynecology, "St Pantelimon" Emergency Hospital, 021661 Bucharest, Romania
* Correspondence: irina.balescu@ponderas-ah.ro; Tel.: +40-72-407-7709
† Authors with equal contribution.

Received: 19 January 2020; Accepted: 21 February 2020; Published: 3 March 2020

Abstract: *Background and objectives:* To identify the risk factors for para-aortic lymph node metastases in cases with presumed early stage ovarian cancer. *Materials and methods*: Between 2014 and 2019, 48 patients with apparent early stage ovarian cancer were submitted to surgery. In all cases, pelvic and para-aortic lymph node dissection was performed for staging purposes. *Results*: Among the 48 cases we identified nine cases with positive pelvic lymph nodes and 11 cases with positive para-aortic lymph nodes. The positivity of the retrieved lymph nodes was significantly correlated with the histopathological subtype represented by serous histology ($p = 0.02$), as well as with the degree of differentiation ($p = 0.004$). *Conclusions*: Patients with serous ovarian carcinomas in association with a poorer degree of differentiation are at risk of associated lymph node metastases even in presumed early stages of the disease. Therefore, lymph node dissection should be performed in such cases in order to provide adequate staging and tailoring of further treatment.

Keywords: early stage; ovarian cancer; para-aortic lymph node metastases

1. Introduction

Ovarian cancer represents a common malignancy affecting women worldwide that unfortunately remains asymptomatic for a long period of time; therefore, most cases are diagnosed in advanced stages of the disease, when dissemination through peritoneal, hematogenous or lymphatic routes is already present [1]. However, a limited number of cases will be diagnosed in presumed early stages of the disease. However, up to 15% of these cases prove to have positive lymph nodes, which will significantly influence the long-term prognosis [2]; in the meantime, routine performance of extended pelvic and para-aortic lymph node dissection in presumed early stage ovarian cancer will lead to an unnecessary surgical procedure in up to 80% of cases who have otherwise negative lymph nodes [3–6]. Moreover, performing such procedures will increase the risk of developing perioperative complications, which might significantly influence the quality of life [7,8]. Therefore, identifying cases which present retroperitoneal para-aortic lymph node metastases will enable the oncologist to provide a better selection of cases that will benefit from adjuvant chemotherapy [2,3,9–11]. The aim of the current paper is to investigate the risk factors for developing para-aortic lymph node metastases in cases diagnosed with a presumed early stage of disease.

2. Materials and Methods

Data of patients submitted to surgery for presumed early stage ovarian cancer between 2014 and 2019 were retrospectively reviewed after receiving the approval of the Ethical Committee (11/January 2020). In all cases, the surgical procedure consisted of total hysterectomy en bloc with bilateral adnexectomy, random peritoneal biopsy, omentectomy, pelvic and para-aortic lymph node dissection, as well as peritoneal washing. Pelvic lymph node dissection consisted of removing the lymph node groups at the level of the common and external iliac vessels and obturatory fossa, while para-aortic lymph node dissection consisted of removing the lymph node groups situated in the close proximity of the abdominal aorta, inferior cava vein and in between the two vessels from the renal vessels to the aortic and caval bifurcation. All cases were classified according to the 2014 International Federation of Obstetrics and Gynecology classification (FIGO 2014) [12]. Statistically significant differences were considered if a p-value lower than 0.05 was obtained. In order to compare different parameters, Fischer's exact test was used due to the relatively low number of cases introduced in the current study.

3. Results

Between 2014 and 2019, 48 patients with presumed early stage ovarian cancer were submitted to surgery with curative intent, the median age at the time of surgery being 43.4 years (range = 28–56 years). According to their menopausal status, there were 13 postmenopausal women. The preoperative diagnostic was suspected based on the detection of higher levels of CA 125 (the median value being 330 U/mL) in association with the imaging detection of ovarian masses/cysts with uncertain aspect. In all cases, surgery consisted of total hysterectomy en bloc with bilateral adnexectomy, pelvic and para-aortic lymph node dissection, omentectomy, serial peritoneal biopsies and also an associated resection of all suspect lesions found at the level of the abdominal cavity and peritoneal washing. Intraoperative details are presented in Table 1.

In all cases, pelvic and para-aortic lymph node dissection was performed, the borders of the lymph node dissection being represented by the origin of the epigastric artery caudally (for the pelvic lymph node dissection) and, respectively, the origin of the renal artery cranially (for the para-aortic lymph node dissection). The median number of retrieved pelvic lymph nodes was 19 while the median number of the retrieved para-aortic lymph nodes was 14. Intraoperative and histopathological details of the lymph node dissection are presented in Table 2.

The median length of the surgical procedure was 130 min (range = 90–160 min), the median estimated blood loss was 350 mL (range = 100–550 mL), while the median length of the hospital stay was 6 days (range = 4–13 days). The histopathological studies confirmed the presence of positive pelvic lymph nodes in 18% of cases and, respectively, positive para-aortic lymph nodes in 22% of cases. However, all cases presenting positive pelvic nodes also had associated positive para-aortic lymph nodes. According to these findings, all cases with positive retroperitoneal lymph nodes were upgraded to FIGO stage III of disease and were therefore confined to the oncology department to be submitted to adjuvant chemotherapy. Patients with positive lymph nodes were further classified as IIIA1 (i) if the dimension of the metastatic deposits was lower than 10 mm (in three cases), IIIA1 (ii) if the dimension of the metastatic deposits was larger than 10 mm (in five cases) and IIIB if macroscopic, lower than 2 cm, extrapelvic peritoneal metastases were encountered (in the remaining three cases). None of these cases presented macroscopic peritoneal metastases larger than 2 cm; therefore, none of them were upstaged to FIGO stage IIIC of disease.

Table 1. Preoperative and intraoperative characteristics of the 48 patients diagnosed with presumed early stage ovarian cancer.

Parameter	No. of Cases
Total number of patients	48
FIGO stage at diagnostic:	
I	23
II	25
Laterality of the tumors:	
Unilateral	19
Bilateral	29
Histopathological findings:	
Serous adenocarcinoma	23
Endometroid carcinoma	13
Clear cell carcinoma	10
Mucinous carcinoma	2
Degree of differentiation:	
Well differentiated	9
Moderately differentiated	29
Poorly differentiated	10

Table 2. Intraoperative and histopathological details of the lymph node dissection.

Parameter	Number
Number of retrieved pelvic lymph nodes (median)	19
Number of positive pelvic lymph nodes (median)	3
Number of retrieved para-aortic lymph nodes (median)	14
Number of positive para-aortic lymph nodes (median)	1
Number of cases with positive pelvic lymph nodes	9 of 48 cases
Number of cases with positive para-aortic lymph nodes	11 of 48 cases

In order to determine the risk factors for developing lymph node metastases in apparently early stage ovarian cancer, we conducted an univariate analysis in which we studied the influence of age, menopausal status, initial FIGO stage at diagnosis, laterality of the tumor, histology and degree of differentiation on the risk of developing node metastases. The univariate analysis demonstrated that the presence of positivity of the retrieved lymph nodes was significantly associated with the serous histopathological subtype as well as with the degree of differentiation. Therefore, patients diagnosed with serous ovarian carcinoma had a significantly higher rate of positive lymph nodes (when compared to the other histopathological subtypes, $p = 0.002$). In the meantime, cases diagnosed with poorly differentiated tumors also exhibited a significantly higher rate of positive lymph nodes when compared to the other degrees of differentiation ($p = 0.004$). Surprisingly, neither the laterality of the tumor nor the presumed FIGO stage at diagnosis influenced the risk of developing such metastases. Data obtained at statistical analysis is presented in the table below (Table 3).

Table 3. Analysis of risk factors for para-aortic lymph node metastases.

Risk Factor	Sample Number (%)	No. of Cases with Positive Para-Aortic Lymph Nodes	Hazard Ratio	95% Confidence Interval	p-Value
Age:					
<50 years	31 (65%)	8 (73%)	1.46	0.751–3.674	p = 0.389
>50 years	17 (35%)	3 (27%)			
Histology:					
Serous	23 (48%)	8 (73%)	2.89	1.623–9.354	p = 0.002
Other histopathological type	25 (52%)	3 (27%)			
Menopausal status:					
Premenopausal	35 (73%)	7 (64%)	0.65	0.522–4.138	p = 0.417
Postmenopausal	13 (27%)	4 (36%)			
Initial FIGO stage at diagnostic:					
I	23 (48%)	6 (54%)	1.3	0.782–3.457	p = 0.276
II	25 (52%)	5 (46%)			
Laterality of the tumor:					
Unilateral	19 (39%)	4 (36%)	0.87	0.673–3.416	p = 0.424
Bilateral	29 (61%)	7 (64%)			
Degree of differentiation:					
Well differentiated	9 (19%)	1 (9%)	0.433	1.773–10.157	p = 0.004
Moderately or poorly differentiated	39 (81%)	10 (91%)			

4. Discussion

The issue of lymph node metastases in presumed early stage ovarian cancer has a particular interest among surgical oncologists, gynecological oncologists and medical oncologists worldwide. It can be observed from the data presented so far that an important number of cases diagnosed with presumed early stage cancer already have, at the time of diagnosis, positive microscopic and even macroscopic lymph nodes, upstaging in this way the disease to a FIGO stage III malignancy. Therefore, all these cases, if submitted to standard treatment for early stage ovarian cancer, are at risk for developing early recurrent disease and a particularly poor long-term prognosis due to mis-staging. In the meantime, routine performance of extended lymph node dissection might predispose a significant number of cases to overtreatment and its secondary early-term and even long-term complications [2,4,13,14].

In order to increase the rates of preoperative detection of potential positive lymph nodes, certain authors proposed routine association of positron emission computed tomography. In the study conducted by Signorelli et al. published in 2013, the authors included 68 patients with presumed early stage ovarian cancer in which routine positron emission tomography, as well as systematic lymph node dissection, was performed. The authors underlined the fact that among the 12 cases who finally presented lymph node metastases at the histopathological studies, 10 cases had been correctly previously identified at the imaging studies. Therefore, the authors concluded that this imaging tool could be safely used in order to identify cases in which systematic lymph node dissection could be avoided, especially based on the high negative predictive value of the method [8]. Another promising method which might provide a more accurate identification of patients who present ovarian cancer lymph node metastases even in apparently early stages of the disease is represented by the sentinel node detection [4]. The method, which has been widely implemented in cases diagnosed with early stage breast cancer, melanoma and even gynecological cancers (such as endometrial cancer or cervical cancer), is still under evaluation in patients with presumed early stage ovarian cancer, further studies being still needed before introducing it as part of the standard therapeutic protocol [4,15–18].

One of the first studies, which designed a nomogram-based analysis in order to identify cases at risk of developing para-aortic lymph node metastases, was conducted by Bogani et al., on 290 patients with presumed early stage disease. According to their study, the authors demonstrated that bilateral lesions as well as high-grade serous histology represent the strongest predictors for para-aortic lymph node metastases even in cases with presumed early stage disease [2].

A similar conclusion was also presented by the study conducted by Zhou et al. [19]. In the paper published in 2016, the Chinese authors came to demonstrate that systematic lymph node dissection should be performed in cases diagnosed with poorly differentiated tumors, with serous histology and higher values of CA125 at the time of diagnosis. Therefore, cases in which the preoperative levels of CA125 surpass 740 U/mL seem to have a higher risk of associated para-aortic lymph node metastases [19].

An interesting study which investigated the effectiveness of surgical staging in cases with apparent early stage ovarian cancer has been recently published by Hengeveld in 2019. The study included all patients submitted to surgery with presumed early stage disease between 2005 and 2017 in Danish and Dutch hospitals [20]. Finally, there were 1234 cases that had been preoperatively presumed to be classified as FIGO stage I disease; in all cases, omentectomy, pelvic and para-aortic lymph node sampling or lymph node dissection, as well as multiple peritoneal biopsies, were retrieved. After analyzing the specimens, the histopathological studies revealed the fact that 20 patients were finally upstaged due to the presence of positive pelvic lymph nodes (in seven cases), positive para-aortic lymph nodes (in 12 cases) and both pelvic and para-aortic lymph nodes (in one case). Moreover, the authors underlined the fact that a total of 207 cases were upstaged after applying this protocol, with other sites of involvement being represented by the omentum, peritoneum or positive cytology. However, the authors underlined the fact that in another 50 cases, the malignant process was down-staged after applying this protocol, as the histopathological analysis of the macroscopically suspect lesions was not able to confirm the disease. This fact was rather explained by the absence of bilateral lesions and the absence of capsular invasion, respectively. Similarly to our study, the presence of serous histology as well as the poorer degree of differentiation significantly impacted on the risk of further upstaging. Other factors that were significantly associated with upstaging were represented by higher age, the postmenopausal status as well as the endometroid histology. Therefore, when it comes to the type of histology that is mainly associated with a poorer prognosis, according to this study, serous and endometroid histology versus any other type of tumor were associated with higher rates of upstaging. Moreover, the authors underlined the fact that upstaging was responsible for changing the plan of treatment in 35.1% of cases. Therefore, the importance of an adequate staging was underlined once again; in the meantime, the study came to demonstrate that a significant proportion of cases that were finally upstaged originated from cases with serous or endometrial histology in association with a lower degree of differentiation [20].

Another extremely interesting study that came to demonstrate the effect of the upstaging of presumed early stage ovarian cancer has been recently published in the *New England Journal of Medicine* in 2019. In this paper, the authors came to demonstrate that seven patients out of the 15 cases that were included in the presumed early stage ovarian cancer group presented in fact para-aortic lymph node metastases and were therefore upstaged to FIGO stage IIIC of disease. Moreover, the authors underlined the fact that performing para-aortic lymph node dissection in presumed early stages of the disease will probably prolong the surgical procedure (which is otherwise a short one) by almost an hour and will not predispose to such important complications when compared to cases diagnosed in advanced stages of the disease. In the meantime, routine association of this procedure in cases with advanced stages will also prolong a more demanding and laborious surgical procedure by another hour and will predispose to significant postoperative complications, such as a larger amount of ascites and lymphorrhea. Moreover, the authors also demonstrated that performing systematic lymph node dissection in patients with clinically negative lymph nodes increases the risk of perioperative complications without improving the long-term outcome [21].

5. Conclusions

Even in cases with presumed early stage ovarian cancer, a certain number of cases present lymph node metastases. Therefore, in such cases, the patients will be automatically upstaged and the therapeutic strategy will be modified. According to our study, the risk of developing para-aortic lymph node metastases seems to be significantly correlated with the serous histology as well as with a poorer degree of differentiation. Other factors that have been proven to modify this risk are represented by the FIGO stage, age at diagnosis and menopausal status. However, in our study none of these parameters seemed to significantly influence the risk of positive para-aortic lymph nodes. However, larger studies are still needed in order to provide a better identification of cases at risk of developing distant lymph node metastases.

Author Contributions: N.B., M.V., S.D., M.D., I.B. performed the surgical procedure, M.V.; A.F. and S.D. reviewed literature data; I.B., C.D., L.I. prepared the draft of the manuscript; I.B. was advisor of the surgical oncology procedures; I.B. reviewed the final version of the manuscript. All authors have read and agreed to the published version of the manuscript.

Funding: This research received no external funding.

Acknowledgments: This work was supported by the project entitled "Multidisciplinary Consortium for Supporting the Research Skills in Diagnosing, Treating and Identifying Predictive Factors of Malignant Gynecologic Disorders", project number PN-III-P1-1.2-PCCDI2017-0833.

Conflicts of Interest: The authors have no conflicts of interest to declare regarding this study.

References

1. American Cancer Society: Ovarian Cancer. Available online: http://www.cancer.org (accessed on 11 December 2016).
2. Bogani, G.; Tagliabue, E.; Ditto, A.; Signorelli, M.; Martinelli, F.; Casarin, J.; Chiappa, V.; Dondi, G.; Leone Roberti, M.U.; Scaffa, C.; et al. Assessing the Risk of Pelvic and Para-Aortic Nodal Involvement in Apparent Early-Stage Ovarian Cancer: A Predictors- and Nomogram-Based Analyses. *Gynecol. Oncol.* **2017**, *147*, 61–65. [CrossRef] [PubMed]
3. Rusu, M.C.; Ilie, A.C.; Brezean, I. Human Anatomic Variations: Common, External Iliac, Origin of the Obturator, Inferior Epigastric and Medial Circumflex Femoral Arteries, and Deep Femoral Artery Course on the Medial Side of the Femoral Vessels. *Surg. Radiol. Anat.* **2017**, *39*, 1285–1288. [CrossRef] [PubMed]
4. Balescu, I.; Bacalbasa, N.; Vilcu, M.; Brasoveanu, V.; Brezean, I. Sentinel lymph node in early stage ovarian cancer; a literature review. *J. Mind Med. Sci.* **2018**, *5*, 184–188. [CrossRef]
5. Bacalbasa, N.; Balescu, I.; Vilcu, M.; Brasoveanu, V.; Tomescu, D.; Dima, S.; Suciu, I.; Suciu, N.; Bodog, A.; Brezean, I. Distal pancreatectomy en bloc with splenectomy as part of tertiary cytoreduction for relapsed ovarian cancer. In Proceedings of the 4th Congress of the Romanian Society for Minimal Invasive Surgery in Ginecology/Annual Days of the National Institute for Mother and Child Health Alessandrescu-Rusescu, Romania, Bucuresti, 1–3 November 2018; pp. 29–32.
6. Brezean, I.; Aldoescu, S.; Catrina, E.; Valcu, M.; Ionut, I.; Predescu, G.; Degeratu, D.; Pantea, I. Pelvic and Abdominal-Wall Actinomycotic Infection by Uterus Gateway Without Genital Lesions. *Chirurgia* **2010**, *105*, 123–125. [PubMed]
7. Gallotta, V.; Ghezzi, F.; Vizza, E.; Chiantera, V.; Ceccaroni, M.; Franchi, M.; Fagotti, A.; Ercoli, A.; Fanfani, F.; Parrino, C.; et al. Laparoscopic Staging of Apparent Early Stage Ovarian Cancer: Results of a Large, Retrospective, Multi-Institutional Series. *Gynecol. Oncol.* **2014**, *135*, 428–434. [CrossRef] [PubMed]
8. Signorelli, M.; Guerra, L.; Pirovano, C.; Crivellaro, C.; Fruscio, R.; Buda, A.; Cuzzucrea, M.; Elisei, F.; Ceppi, L.; Messa, C. Detection of Nodal Metastases by 18F-FDG PET/CT in Apparent Early Stage Ovarian Cancer: A Prospective Study. *Gynecol. Oncol.* **2013**, *131*, 395–399. [CrossRef] [PubMed]
9. Bacalbasa, N.; Balescu, I.; Dima, S.; Herlea, V.; David, L.; Brasoveanu, V.; Popescu, I. Initial Incomplete Surgery Modifies Prognosis in Advanced Ovarian Cancer Regardless of Subsequent Management. *Anticancer Res.* **2015**, *35*, 2315–2320. [PubMed]

10. Bacalbasa, N.; Balescu, I.; Dima, S.; Popescu, I. Ovarian Sarcoma Carries a Poorer Prognosis Than Ovarian Epithelial Cancer Throughout All FIGO Stages: A Single-Center Case-Control Matched Study. *Anticancer Res.* **2014**, *34*, 7303–7308. [PubMed]
11. Bacalbasa, N.; Taras, C.; Orban, C.; Iliescu, L.; Hurjui, I.; Hurjui, M.; Niculescu, N.; Cristea, M.; Balescu, I. Atypical Right Hepatectomy for Liver Metastasis From Ovarian Leiomyosarcoma—A Case Report and Literature Review. *Anticancer Res.* **2016**, *36*, 1835–1840. [PubMed]
12. Society of Gynecologic Oncology. Available online: https://www.sgo.org/wp-content/uploads/2012/09/FIGO-Ovarian-Cancer-Staging_1.10.14.pdf (accessed on 11 December 2016).
13. Fotopoulou, C.; Swart, A.M.; Coleman, R.L. Controversies in the Treatment of Women with Early-Stage Epithelial Ovarian Cancer. In *Controversies in the Management of Gynecological Cancers*; Ledermann, J.A., Creutzberg, C.L., Quinn, M.A., Eds.; Springer-Verlag: London, UK, 2014; Volume 1.
14. Maggioni, A.; Benedetti, P.P.; Dell'Anna, T.; Landoni, F.; Lissoni, A.; Pellegrino, A.; Rossi, R.S.; Chiari, S.; Campagnutta, E.; Greggi, S.; et al. Randomised Study of Systematic Lymphadenectomy in Patients With Epithelial Ovarian Cancer Macroscopically Confined to the Pelvis. *Br. J. Cancer* **2006**, *95*, 699–704. [CrossRef] [PubMed]
15. Zahoor, S.; Haji, A.; Battoo, A.; Qurieshi, M.; Mir, W.; Shah, M. Sentinel Lymph Node Biopsy in Breast Cancer: A Clinical Review and Update. *J. Breast Cancer* **2017**, *20*, 217–227. [CrossRef] [PubMed]
16. Lee, S.; Kim, E.Y.; Kang, S.H.; Kim, S.W.; Kim, S.K.; Kang, K.W.; Kwon, Y.; Shin, K.H.; Kang, H.S.; Ro, J.; et al. Sentinel Node Identification Rate, but Not Accuracy, Is Significantly Decreased After Pre-Operative Chemotherapy in Axillary Node-Positive Breast Cancer Patients. *Breast Cancer Res. Treat.* **2007**, *102*, 283–288. [CrossRef] [PubMed]
17. Abdelazim, I.A.; Abu-Faza, M.; Zhurabekova, G.; Shikanova, S.; Karimova, B.; Sarsembayev, M.; Starchenko, T.; Mukhambetalyeva, G. Sentinel Lymph Nodes in Endometrial Cancer Update 2018. *Gynecol. Minim. Invasive Ther.* **2019**, *8*, 94–100. [CrossRef] [PubMed]
18. Wu, Y.; Li, Z.; Wu, H.; Yu, J. Sentinel Lymph Node Biopsy in Cervical Cancer: A Meta-Analysis. *Mol. Clin. Oncol.* **2013**, *1*, 1025–1030. [CrossRef] [PubMed]
19. Zhou, J.; Sun, J.Y.; Wu, S.G.; Wang, X.; He, Z.Y.; Chen, Q.H.; Li, F.Y. Risk factors for lymph node metastasis in ovarian cancer: Implications for systematic lymphadenectomy. *Int. J. Surg.* **2016**, *29*, 123–127. [CrossRef] [PubMed]
20. Hengeveld, E.M.; Zusterzeel, P.L.M.; Lajer, H.; Hogdall, C.K.; Rosendahl, M. The value of surgical staging in patients with apparent early stage epithelial ovarian carcinoma. *Gynecol. Oncol.* **2019**, *154*, 308–313. [CrossRef] [PubMed]
21. Harter, P.; Sehouli, J.; Lorusso, D.; Reuss, A.; Vergote, I.; Marth, C.; Kim, J.W.; Raspagliesi, F.; Lampe, B.; Aletti, G.; et al. A Randomized Trial of Lymphadenectomy in Patients With Advanced Ovarian Neoplasms. *N. Engl. J. Med.* **2019**, *380*, 822–832. [CrossRef] [PubMed]

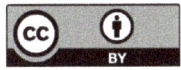

© 2020 by the authors. Licensee MDPI, Basel, Switzerland. This article is an open access article distributed under the terms and conditions of the Creative Commons Attribution (CC BY) license (http://creativecommons.org/licenses/by/4.0/).

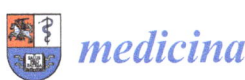

Article

Dietary Attitude of Adults with Type 2 Diabetes Mellitus in the Kingdom of Saudi Arabia: A Cross-Sectional Study

Waqas Sami [1,*], Khalid M Alabdulwahhab [2], Mohd Rashid Ab Hamid [3], Tariq A. Alasbali [4], Fahd Al Alwadani [5] and Mohammad Shakil Ahmad [1]

[1] Department of Community Medicine and Public Health, College of Medicine, Majmaah University, Al-Majmaah 11952, Saudi Arabia; m.shakil@mu.edu.sa
[2] Department of Ophthalmology, College of Medicine, Majmaah University, Al-Majmaah 11952, Saudi Arabia; k.alabdulwahhab@mu.edu.sa
[3] Centre for Mathematical Sciences, Universiti Malaysia Pahang, Lebuhraya Tun Razak, Gambang, Kuantan, Pahang 26300, Malaysia; rashid@ump.edu.my
[4] Department of Ophthalmology, College of Medicine, Al-Imam Mohammad Ibn Saud Islamic University, Riyadh 7544, Saudi Arabia; taalasbali@imamu.edu.sa
[5] Department of Ophthalmology, College of Medicine, King Faisal University, Hofuf 31982, Saudi Arabia; dr_wadani@yahoo.com
* Correspondence: w.mahmood@mu.edu.sa

Received: 7 February 2020; Accepted: 23 February 2020; Published: 24 February 2020

Abstract: *Background and Objectives:* There is a paucity of literature on the dietary attitude (DA) of patients with type 2 diabetes in the Kingdom of Saudi Arabia (KSA). Although the prevalence of diabetes mellitus (DM) is high in Gulf countries, there remains a lack of understanding of the importance of dietary behavior in diabetes management among patients. Understanding the behavior of patients with diabetes towards the disease requires knowledge of their DA. Therefore, this study aimed to assess and evaluate the DA of type 2 diabetes patients, and it is the first of its kind in the KSA. *Material and Methods:* An analytical cross-sectional study was conducted among 350 patients with type 2 diabetes. A self-administered DA questionnaire was used to collect the data. Psychometric properties of the questionnaire were assessed by face validity, content validity, exploratory factor analysis, and internal consistency reliability. The data were collected using a systematic random sampling technique. *Results:* The overall DA of the patients was inappropriate ($p = 0.014$). Patients had an inappropriate DA towards food selection ($p = 0.003$), healthy choices ($p = 0.005$), food restraint ($p < 0.001$), health impact ($p < 0.001$), and food categorization ($p = 0.033$). A poor DA was also observed in relation to the consumption of red meat ($p < 0.001$), rice ($p < 0.001$), soup and sauces ($p = 0.040$), dairy products ($p = 0.015$), and junk food ($p < 0.001$). *Conclusions:* It is highly recommended that patients with diabetes receive counseling with an empowerment approach, as this can bring about changes in their dietary behavior, which is deeply rooted in their daily routine. Healthcare providers should also be well-informed about patients' attitudes and beliefs towards diabetes to design tailored educational and salutary programs for this specific community. Diabetes self-management educational programs should also be provided on a regular basis with a special emphasis on diet and its related components.

Keywords: dietary attitude; type 2 diabetes mellitus; diabetes self-management; empowerment approach; dietary behavior

1. Introduction

Dietary attitude (DA) is defined as beliefs, thoughts, and feelings about, behaviors toward, and relationships with food. It can influence people's food choices and their health status [1]. Different DAs affect human health in noncommunicable diseases and play a great role in determining cultural differences [2,3]. Local and international literature assessing the DA of patients with type 2 diabetes is very scarce. However, some studies have shown that assessing patients' DA may have a considerable benefit for treatment compliance and decreases the occurrence rate of complications as well [4]. Unhealthy eating habits, failure to follow a strict diet plan, and physical inactivity are the leading causes of complications among patients with type 2 diabetes mellitus (T2DM) [5]. A study conducted in Egypt reported that the attitude of patients towards food, compliance with treatment, food control with and without drug use, and foot care was inadequate [6]. Another study indicated that only one-third of diabetic patients were aware of the importance of diet planning and limiting cholesterol intake to prevent cardiovascular disease (CVD) [7]. A study conducted in the Kingdom of Saudi Arabia (KSA) reported that diabetic patients do not regard the advice given by their physicians regularly for diet planning, diet modification, and exercise [8]. There is a need for patients with diabetes to develop a positive attitude towards diet that would help improve glycemic control, and eventually increase their health-related quality of life [9].

Although the prevalence of diabetes mellitus (DM) is high in Gulf countries (Kuwait, Qatar, Bahrain, United Arab Emirates, and Oman), there remains a lack of understanding of the importance of dietary behavior in diabetes management among patients [10]. Understanding the behavior of patients with diabetes towards the disease requires knowledge of their DA. Therefore, this study aimed to assess and evaluate the DA of type 2 diabetes patients. Since this is the first study in the KSA to focus on this issue, the results can therefore serve as a baseline for similar studies conducted in the KSA and in the neighboring Gulf countries.

2. Materials and Methods

The study was performed using an analytical cross-sectional design. Data were collected from the patients visiting the Primary Healthcare Centers (PHCs) in Majmaah City, KSA from February to April 2017. A systematic random sampling technique was used for the selection of patients based on the inclusion criteria, which were: clinically diagnosed cases of type 2 diabetes mellitus of either gender and in the age range of 35–55 years. The DM prevalence value of 23.7% [11] was used for sample size calculation, and the values were placed in the level of precision formula that yielded a sample size of 278. To compensate for potential missing observations/patients withdrawing from the study, the sample size was increased to 350. Each patient's consent was obtained prior to data collection. This research was approved by the ethical review committee of Majmaah University, KSA vides reference number: MURECApril.02/COM-2016.

The dietary attitude questionnaire (DAQ) was prepared following a thorough review of the literature and based on meetings with local experts to determine the pattern of questions suitable for assessing and evaluating the DA of patients with type 2 diabetes. The self-administered valid and reliable questionnaire was divided into three sections (Section A, B, and C). We have discussed the psychometric properties (face validity, content validity, exploratory factor analysis (EFA), and reliability) of the DAQ in a separate article [12]. The internal consistency reliability of the DAQ was excellent (Cronbach Alpha = 0.841). Based on the pilot study results of the EFA, the five factors were labelled as "food selection", "health impact", "healthy choices", "food restraint", and "food categorization" [12].

Section A contained questions related to demographic characteristics. Section B was comprised of 16 questions that assessed patients' general DA towards food. All of the questions were measured on a seven-point Likert scale (strongly agree, agree, somewhat agree, neutral, disagree, somewhat disagree, and strongly disagree). The DA was further classified as positive and negative based on mean values. Values at or above the mean were classified as having a positive DA, and values below the mean were referred to as having a negative DA [13,14]. Section C was also comprised of 16 questions: The first

15 questions assessed patients' DA towards specific food items with categories ("not" eating this food is healthy and necessary, eating this food "occasionally" is healthy and necessary, and eating this food "often" is healthy and necessary), and the last question was about "opinion regarding healthy diet" with the options "yes" and "no".

The data were entered and analyzed using IBM SPSS version 25 (IBM Corp., Armonk, N.Y., USA). Normality of the quantitative variables was assessed through a One-Sample Kolmogorov–Smirnov (KS) test. A univariate method (z-score) was used for the detection of outliers. Qualitative variables are expressed as frequencies and percentages, while a median and quartiles (25th–75th) are given for non-normally distributed variables. A one-sample non-parametric chi-squared test was used to assess the significance of overall and subgroup positive and negative DA. Pearson's chi-squared test was applied to compare the overall positive and negative DA between gender, body mass index (BMI), education status, and marital status. Binary logistic regression with the backward conditional approach was used to predict the set of variables assessing the DA of patients towards specific food items. The odds ratios were further converted into probabilities by using the equation ($\hat{y}$ = odds/1 + odds). The statistical significance value was set at $p < 0.05$.

3. Results

3.1. Demographic Characteristics of Patients—Section A

The data were collected from 350 patients with a median age of 45 years (range: 40–51 years). The results presented in Table 1 show that there were more male patients ($n = 202$; 57.7%) than female patients ($n = 148$; 42.3%). More than 90% of the patients were married. A majority of patients had received a secondary education ($n = 200$; 57.14%), while some were illiterate ($n = 69$; 19.7%), and others were graduates and postgraduates ($n = 81$; 23.14%). A majority of patients in the study were overweight ($n = 167$; 47.7%), some were obese ($n = 115$; 32.9%), some had a normal weight ($n = 56$; 16%), and others were underweight ($n = 12$; 3.4%). A significant association was observed between the overall DA of patients and their educational status ($p = 0.034$). However, the overall DA was not significantly associated with gender ($p = 0.142$), marital status ($p = 0.413$), or BMI ($p = 0.666$). The frequency, percentage, and ranked mean score for each item are presented in Table 2.

Table 1. Sociodemographic Characteristics.

	n(%)		n(%)
Gender		**Education Status**	
		Illiterate	69 (19.7)
Male	202 (57.7)	Primary	115 (32.9)
		Secondary	85 (24.3)
		Graduates	51 (14.6)
Female	148 (42.3)	Postgraduates	30 (8.6)
Marital Status		**BMI**	
Married	322 (92.0)	Underweight	12 (3.4)
Single	11 (3.1)	Normal weight	56 (16.0)
Widow	06 (1.7)	Overweight	167 (47.7)
Divorced/Separated	11 (3.1)	Obese	115 (32.9)

BMI, Body mass index.

Table 2. General dietary attitude of patients with type 2 diabetes based on ranking analysis.

Items	Strongly Disagree n (%)	Somewhat Disagree n (%)	Disagree n (%)	Neutral n (%)	Agree n (%)	Somewhat Agree n (%)	Strongly Agree n (%)	Mean Score Mean ± SD
It is important that the food you eat keeps you healthy and energetic	6 (1.7)	32 (9.1)	61 (17.4)	24 (6.9)	109 (31.1)	75 (21.4)	73 (12.3)	4.70 ± 1.77
You are aware of the energetic (caloric) content in the food that you eat	0 (0.0)	32 (9.1)	81 (23.1)	45 (12.9)	68 (19.4)	75 (21.4)	49 (14.0)	4.63 ± 1.58
It is important that the food that you eat contains vitamin and minerals	13 (3.7)	53 (15.1)	37 (10.6)	71 (20.3)	99 (28.3)	47 (13.4)	30 (8.6)	4.29 ± 1.60
You feel guilty after eating oily foods	16 (4.6)	36 (10.3)	84 (24.0)	60 (17.1)	77 (22.0)	47 (13.4)	30 (8.6)	4.16 ± 1.60
The healthiness of food has little impact on your food choices	0 (0.0)	38 (10.9)	93 (26.6)	59 (16.9)	97 (27.7)	63 (18.0)	0 (0.0)	4.15 ± 1.29
You generally feel comfortable after eating sweets	0 (0.0)	71 (20.3)	42 (12.0)	108 (30.9)	25 (7.1)	104 (29.7)	0 (0.0)	4.14 ± 1.47
You give too much time and thought to food selection	35 (10.0)	43 (12.3)	37 (10.6)	68 (19.4)	90 (25.7)	47 (13.4)	30 (8.6)	4.13 ± 1.74
It is important that the food you eat helps you control your weight	23 (6.6)	67 (19.1)	61 (17.4)	28 (8.0)	72 (20.6)	83 (23.7)	16 (4.6)	4.06 ± 1.76
You enjoy trying new, rich, nutritious food	0 (0.0)	37 (10.6)	87 (24.9)	106 (30.3)	74 (21.1)	46 (13.1)	0 (0.0)	4.01 ± 1.18
You like to consume food cooked in olive oil (virgin, extra, etc.)	38 (10.9)	45 (12.9)	62 (17.7)	48 (13.7)	115 (32.9)	13 (3.7)	29 (8.3)	3.89 ± 1.69
You can show self-control around food	26 (7.4)	62 (17.7)	62 (17.7)	42 (12.0)	122 (34.9)	21 (6.0)	15 (4.3)	3.84 ± 1.58
You try to stay away from foods such as bread, potato, and rice	0 (0.0)	106 (30.3)	102 (29.1)	12 (3.4)	36 (10.3)	94 (26.9)	0 (0.0)	3.74 ± 1.61
You eat what you like to eat and do not worry about the healthiness of food	50 (14.3)	58 (16.6)	57 (16.3)	42 (12.0)	105 (30.0)	38 (12.9)	0 (0.0)	3.59 ± 1.64
You stay away from foods that contain sugar	41 (11.7)	103 (29.1)	37 (10.6)	56 (16.0)	52 (14.9)	32 (9.1)	30 (8.6)	3.55 ± 1.84
Do you think that eating healthy food influences the outcomes of DM?	50 (14.3)	58 (16.6)	71 (20.3)	69 (19.7)	57 (16.3)	45 (12.9)	0 (0.0)	3.46 ± 1.59
You like to eat diet food	74 (21.1)	62 (17.7)	62 (17.7)	30 (8.6)	97 (27.7)	25 (7.1)	0 (0.0)	3.25 ± 1.67

DM, Diabetes mellitus; SD, Standard deviation.

3.2. Patients' General Dietary Attitude Towards Food—Section B

No outlier problem was detected in the overall DA score variable as z-score values (−2.30–2.22) were less than the absolute value of 4. The mean DA score of 16 items was 3.94 + 0.87. Based on the mean score, the DA was categorized into having a positive attitude and having a negative attitude. There was a majority of patients with a negative DA (n = 198; 56.6%) compared with those with a positive DA (n = 152; 43.4%). The result of the one-sample chi-squared test showed that the overall DA of patients with type 2 diabetes was inappropriate (χ^2 = 6.04 (1), p = 0.014). The positive and negative attitude when compared within the subgroups (identified by EFA) showed that the patients also had an inappropriate DA towards food selection (p = 0.003), healthy choices (p = 0.005), food restraint (p < 0.001), health impact (p < 0.001), and food categorization (p = 0.033). These results are presented in Table 3.

Table 3. Comparison of Positive and Negative Dietary Attitude in Subgroups identified by exploratory factor analysis (EFA).

Food Selection	Health Impact	Healthy Choices	Food Restraint	Food Categorization
It is important that the food you eat contains vitamin and minerals	It is important that the food you eat keeps you healthy and energetic	You like to eat diet food	You eat what you like to eat and do not worry about the healthiness of food	The healthiness of food has little impact on your food choices
You stay away from foods that contain sugar	It is important that the food you eat helps you control your weight	You like to consume food cooked in olive oil (virgin, extra, etc.)	You can show self-control around food	You try to stay away from foods such as bread, potato, and rice
You give too much time and thought to food selection	You are aware of the energetic (caloric) content in the food that you eat	Do you think that eating healthy food has an effect on the outcomes of DM?	-	You enjoy trying new, rich, nutritious food
You feel guilty after eating oily foods	You generally feel comfortable after eating sweets	-	-	-
PDA = 147 (42.0%)	PDA = 149 (42.6%)	PDA = 140 (40%)	PDA = 126 (36%)	PDA = 155 (44.3)
NDA = 203 (58.0%)	NDA = 201 (57.4%)	NDA = 210 (60%)	NDA = 224 (64%)	NDA = 195 (55.7)
$\chi^2 = 8.98, p = 0.003$ *	$\chi^2 = 7.72, p = 0.005$ *	$\chi^2 = 14.0, p < 0.001$ *	$\chi^2 = 27.4, p < 0.001$ *	$\chi^2 = 4.57, p = 0.033$ *

DM, Diabetes mellitus; PDA, Positive Dietary Attitude; NDA, Negative Dietary Attitude; * statistically significant at the 5% level of significance.

3.3. Patients' General Dietary Attitude Towards Food—Section B

Backward elimination with the conditional approach retained six items in the final model. The values of model chi-squared and Hosmer–Lemeshow tests were 81.80 ($p < 0.001$) and 20.02 ($p < 0.001$), respectively, which showed that the fitted model was appropriate at the 95% confidence interval (CI). Overall, the model correctly classified 71.4% of patients. The odds ratio for red meat was 2.43 ($p < 0.001$). Converting the odds ratio into a probability showed that the consumption of red meat was 70.84% greater in patients who said "yes" they are eating a healthy diet. Dairy products had an odds ratio of 1.408 ($p = 0.015$), which showed that the consumption of dairy products was 58.38% greater in patients who said "yes" they are eating a healthy diet. The odds ratio for rice was 3.472 ($p < 0.001$). The probability results showed that consumption of rice was 77.63% greater in patients who said "yes" they are eating a healthy diet. Junk food had an odds ratio of 2.347 ($p < 0.001$), showing that the consumption of junk food was 70.12% greater in patients who said "yes" they are eating a healthy diet. The odds ratio for soups and sauces was 1.383 ($p = 0.040$). The probability results showed that the consumption of soups and sauces was 58.03% greater in patients who said "yes" they are eating a healthy diet. Fruits had an odds ratio of 1.416 ($p = 0.024$). Converting the odds ratio into a probability showed that the consumption of fruits was 58.60% greater in patients who said "yes" they are eating a healthy diet. However, for foods such as white meat, bakery products, cereals, sweets and snacks, drinks, vegetables, boiled or grilled meals, olive oil, and canned food, there was no statistical significance ($p > 0.05$). These results are presented in Table 4.

Table 4. Binary Logistic Regression Analysis using the Backward Conditional Approach for the Dietary Attitude of Patients with Type 2 Diabetes towards Specific Food Items.

Food Item	β	Wald	p-Value	Adjusted Odds Ratio	95% CI for Odds	
					Lower	Upper
White Meat	0.098	0.345	0.557 †	0.907	0.654	1.257
Red Meat	0.888	0.175	0.000 *	2.430	1.726	3.422
Dairy Products	0.342	0.140	0.015 *	1.408	1.070	1.853
Bakery Products	0.136	0.611	0.434 †	0.873	0.662	1.227
Rice	1.245	0.209	0.000 *	3.472	2.303	5.233
Cereals	0.032	0.040	0.842 †	0.958	0.705	1.330
Junk Food	0.853	0.189	0.000 *	2.347	1.621	3.399
Soups and Sauces	0.324	0.158	0.040 *	1.383	1.015	1.884
Sweets and Snacks	0.060	0.136	0.712 †	1.062	0.772	1.460
Drinks	0.303	2.769	0.096 †	0.739	0.517	1.055
Fruits	0.348	0.154	0.024 *	1.416	1.047	1.914
Vegetables	0.074	0.180	0.671 †	1.077	0.765	1.515
Boiled or Grilled Meals	0.015	0.009	0.924 †	0.985	0.719	1.349
Olive Oil	0.079	0.210	0.647 †	0.924	0.660	1.295
Canned Food	0.223	1.696	0.193 †	0.800	0.573	1.119

* Significant at the 5% level of significance; † non-significant variables.

4. Discussion

Our study showed that patients with type 2 diabetes had an overall inappropriate DA. Subgroup analysis also showed an inappropriate DA of patients towards food selection, health impact of food, healthy choices, food restraint, and food categorization. In addition, the patients had a poor DA towards the consumption of red meat, rice, soup and sauces, dairy products, and junk food. The results of our study also showed that for the majority of patients, food selection and health impact of food were not important, and this is consistent with the findings of a study conducted in Egypt [6]. This may be because of deeply rooted cultural beliefs and values, which may pose a difficulty for patients' adherence to food selection and consumption of foods having a health impact. The role of cultural attitudes and behaviors towards food in the management of diabetes cannot be neglected [15]. This is consistent with our study results, as the attitude of patients with diabetes towards food is influenced by a strong cultural attitude. Most of them stated that the selection of food, its health impact, healthy choices, food restriction, and food categorization are not important to them. The Saudi cultural barrier factor towards food selection and its consumption and health impact has also been supported by a local study [16]. In our study, a majority of the patients stated that they do not like to eat diet food, nor do they like to stay away from foods that contain sugar. Moreover, only one-fifth of the patients indicated that they feel guilty after eating oily foods. These findings are supported by research conducted by Buttar et al. [17].

A study conducted by Ntaate [18] among patients with type 2 diabetes from Uganda reported a positive DA (82%) towards diet. In contrast, in our study, the patients not only had an overall inappropriate DA, but also an inappropriate DA towards the consumption of red meat, rice, soup and sauces, dairy products, and junk food. Most of the patients in our study were unaware of the caloric content in the food they were consuming. This can be attributed to their literacy level; in our study, 57.2% of the patients had received a primary and secondary education, while approximately 20% were illiterate. This fact is supported by studies that also stated that literacy is an important influential factor, because patients with low literacy have difficulty reading food labels and estimating potion sizes [19–21].

Therefore, to achieve the DA goals, a patient empowerment approach should be used. Since an empowerment approach is a social phenomenon, when a patient is empowered with necessary knowledge about lifestyle modification, outcomes of disease if not controlled, etc., he/she shows a more responsible attitude with better self-efficacy towards diabetes care [22,23]. The empowerment approach in dealing with type 2 diabetes is highly recommendable because it brings about changes in the behavior of the patient that is deeply rooted in their daily routine. Healthcare providers should be well-informed about patient attitudes and beliefs towards diabetes to design tailored educational and salutary programs for a specific community [24].

Imparting nutritional education is a perilous component of diabetes care, especially for the self-management of the disease. Thus, for better diabetes care, patients should be referred to dietitians who should assess their attitude towards food in general, and towards various foods such as meat, rice, junk food, etc., and suggest tailored dietary self-management strategies. To facilitate behavioral dietary changes, this assessment should be individualized and patient-centered, and it must be based on a patient's cultural beliefs, norms, psychosocial status, and literacy, as these factors have been identified as a barrier to reaching nutritional therapy goals [25]. Along with these efforts, the authorities in the Kingdom of Saudi Arabia should provide diabetes self-management educational programs on a regular basis, with special emphasis on diet and its related components. Such educational programs have been found to have an encouraging impact on patient behaviors. However, to achieve a long-term positive effect on behavior modification, sustained reinforcement is needed, which can be achieved using a patient empowerment approach [26].

There are some limitations to this study. The research design was cross-sectional, which itself has methodological limitations, so it cannot be used to analyze behavior over a period of time. The study was conducted in the central region of the KSA, and although the eating habits do not vary much within the eastern, southern and northern regions of the KSA, there is still a need for a national DA assessment program. Another limitation is that we were unable to compare the self-prepared DAQ with the gold standard; doing so might have helped us to study the DA of the patients with diabetes in more detail to devise strategies for better patient care. Nonetheless, the study provided important points: The results can be generalized as we used a systematic random sampling technique for the selection of patients, the DA questionnaire was reviewed by experts in the field, it successfully passed the psychometric analysis, and we can say that it is a valid and reliable questionnaire for assessing and evaluating the DA of patients with type 2 diabetes. This is the first study conducted in the KSA related to assessing and evaluating the DA of patients with type 2 diabetes. Therefore, the results can serve as a baseline for similar studies conducted in the KSA and references can be extended to the neighboring Gulf Cooperation Council (GCC) countries.

5. Conclusions

Patients with type 2 diabetes had an overall inappropriate dietary attitude. It is highly recommended that these patients be counseled with an empowerment approach as it can bring about changes in their dietary behavior that is deeply rooted in their daily routine. Healthcare providers should also be well-informed about patients' attitudes and beliefs towards diabetes to plan tailored educational and salutary programs for this specific community. Diabetes self-management educational programs should also be provided on a regular basis with a special emphasis on diet and its related components.

Author Contributions: Conceptualization, W.S.; Methodology, W.S.; Software, M.R.A.H.; Validation, K.M.A.; Formal analysis, M.R.A.H.; Investigation, M.S.A.; Resources, W.S.; Data curation, M.S.A.; Writing—Original draft preparation, K.M.A.; Writing—Review and editing, T.A.A.; Visualization, W.S.; Supervision, F.A.A.; Project administration, K.M.A.; Funding acquisition, W.S. All authors have read and agreed to the published version of the manuscript.

Funding: The authors extend their appreciation to the Deanship of Scientific Research at Majmaah University for funding this work under project number (No. RGP-2019-36).

Conflicts of Interest: The authors declare no conflicts of interest.

References

1. Alvarenga, M.D.S.; Scagliusi, F.B.; Philippi, S.T. Comparison of eating attitudes among university students from the five Brazilian regions. *Cien. Saude. Colet.* **2012**, *17*, 435–444. [CrossRef]
2. Roininen, K.; Tuorila, H.; Zandstra, E.; De, G.C.; Vehkalahti, K.; Stubenitsky, K.; Mela, D.J. Differences in health and taste attitudes and reported behaviour among Finnish, Dutch and British consumers: A cross-national validation of the Health and Taste Attitude Scales (HTAS). *Appetite* **2001**, *37*, 33–45. [CrossRef] [PubMed]
3. Rozin, P.; Fischler, C.; Imada, S.; Sarubin, A.; Wrzesniewski, A. Attitudes to food and the role of food in life in the USA, Japan, Flemish Belgium and France: Possible implications for the diet–health debate. *Appetite* **1999**, *33*, 163–180. [CrossRef] [PubMed]
4. El-Khawaga, G.; Abdel-Wahab, F. Knowledge, attitudes, practice and compliance of diabetic patients in Dakahlia, Egypt. *Eur. J. Res. Med. Sci.* **2015**, *3*, 40–53.
5. Gæde, P.; Lund-Andersen, H.; Parving, H.H.; Pedersen, O. Effect of a multifactorial intervention on mortality in type 2 diabetes. *N. Engl. J. Med.* **2008**, *358*, 580–591. [CrossRef] [PubMed]
6. Majed Isleem, E.A.; Aljeesh, Y. Evaluation of Diabetic Foot Management in the Gaza Strip. *Eval. Diabet. Foot Manag. Gaza Strip* **2015**, *4*, 73–79.
7. Willett, W.C.; Koplan, J.P.; Nugent, R.; Dusenbury, C.; Puska, P.; Gaziano, T.A. Prevention of chronic disease by means of diet and lifestyle changes. In *Disease Control Priorities in Developing Countries*, 2nd ed.; The International Bank for Reconstruction and Development/The World Bank: Washington, DC, USA, 2006.
8. Midhet, F.M.; Al-Mohaimeed, A.A.; Sharaf, F.K. Lifestyle related risk factors of type 2 diabetes mellitus in Saudi Arabia. *Saudi. Med. J.* **2010**, *31*, 768–774.
9. Grey, M.; Boland, E.A.; Davidson, M.; Li, J.; Tamborlane, W.V. Coping skills training for youth with diabetes mellitus has long-lasting effects on metabolic control and quality of life. *J. Pediatr.* **2000**, *137*, 107–113. [CrossRef]
10. Sami, W.; Alabdulwahhab, K.M.; Ab Hamid, M.R.; Alasbali, T.A.; Alwadani, F.A.; Ahmad, M.S. Dietary Knowledge among Adults with Type 2 Diabetes—Kingdom of Saudi Arabia. *Int. J. Environ. Res. Public Health* **2020**, *17*, 858. [CrossRef]
11. Alsulaiman, T.A.; Al-Ajmi, H.A.; Al-Qahtani, S.M.; Fadlallah, I.M.; Nawar, N.E.; Shukerallah, R.E.; Nadeem, S.R.; Al-weheedy, N.M.; Al-sulaiman, K.A.; Hassan, A.A.; et al. Control of type 2 diabetes in King Abdulaziz Housing City (Iskan) population, Saudi Arabia. *J. Fam. Community. Med.* **2016**, *23*, 1–5. [CrossRef]
12. Sami, W.; Ansari, T.; Butt, N.; Ab Hamid, M. Psychometric evaluation of dietary habits questionnaire for type 2 diabetes mellitus. *J. Phys. Conf.* **2017**, *890*, 012151. [CrossRef]
13. Chin, W.Y.; Lai, M.P.S.; Chia, C.Y. The validity and reliability of the English version of the diabetes distress scale for type 2 diabetes patients in Malaysia. *BMC Fam. Pract.* **2017**, *18*, 25–33. [CrossRef] [PubMed]
14. Chotisiri, L.; Yamarat, K.; Taneepanichskul, S. Exploring knowledge, attitudes, and practices toward older adults with hypertension in primary care. *J. Multidiscip. Healthc.* **2016**, *9*, 559–564. [CrossRef] [PubMed]
15. Naeem, A. The role of culture and religion in the management of diabetes: A study of Kashmiri men in Leeds. *Royal. Society. Promot. Health. J.* **2003**, *123*, 110–116. [CrossRef]
16. Mohamed, B.A.; Almajwal, A.M.; Saeed, A.A.; Bani, I.A. Dietary practices among patients with type 2 diabetes in Riyadh, Saudi Arabia. *J. Food Agric. Environ.* **2013**, *11*, 110–114.
17. Buttar, H.S.; Li, T.; Ravi, N. Prevention of cardiovascular diseases: Role of exercise, dietary interventions, obesity and smoking cessation. *Exp. Clin. Cardiol.* **2005**, *10*, 229–249.
18. Ntaate, C. Dietary knowledge, attitude and practices of diabetic patients at Nsambya Hospital Kampala, Uganda. Ph.D. Thesis, University of Stellenbosch, Stellenbosch, South Africa, 2015.
19. Aikman, S.N.; Min, K.E.; Graham, D. Food attitudes, eating behavior, and the information underlying food attitudes. *Appetite* **2006**, *47*, 111–114. [CrossRef]
20. Huizinga, M.M.; Carlisle, A.J.; Cavanaugh, K.L.; Davis, D.L.; Gregory, R.P.; Schlundt, D.G.; Rothman, R.L. Literacy, numeracy, and portion-size estimation skills. *Am. J. Prev. Med.* **2009**, *36*, 324–328. [CrossRef]

21. Rothman, R.L.; Housam, R.; Weiss, H.; Davis, D.; Gregory, R.; Gebretsadik, T.; Shintani, A.; Elasy, T.A. Patient understanding of food labels: The role of literacy and numeracy. *Am. J. Prev. Med.* **2006**, *31*, 391–398. [CrossRef]
22. Bandura, A. *Self-Efficacy: The Exercise of Control*; Macmillan: New York, NY, USA, 1997.
23. Tones, K.; Tilford, S. *Health Promotion: Effectiveness, Efficiency and Equity*; Nelson Thornes: Cheltenham, UK, 2001.
24. Abolghasemi, R.; Sedaghat, M. The patient's attitude toward type 2 diabetes mellitus, a qualitative study. *J. Relig. Health* **2015**, *54*, 1191–1205. [CrossRef]
25. Haas, L.; Maryniuk, M.; Beck, J.; Cox, C.E.; Duker, P.; Edwards, L.; Fisher, E.; Hanson, L.; Kent, D.; Kolb, L.; et al. National standards for diabetes self-management education and support. *Diabetes Educ.* **2012**, *38*, 619–629. [CrossRef] [PubMed]
26. Klein, H.A.; Jackson, S.M.; Street, K.; Whitacre, J.C.; Klein, G. Diabetes self-management education: Miles to go. *Nurs. Res. Pract.* **2013**, *2013*, 1–15. [CrossRef] [PubMed]

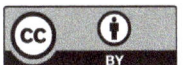

© 2020 by the authors. Licensee MDPI, Basel, Switzerland. This article is an open access article distributed under the terms and conditions of the Creative Commons Attribution (CC BY) license (http://creativecommons.org/licenses/by/4.0/).

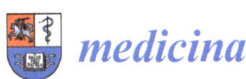

Review

State of the Art in Fertility Preservation for Female Patients Prior to Oncologic Therapies

Călin Bogdan Chibelean [1,2,†], Răzvan-Cosmin Petca [3,4,*], Dan Cristian Radu [5,†] and Aida Petca [3,6]

1. Department of Urology, George Emil Palade University of Medicine, Pharmacy, Science, and Technology of Targu-Mures, 540139 Targu-Mures, Romania; calinchibelean@yahoo.com
2. Mureș County Hospital, 540136 Targu-Mures, Romania
3. "Carol Davila" University of Medicine and Pharmacy, 050471 Bucharest, Romania; aidapetca@gmail.com
4. Department of Urology, "Prof. Dr. Th. Burghele" Clinical Hospital, 050659 Bucharest, Romania
5. Neolife Medical Center, 077190 Bucharest, Romania; dan.c.radu@gmail.com
6. Department of Obstetrics and Gynecology, Elias University Emergency Hospital, 011461 Bucharest, Romania
* Correspondence: drpetca@gmail.com; Tel.: +40-722-224492
† These authors contributed equally to this work.

Received: 27 December 2019; Accepted: 18 February 2020; Published: 23 February 2020

Abstract: Quality of life improvement stands as one of the main goals of the medical sciences. Increasing cancer survival rates associated with better early detection and extended therapeutic options led to the specific modeling of patients' choices, comprising aspects of reproductive life that correlated with the evolution of modern society, and requires better assessment. Of these, fertility preservation and ovarian function conservation for pre-menopause female oncologic patients pose a contemporary challenge due to procreation age advance in evolved societies and to the growing expectations regarding cancer treatment. Progress made in cell and tissue-freezing technologies brought hope and shed new light on the onco-fertility field. Additionally, crossing roads with general fertility and senescence studies proved highly beneficial due to the enlarged scope and better synergies and funding. We here strive to bring attention to this domain of care and to sensitize all medical specialties towards a more cohesive approach and to better communication among caregivers and patients.

Keywords: fertility preservation; cryo-preservation; vitrification; breast cancer

---

1. Introduction

The female perspective on fertility after cancer treatment is, nowadays, an important issue. A 2012 study that analyses the information received from cancer survivors has found that there is a sex bias. Thus, men received more information regarding the influence of treatment on fertility 80% vs. 48%, and more men also received information about options to preserve fertility—68%, compared to 14% for women [1]. Statistics show that over 50% of men opted to cryopreserve sperm; only 2% of women undertook any means of fertility preservation [1]. The onco-fertility preservation necessity arises as 8% to 12% of all breast cancers occur before the age of 35 [2,3] and the tally rises to 15% for women 40 years old [4,5], in the backdrop of breast cancer being the most frequent of all cancers among women of childbearing age—affecting one-third of the young with cancer [6]. If we look at the breast cancer incidence in patients between the ages of 20 and 34 years, it stands at 1.9% of all newly diagnosed breast cancers and rises to 10.5% for breast cancers occurring in 35 and 44 year old women [7,8]. Breast cancer in young patients has special traits, characterized by specific oncogenic signaling pathways and associates a higher incidence of hormone receptor-negative, higher grade, and human EGF2 receptor-overexpressing tumors [9]. Advances in breast cancer early detection rates and treatment options have led to a five-year breast cancer survival rate of over 80% [10]. As greater survival rates are obtained, there is also a greater focus on achieving goals of motherhood and family completeness.

Young Women's Breast Cancer Study concluded that 50% of women younger than 40 years have concerns about future fertility and pregnancy options, following chemotherapy and radiotherapy [11]. There is also a psychological burden upon cancer survivors as a result of the fertility concern, and there are wide-spread studies to attest to the rising awareness of such instances [12].

A 2012 review of fertility demographics in USA showed an increase in the number of women giving birth after 30 years of age, with a peak for white women at 35 years [13]. The infertility risk of a woman in her teens is 0.2%, which will rise to 2% by her twenties, and reach 20% in her early thirties, which thus acknowledges only the number and quality of oocytes—by the time that most women will consider getting pregnant, they are already 20% infertile [14], resembling an infertility pandemic in developed countries. Adding to this is the increased incidence of cancer in young women, which will increase the cost of treatment and frequently implies infertility. Up to 6% of fertile age women are cancer survivors, and the incidence of cancer increases from about 1 in 10,000 shortly after birth to about 1 in 300 by mid-forties [15]. Depending on the source, ovarian failure characterizes 6.3% up to 12% of women that are childhood cancer survivors [16] and up to 50% of the patients that receive oncologic treatment at 40 years old will suffer early ovarian failure [17]. Most studies take account of the abrupt onset of menopause five years from chemotherapy, as evidence of ovarian failure, underestimating subtler manifestations such as subfertility and diminished ovarian reserve.

Chemo-therapeutic agents, known for deleterious effects, include alkylating agents that are considered high risk, such as Cyclophosphamide, Mechlorethamine, Chlorambucil, Busulfan, and Melphalan, whose active metabolites form DNA crosslinks leading to its function and synthesis arrest [18]. They produce DNA double-strand breakage, followed by P63 mediated apoptosis. Platinum-based compounds, Cisplatin and Carboplatin covalently binds DNA and forms intra and interstrand bonds that produce DNA strands breakage during replication. DNA transcription, synthesis, and function are, thus, inhibited. They are considered intermediate risk, though there was no demonstrated specific toxicity upon human primordial follicles [15,19]. Antimetabolites include Methotrexate, 5-fluorouracil, and Cytarabine and inhibit DNS synthesis and ARN purines and Thymidylate synthesis, being considered of low risk. Vinca alkaloids, Vincristine and Vinblastine inhibit tubulin polymerization, producing microtubules disruption during mitosis with mitosis arrest in metaphase and consecutive cellular death [3,18]. It is labeled as low risk. Anthracyclines, Daunorubicin, Bleomycin, Adriamycin (doxorubicin) inhibit DNA synthesis and function and inhibit Topoisomerase II leading to DNA breakage. They also form free oxygen radicals that also affect DNA synthesis and function by DNA breakage. Doxorubicin determines DNA double-strand breakage and human primordial follicles P63 mediated apoptosis. Except for Doxorubicin, which is considered of medium risk, they are low risk [18].

2. Current Fertility Preservation Methods

The 2018 American Society of Clinical Oncology (ASCO) recommendations paint a clear image of current onco-fertility focusing and emerging possibilities. While patients will first be taken aback by a cancer diagnosis, it is recommended that, early in the therapeutic process, discussions be initiated with the fertile patients concerning the risk of diminished fertility induced by specific treatment and about the options available for fertility preservation. Oocytes and embryo freezing, due to technological progress, are considered the standard of care and are widely available. Considering the conflicting evidence concerning GnRH agonist use to protect ovarian reserve during oncologic treatment [19], ASCO recommends only using GnRH agonists in young patients that are not fit for other methods. Embryo cryo-preserving is routinely used to preserve embryos that were not used for fresh embryo transfer after IVF. Oocyte freezing may be an adequate option for patients currently without a male partner, for those who do not want to use donor sperm or have ethical or religious objections regarding embryo cryopreservation. As of 2012, ASCO no longer considers oocyte cryopreservation experimental. As multiple ovarian stimulation protocols are available, there is no longer a need to delay ovarian stimulation depending on the menstrual cycle, favoring oocyte retrieval. For estrogen receptor-positive breast cancer patients that may be at risk due to the elevated estrogen levels in classic stimulation protocols, ASCO recommends aromatase inhibitors stimulation protocols as current studies do not show evidence of increased recurrence risk [20].

In this context of social pressure, and ultimately, financial stimulus, assisted reproduction technologies had a steep curve of evolution. In this process, IVF has greater visibility and striving for successful pregnancies produced more embryos. A limited number of the better-quality embryos are being selected for intrauterine embryo-transfer, while the remaining good quality embryos were frozen for cryopreservation. The resulting technological prowess led to increasing rates of embryo survival after freeze-thaw, and in turn, to a greater number of pregnancies, similar rates of pregnancies being obtained for fresh embryos and frozen ones. This highlighted the idea that all embryo-transfers should be realized with frozen embryos in a subsequent cycle; in favor of this judgment is the standing lower risk of ovarian hyperstimulation syndrome and a higher endometrial receptivity due to different gene expressions in stimulated versus unstimulated endometrium [21,22]. It seems that the cryo-preservation only strategy sustains a better chance for a viable pregnancy and lower abortion rates, and ovarian hyperstimulation has a 7% occurrence rate for fresh embryo pregnancies versus 1–3% for pregnancies with cryo-preserved embryos [23]. Frozen embryo pregnancies grew steadily, for example, from 28% in 2010 to 32% in 2011. Current trends contribute already by the discussed segmentation of IVF cycles, and pre-implantation genetic testing indicated the necessity by the advancing age of motherhood to the growing proportion of freeze-thaw cycles. Some countries like Switzerland, Finland, Holland, Iceland, and Sweden were fast to achieve 50% pregnancies from cryo-preserved embryos [24], mainly due to differences in embryo-transfer legislation and by the number limitation, which, in turn, increased the number of frozen embryos. As an answer to restrictive legislation like in Germany, Swiss, and Austria, or even interdiction as in Italy 2004–2009, oocyte-preserving techniques were fast emerging. Two types of cooling are used: slow freeze, which allows for cell dehydration, thus lowering ice formation and vitrification, creating a glass-like state by very fast cooling without ice formation. When cells are frozen very slow, excessive dehydration and shrinkage also lead to cellular death, and to avoid such an instance, cryo-protectants are typically used. Non-permeating cryo-protectants remain in the extracellular space, leading to the rising osmolality of the extracellular solution before freezing, and thus, preventing intracellular ice formation. The most used slow freezing cryoprotectant is a permeating agent, dimethyl sulfoxide—DMSO, and it was used as a cryo-protective agent for the first frozen-thaw human cleavage embryo transferred. DMSO displaces intracellular water; its cryo-protectant effect augments it with concentration but also increases cytotoxicity and clinical practice, as demonstrated by the toxic effect on patients [25]. The first successful mammalian embryo cryo-preservation was realized in 1972 by applying a cooling rate of ~1 °C/min up to −70 °C. This type of cooling is labeled equilibrium freezing, and the target is to maintain a sufficient intracellular dehydration rate to maintain intracellular water chemical potential in equilibrium with extracellular, partially frozen water. Mostly, ice formation occurs in the extracellular space with subsequent increases in cellular membrane osmotic pressure that accentuates after ice formation continues following nucleation due to the ice lattice excluding solvates that concentrate in the extracellular medium. Less permeable cell membranes rupture due to the abrupt rise in osmotic pressure if they cannot dehydrate fast enough. Intracellular ice formation may be lethal, and exposure to high concentrations of electrolytes may also cause cellular death [26]. Cryogenic injury is related to the cellular membrane permeability, and as a consequence, cells with higher membrane permeability have better survival rates at fast freezing rates, and cells with less permeable membranes need slower cooling. Vitrification was first used for mouse embryo cryopreservation, and became a viable alternative to conventional protocols, as it was shown to reduce cellular damage. During vitrification procedures, cells and tissues are exposed to cryo-protectants that dehydrate cells before commencing cooling. The most frequent method for embryo vitrification necessitates small specimen volumes to be exposed to super-fast cooling and warming rates. This technique was first used in human embryology by 1998 for cleavage stage embryos and then in 1999 for oocytes and pronuclear embryos. In the last 20 years, more vitrification methods were described, which involved a large array of cryo-preservers combinations such as Ethylene glycol (EG), DMSO, PROH

(1,2-propanediol) and sucrose, Ficoll (polysaccharide solution), Trehalose, with varying parameters of dilution and equilibrium, support and cooling systems, storage and warming devices [27]. In 2005, Kuwayama M. et al. considered that the usual embryo and oocyte vitrification implied using a 15% solution of DMSO, 15% Ethylene Glycol, and 0.5 M sucrose in a very small volume ≤1 µL [28]. The fast cooling in vitrification is achieved by immersing the specimen in liquid nitrogen, and from this, two techniques are realized: open and closed vitrification. The majority of embryos and oocytes are vitrified by direct exposure to liquid nitrogen in the open system, favored because of its fast cooling and warming rates, increasing the method's success [29]. The alternative is represented by the use of devices that mediate direct contact with liquid nitrogen-closed systems, presumably marred by lower cooling and thawing rates. It is currently considered that successful vitrification is closely dependent on successful cellular osmotic dehydration before cooling and on the warming rate than on the type and concentration of the cryo-preserving agent, so as to avoid water re-crystallization in the thawing cycle where very fast warming is a requisite. To highlight these conclusions, a recent study performed by a team that included Peter Mazur, one of the pioneers in the field, has demonstrated high survival rates after oocytes and embryos were vitrified without permeating cryoprotectants, and the thawing procedure was realized by ultra-fast warming by an infrared laser pulse [30]. Another study aimed to use a laser beam to dehydrate the blastocoel before vitrification and found substantial improvement in the clinical outcome by lowering the risk of ice recrystallization [31]. Vitrification is now considered the gold standard for oocyte and embryo cryopreservation [30]. Fast freezing protocols need a cell dehydration stage by cryo-protective agents to prevent ice formation, though the direct correlation between intracellular ice formation and cell death has yet to be well defined [26]. It seems that cell survival following cryo-preservation depends on the rate the cells are warmed during the thawing process, as cell damage does not occur during initial ice nucleation, but by another process during thawing and ice recrystallization [32] seems to be the main culprit. Among the first observations are the studies on organisms that naturally survive freezing and physiologically produce recrystallization inhibitors in large amounts [33]. Cryo-protectants based on carbohydrates represent an alternative to DMSO and have minimal or no toxicity; they act like glycerol, which is known to influence ice formation [34]. Ice recrystallization is inhibited by mono and poli-disaccharides, thus suggesting possible use in human cell cryopreservation. One study compared cellular viability after cryopreservation with mono and poli-disaccharides, and with the DMSO control. They found that the most powerful ice recrystallization inhibitors were 220 mM disaccharides solution, and the best viability was obtained with D-galactose 200 mM. It seems that the protective effect of D-galactose resides in its internalization, consequently lowering cellular osmotic stress [35]. Several studies used carbohydrates in the cryopreservation media, but did not strive to evaluate their efficiency, while in others, the success seemed dependent on the chemical structure or correlated carbohydrate efficiency with dehydration level of the milieu [36]. As recrystallization seems to be involved in cellular death derived from cryo-preservation [26,32], the intimate structural characteristic that is involved in recrystallization inhibition is not yet known. It is considered essential for the vitrification process's success to limit to the minimum the amount of vitrification specimen to obtain a high rate of cooling and warming, thus preventing ice formation, and in this respect, oocytes are suitable freeze due to the low surface volume ratio that makes the cell membrane difficult to traverse for water and cryo-protectants [37]. Further, mature oocyte vitrification in metaphase meiosis (MII) may disrupt and deregulate the meiosis spindle, increasing the risk of chromosomal aberrations [38]. Unlike oocytes, embryos are more tolerant of freezing because membrane characteristics change after fertilization, favoring dehydration during cryo-preservation [39]. Embryo cryo-conservation led to the development of numerous devices that facilitate cooling and warming procedures, such as Cryoloop, nylon loop, Hemi-straw system, electron microscope plate, glass capillary, and Cryotop. Open Pulled Straw (OPS) was the first device specifically conceived for ultrafast vitrification, which was introduced by Vajta in 1998, and is still considered to be one of the best devices. The Cryotop is considered to be one of the most efficient vitrification methods both for oocytes and embryos, providing high rates of survival for both humans and animal models, and like other open cryo-preservation systems, directly contacts liquid nitrogen, increasing the risk of viral contamination [40]. Alternative methods were devised, such as micro-volume air-cooling (MVAC) that focused on preventing direct contact of the specimen with the liquid nitrogen [41].

There are patients for whom embryo cryo-preservation was not an option, and because oocyte cryo-preservation techniques had slower progress, ovarian tissue-slow-freeze represented the only fertility preservation method. Lately, oocyte cryo-preservation methods achieved good results, and the Practice Committee of the American Society for Reproductive Medicine (ASRM) reclassified oocyte cryopreservation technology as "nonexperimental" in 2013 [42]. While many oocyte preservation programs do not have long term data on oocyte preservation, especially for patients that received chemotherapy and radiotherapy treatment. Lastly, for increased chances of pregnancy, a few stimulation cycles could be necessary for oocyte preservation in light of evidence that using fresh oocytes only increases the chance of pregnancy by 5% [43].

3. New Techniques of Fertility Preservation

Ovarian tissue cryo-preservation may be an alternative to oocyte preservation, because for some patients' ovarian tissue cryo-preservation, it may eliminate the need for the oncologic treatment delay needed for stimulation cycles for oocyte retrieval. There is hope that ovarian tissue transplant reinstates not only fertility, but also endocrine function. The slow freeze was compared with vitrification methods for the ovarian tissue [44] and some authors consider slow freezing a better method due to greater primordial follicle density and viability, less apoptotic cells and better morpho-functional aspects [44], while others did not find a significant difference in regards to these characteristics [45]. Shi et al. [46] showed that vitrification produces less DNA fragmentation regarding primordial follicles, and vitrification also produces superior results for the granulosa and stromal cells ultra-structure after vitrification. The large variety and the array of conflicting results stem from lack of standardization of the cryo-preservation protocols, the large spread of cryoprotective agents concentration, the variety of experimental animals, the varying implanting sites of the ovarian tissue, the different duration of observation protocols, and last but not least, the varying methods of success measurement. Clinical benefits of ovarian transplantation may be disputed, but, for sure, it benefits fundamental science on ovarian function, primordial follicle activation and development arrest as provided by studies such as those of Winkler et al., and more recently, Silber et al. and Hayashi et al. [47,48]. ASCO acknowledges that ovarian tissue cryopreservation and transplantation does not need ovarian stimulation and may be immediately performed. The added benefit resides in that it does not need sexual maturity, being the only method fit for children in the scope of fertility preservation and being able to restore the global ovarian function. As of 2018, ASCO considers ovarian tissue preservation still experimental, but keeps it open for evidence that can change this status [20]. Improving techniques led to an estimated 35%–40% live birth [49], since the first alive human baby, obtained as a result of ovarian cortex auto-transplant, was reported in 2004, and there were more than 100 live births worldwide; however, global reach of the procedure remains low, limiting further progress [49]. There are growing numbers of studies trying to discern how the best results can be obtained, by ovarian strip vitrification, or slow freezing, whole ovary versus ovarian strip, or the best place to insert the implant as one study concluded that implant location could significantly affect the results [50]. One group [51] compared whole ovary vitrification vs. slow freezing and concluded that the efficacy of whole ovaries cryopreservation by vitrification was higher than those by conventional freezing and rapid freezing, and that conventional freezing of ovarian cortical strips was more effective than cryopreservation of whole ovaries, independent of the way of whole ovary cryopreservation. Most of the live births after ovarian tissue cryopreservation, so far, have been achieved by slow controlled freezing, and only two teams achieved live births from ovarian tissue vitrification [52,53], while others still use the slow freezing method. Laboratories are striving to find the optimal concentration of cryo-protectants for the best results in ovarian tissue cryopreservation by vitrification. One of the pioneers of ovarian tissue vitrification, Silber S [53], reported that he and his team have used only ovarian tissue vitrification since 2008, after 11 years of slow freezing use.

Vitrification may overcome the negative effects of freezing by inhibiting ice crystal formation, and also, vitrification has advantages related to its relatively lower cost, and does not require sophisticated freezing machines or ultra-specialized laboratory staff.

During the antenatal period, human ovaries lose to follicular atresia 80% of its germinal cells to roughly 500,000–1,000,000 at birth [54] and reaching puberty with only 300,000 to 500,000 oocytes; of these, just 400–500 will be selected for ovulation in the following 30–40 years and the rest will be extinguished. The 1% selected for ovulation is subjected to an FSH dependent process that leads to a dominant follicle that produces ovulation during the same cycle. It is considered that follicular activation in humans takes place in a wave pattern, taking effect even during pregnancy or contraceptive medication [54,55]. Follicular recruitment varies with age, from more than 1400 at the beginning of the third decade of life to less than 30 towards the end of the fifth decade and follicular destruction takes place in great numbers before or after follicular recruitment dependent or not on the menstrual cycle, with a decreasing rate during the lifetime, with more follicular loss occurring in young women [56]. The remaining ovarian follicle cohort thus declines in number throughout the lifetime, leading to reduced fertility in the fourth decade, irregular menses by the middle of the fifth decade, and menopause at around 50 years of age. This process remains in a mysterious equilibrium of reproductive aging and organismal aging as it is one of the most precocious aging phenomena in women, but new studies are bringing fresh hypotheses on how ovarian follicles are being activated. Some authors realized that following auto-transplant of ovary tissue after a very marked spike in AMH, the values stabilized at low levels. It has been described as a 'burn out effect', and there is still debate around the implicated mechanisms. One study concluded that the increased number of growing follicles versus resting follicles might be due to the downregulation of PTEN gene expression and subsequent augmentation of follicular recruitment [57]. A Japanese team led by Kawamura [58] recently proposed a premature ovarian insufficiency treatment by Hippo signaling dysregulation, realized by fragmenting ovarian tissue followed by Akt application and autografting. The serine/threonine kinase Akt (protein kinase B or PKB) has become a major focus of attention because of its critical role in regulating diverse cellular functions, including metabolism, growth, proliferation, survival, transcription and protein synthesis, while Hippo signaling is a conserved pathway regulating organ size by cell proliferation, apoptosis, and stem cell activity. It is thought that the disruption of the Hippo pathway contributes to cancer development. Other authors consider that follicle activation and 'burn-out' have an important contribution to post-implantation follicular depletion affecting ovarian tissue grafts [59]. SonerCelik et al. [60] research team's findings regarding ovarian cryo-preservation and auto-transplantation demonstrate that expression of inhibitor proteins that control primordial follicle reserve decreases in cryopreserved ovaries after transplantation. The observation is consistent with the ovarian activity rush observed by others [61,62], and thus they debate the recommendation of follicular activation prior (in vitro activation IVA) to transplantation [58,63]. The longevity of the transplanted ovarian tissue varies widely and may depend on the age of the woman at cryo-preservation [64], some blaming the revascularization rate after transplantation as an important issue [65]; however, long functioning viability of more than ten years has been reported [66]. This success has promoted ovary cryo-preservation for potential use in severe genetic conditions with a risk of primary ovarian insufficiency like sickle cell anemia, thalassemia, Turner syndrome, and galactosemia [67]. A study performed mathematical modeling after losing 50% of the ovarian reserve after mono ovariectomy and concluded that the maintenance of ovarian function suggests an extra-ovarian, probably an age-dependent regulation agent of reproductive decline [68]. A review of cases comprising women with unilateral oophorectomy concluded that the menopause age was lowered by only 1.8 years [69]. By the same logic, it has been suggested that extracting ovarian strips early in life would not substantially affect menopause age, but by cryo-preservation, the ovarian tissue would later be re-implanted, thus conveniently delaying menopause [70]. A proposed mechanism for this ovarian function refers to the downregulation of follicular activation as the follicle pool is diminishing [71]. Another method described for fertility augmentation refers to autologous stem cell ovarian transplantation with, seemingly, relative success [72]. Tilly et al. have long provoked the fertility dogma that women dispose from birth of a fixed, limited number of follicles, by affirming the existence of oogonial stem cells that can be activated, thus jumpstarting fertility [73]. There are reports that sphingosine-1-phosphate has cytoprotective functions in human ovaries, two studies showing that S1P reduces primordial follicle loss in human ovarian tissue xenografted in mice and exposed to cyclophosphamide as an in-vivo model of chemotherapy-induced ovarian damage [74,75]. Another study suggested the use of Sphingosine-1-phosphate to reduce the follicular atresia occurring during the freeze-thawing procedure [76].

As an alternative to ovarian tissue transplants, probing the hypotheses that limited success with ovarian tissue strips is due to the limited and late graft vascularization, there were animal and human trials with whole ovary transplants with limited success [77]. Some limitations were linked to the sheer mass of the ovary (sometimes animal trial included bovine ovaries) posing difficulties in the freezing process, being slow or exhibiting vitrification even after cannulation of the main vessels with cryo-protectants and likely experiencing ice recrystallization in the thawing [78]. Another obstacle is presented by the reperfusion lesions for the prevention, for which some authors tried edaravone, as it is supposed to relieve oxidative stress [79]. An observed supplemental difficulty results from the extensive dissection needed for extraction, but mostly for the ovarian implant, especially venous anastomosis due to the thin venous walls even for experienced teams like M Brännström's that is pioneering uterus transplantation [80].

Owing to the dispute that entangles the use of GnRH agonists [19], alternatives are looked for with the scope to protect ovarian function during chemotherapy. One example of such a protecting agent is represented by Sphingosine-1-phosphate [74,75], others examined co-administration of imatinib, (a 2-phenyl amino pyrimidine derivative that inhibits activity of the tyrosine kinase domains of c-Abl, c-Kit) and platelet-derived growth factor receptor, as they have been reported to attenuate follicle depletion in mice caused by cytotoxic treatments [81], although other studies failed to evidence the protective effect [82]. Anti-Müllerian hormone (AMH) represents another example of hopeful agents to be used in fertility preservation. AMH is part of the transforming growth factor (TGF)-beta family, with a central role in the control of sexual differentiation and follicular genesis, and while serum AMH levels have long been used in reproductive medicine as an indicator of ovarian reserve, it is now investigated as a protective agent [83].

The advent of new technologies brought new fields of research, and while ovarian strip auto-transplant harbors hope for both fertility preservation after oncologic therapy and menopause delay, studies searching for artificial support or even fully artificial ovaries are in full stride. A team is proposing a bioprosthetic ovary that was assembled using 3D printed microporous scaffolds in order to restore ovarian function [84]. Additionally, this is not a singular example since the oncofertility field is evolving; meanwhile, eager bioengineers have sought to create artificial ovaries with biomaterials and isolated follicles [85].

4. Conclusions

Societal pressures pushed forward the long and successful experience with ART due to the increasing age of childbearing, which, in turn, exposed women intending to procreate to a higher risk of malign conditions. This is coupled with the better chance and longer disease-free survival by novel chemotherapy schemes that produce a growing population of women trying to conceive at increasing ages, often after oncologic treatment. Oncofertility studies crosslink with female aging studies and general fertility. There are promising technologies from oogonial stem cells activation, artificial scaffold bioprosthetic ovaries, and proactive ovarian tissue extraction for future use that could push female fertility farther away into what is now senescence.

Author Contributions: Conceptualization, C.B.C. and D.C.R.; methodology, C.B.C., D.C.R. and A.P.; validation, R.-C.P.; investigation, R.-C.P.; writing—original draft, C.B.C. and D.C.R.; writing—review & editing, R.-C.P., D.C.R. and A.P.; visualization, A.P.; supervision, C.B.C. and A.P. All authors have read and agreed to the published version of the manuscript.

Funding: This research received no external funding.

Conflicts of Interest: The authors declare no conflict of interest.

References

1. Armuand, G.M.; Rodriguez-Wallberg, K.A.; Wettergren, L.; Ahlgren, J.; Enblad, G.; Höglund, M.; Lampic, C. Sex differences in fertility-related information received by young adult cancer survivors. *J. Clin. Oncol.* **2012**, *30*, 2147–2153. [CrossRef]
2. Petru, E. MaligneTumoren der Mamma: Fertilität, Kontrazeption und Hormonersatz. In *Praxisbuch Gynäkologische Onkologie*; Petru, E., Fink, D., Köchli, O.R., Loibl, S., Eds.; Springer-Verlag: Berlin/Heidelberg, Germany, 2019; pp. 33–38.
3. Mehedintu, C.; Bratila, E.; Berceanu, C.; Cirstoiu, M.M.; Barac, R.I.; Andreescu, C.V.; Badiu, D.C.; Gales, L.; Zgura, A.; Bumbu, A.G. Comparison of Tumor - Infiltrating Lymphocytes Between Primary and Metastatic Tumors in Her2+and HER2-Breast Cancer Patients. *Rev. Chim. Buchar.* **2018**, *69*, 4033–4037. [CrossRef]
4. Hankey, B.F.; Miller, B.; Curtis, R.; Kosary, C. Trends in breast cancer in younger women in contrast to older women. *J. Natl. Cancer. Inst. Monogr.* **1994**, *16*, 7–14.
5. Voinea, O.C.; Sajin, M.; Dumitru, A.V.; Patrascu, O.M.; Georgescu, T.A.; Cirstoiu, M.M.; Jinga, D.C.; Nica, A.E. Emerging concepts regarding the molecular profile of breast carcinoma: One-year experience in a University Center. *Rom. J. Mil. Med.* **2018**, *121*, 17–24.
6. Jemal, A.; Tiwari, R.C.; Murray, T.; Ghafoor, A.; Samuels, A.; Ward, E.; Feuer, E.J.; Thun, M.J.; American Cancer Society. Cancer statistics, 2004. *CA Cancer J. Clin.* **2004**, *54*, 8–29. [CrossRef]
7. Hankey, B.F.; Ries, L.A.; Edwards, B.K. The surveillance, epidemiology, and end results program: A national resource. *Cancer Epidemiol. Biomark. Prev.* **1999**, *8*, 1117–1121.
8. Zgura, A.; Gales, L.; Haineala, B.; Bratila, E.; Mehedintu, C.; Andreescu, C.V.; Berceanu, C.; Petca, A.; Barac, R.I.; Ionescu, A.; et al. Correlations Between Known Prognostic Markers and Tumor - infiltrating Lymphocytes in Breast Cancer. *Rev. Chim. Buchar.* **2019**, *70*, 2362–2366. [CrossRef]
9. Anders, C.K.; Hsu, D.S.; Broadwater, G.; Acharya, C.R.; Foekens, J.A.; Zhang, Y.; Wang, Y.; Marcom, P.K.; Marks, J.R.; Febbo, P.G.; et al. Young age at diagnosis correlates with worse prognosis and defines a subset of breast cancers with shared patterns of gene expression. *J. Clin. Oncol.* **2008**, *26*, 3324–3330. [CrossRef]
10. McGuire, S. *World Cancer Report 2014*; World Health Organization: Geneva, Switzerland, 2015.
11. Pagani, O.; Partridge, A.; Korde, L.; Badve, S.; Bartlett, J.; Albain, K.; Gelber, R.; Goldhirsch, A.; Breast International Group; North American Breast Cancer Group; et al. Pregnancy after breast cancer: If you wish, ma'am. *Breast Cancer Res. Treat.* **2011**, *129*, 309–317. [CrossRef]
12. Logan, S.; Perz, J.; Ussher, J.M.; Peate, M.; Anazodo, A. Systematic review of fertility-related psychological distress in cancer patients: Informing on an improved model of care. *Psychol. Oncol.* **2019**, *28*, 22–30. [CrossRef]
13. Monte, L.M.; Ellis, R.R. Fertility of women in the United States: 2012. *Econ* **2014**, *24*, 1071–1100.
14. Te Velde, E.R.; Pearson, P.L. The variability of female reproductive ageing. *Hum. Reprod. Update* **2002**, *8*, 141–154. [CrossRef] [PubMed]
15. Anderson, R.; Themmen, A.; Al-Qahtani, A.; Groome, N.; Cameron, D. The effects of chemotherapy and long-term gonadotrophin suppression on the ovarian reserve in premenopausal women with breast cancer. *Hum. Reprod.* **2006**, *21*, 2583–2592. [CrossRef] [PubMed]
16. Chemaitilly, W.; Mertens, A.C.; Mitby, P.; Whitton, J.; Stovall, M.; Yasui, Y.; Robison, L.L.; Sklar, C.A. Acute ovarian failure in the childhood cancer survivor study. *J. Clin. Endocrinol. Metab.* **2006**, *91*, 1723–1728. [CrossRef] [PubMed]
17. Goodwin, P.J.; Ennis, M.; Pritchard, K.I.; Trudeau, M.; Hood, N. Risk of menopause during the first year after breast cancer diagnosis. *J. Clin. Oncol.* **1999**, *17*, 2365–2370. [CrossRef] [PubMed]
18. Soleimani, R.; Heytens, E.; Darzynkiewicz, Z.; Oktay, K. Mechanisms of chemotherapy-induced human ovarian aging: Double strand DNA breaks and microvascular compromise. *Aging Albany NY* **2011**, *3*, 782–793. [CrossRef]
19. Moore, H.C.; Unger, J.M.; Phillips, K.-A.; Boyle, F.; Hitre, E.; Porter, D.; Francis, P.A.; Goldstein, L.J.; Gomez, H.L.; Vallejos, C.S.; et al. Goserelin for ovarian protection during breast-cancer adjuvant chemotherapy. *N. Engl. J. Med.* **2015**, *372*, 923–932. [CrossRef]
20. Oktay, K.; Harvey, B.E.; Loren, A.W. Fertility preservation in patients with cancer: ASCO clinical practice guideline update summary. *J. Oncol. Pract.* **2018**, *14*, 381–385. [CrossRef]
21. Wong, K.M.; Mastenbroek, S.; Repping, S. Cryopreservation of human embryos and its contribution to in vitro fertilization success rates. *Fertil. Steril.* **2014**, *102*, 19–26. [CrossRef]

22. Haouzi, D.; Assou, S.; Mahmoud, K.; Tondeur, S.; Rème, T.; Hedon, B.; De Vos, J.; Hamamah, S. Gene expression profile of human endometrial receptivity: Comparison between natural and stimulated cycles for the same patients. *Hum. Reprod.* **2009**, *24*, 1436–1445. [CrossRef]
23. Wong, K.M.; van Wely, M.; Mol, F.; Repping, S.; Mastenbroek, S. Fresh versus frozen embryo transfers in assisted reproduction. *Cochrane Database Syst. Rev.* **2017**, *3*, CD011184. [CrossRef] [PubMed]
24. European IVF-Monitoring Consortium (EIM); European Society of Human Reproduction and Embryology (ESHRE); Kupka, M.S.; D'Hooghe, T.; Ferraretti, A.P.; de Mouzon, J.; Erb, K.; Castilla, J.A.; Calhaz-Jorge, C.; De Geyter, C.H.; et al. Assisted reproductive technology in Europe, 2011: Results generated from European registers by ESHRE. *Hum. Reprod.* **2016**, *31*, 233–248. [PubMed]
25. Liseth, K.; Foss Abrahamsen, J.; Bjørsvik, S.; Grøttebø, K.; Bruserud, Ø. The viability of cryopreserved PBPC depends on the DMSO concentration and the concentration of nucleated cells in the graft. *Cytotherapy* **2005**, *7*, 328–333. [CrossRef]
26. Fowler, A.; Toner, M. Cryo-injury and biopreservation. *Ann. N. Y. Acad. Sci.* **2006**, *1066*, 119–135. [CrossRef] [PubMed]
27. Vajta, G.; Nagy, Z.P. Are programmable freezers still needed in the embryo laboratory? Review on vitrification. *Reprod. Biomed. Online* **2006**, *12*, 779–796. [CrossRef]
28. Kuwayama, M.; Vajta, G.; Kato, O.; Leibo, S.P. Highly efficient vitrification method for cryopreservation of human oocytes. *Reprod. Biomed. Online* **2005**, *11*, 300–308. [CrossRef]
29. Vajta, G.; Rienzi, L.; Ubaldi, F.M. Open versus closed systems for vitrification of human oocytes and embryos. *Reprod. Biomed. Online* **2015**, *30*, 325–333. [CrossRef]
30. Jin, B.; Mazur, P. High survival of mouse oocytes/embryos after vitrification without permeating cryoprotectants followed by ultra-rapid warming with an IR laser pulse. *Sci. Rep.* **2015**, *5*, 9271. [CrossRef]
31. Darwish, E.; Magdi, Y. Artificial shrinkage of blastocoel using a laser pulse prior to vitrification improves clinical outcome. *J. Assist. Reprod. Genet.* **2016**, *33*, 467–471. [CrossRef]
32. Mazur, P. Principles of cryobiology. In *Life in the Frozen State*; Fuller, B.J., Lane, N., Benson, E.E., Eds.; CRC Press: Boca Raton, FL, USA, 2004; pp. 3–65.
33. Ramløv, H.; Wharton, D.A.; Wilson, P.W. Recrystallization in a freezing tolerant Antarctic nematode, Panagrolaimusdavidi, and an alpine weta, Hemideinamaori (Orthoptera; Stenopelmatidae). *Cryobiology* **1996**, *33*, 607–613. [CrossRef]
34. Dashnau, J.; Vanderkooi, J. Computational approaches to investigate how biological macromolecules can be protected in extreme conditions. *J. Food Sci.* **2007**, *72*, R001–R010. [CrossRef]
35. Chaytor, J.L.; Tokarew, J.M.; Wu, L.K.; Leclère, M.; Tam, R.Y.; Capicciotti, C.J.; Guolla, L.; von Moos, E.; Findlay, C.S.; Allan, D.S.; et al. Inhibiting ice recrystallization and optimization of cell viability after cryopreservation. *Glycobiology* **2011**, *22*, 123–133. [CrossRef]
36. Tam, R.Y.; Ferreira, S.S.; Czechura, P.; Chaytor, J.L.; Ben, R.N. Hydration Index-A Better Parameter for Explaining Small Molecule Hydration in Inhibition of Ice Recrystallization. *J. Am. Chem. Soc.* **2008**, *130*, 17494–17501. [CrossRef]
37. Pereira, R.; Marques, C. Animal oocyte and embryo cryopreservation. *Cell Tissue Bank.* **2008**, *9*, 267–277. [CrossRef]
38. Arav, A.; Zeron, Y.; Leslie, S.; Behboodi, E.; Anderson, G.; Crowe, J. Phase transition temperature and chilling sensitivity of bovine oocytes. *Cryobiology* **1996**, *33*, 589–599. [CrossRef]
39. Chen, S.; Lien, Y.; Chao, K.; Ho, H.-N.; Yang, Y.; Lee, T. Effects of cryopreservation on meiotic spindles of oocytes and its dynamics after thawing: Clinical implications in oocyte freezing-a review article. *Mol. Cell. Endocrinol.* **2003**, *202*, 101–107. [CrossRef]
40. AbdelHafez, F.; Xu, J.; Goldberg, J.; Desai, N. Vitrification in open and closed carriers at different cell stages: Assessment of embryo survival, development, DNA integrity and stability during vapor phase storage for transport. *BMC Biotechnol.* **2011**, *11*, 29. [CrossRef]
41. Punyawai, K.; Anakkul, N.; Srirattana, K.; Aikawa, Y.; Sangsritavong, S.; Nagai, T.; Imai, K.; Parnpai, R. Comparison of Cryotop and micro volume air cooling methods for cryopreservation of bovine matured oocytes and blastocysts. *J. Reprod. Dev.* **2015**, *61*, 431–437. [CrossRef]
42. Practice Committees of American Society for Reproductive Medicine; Society for Assisted Reproductive Technology. Mature oocyte cryopreservation: A guideline. *Fertil. Steril.* **2013**, *99*, 37–43. [CrossRef]

43. Patrizio, P.; Sakkas, D. From oocyte to baby: A clinical evaluation of the biological efficiency of in vitro fertilization. *Fertil. Steril.* **2009**, *91*, 1061–1066. [CrossRef]
44. Isachenko, V.; Isachenko, E.; Weiss, J.M.; Todorov, P.; Kreienberg, R. Cryobanking of human ovarian tissue for anti-cancer treatment: Comparison of vitrification and conventional freezing. *CryoLetters* **2009**, *30*, 449–454.
45. Klocke, S.; Bündgen, N.; Köster, F.; Eichenlaub-Ritter, U.; Griesinger, G. Slow-freezing versus vitrification for human ovarian tissue cryopreservation. *Arch. Gynecol. Obstet.* **2015**, *291*, 419–426. [CrossRef] [PubMed]
46. Shi, Q.; Xie, Y.; Wang, Y.; Li, S. Vitrification versus slow freezing for human ovarian tissue cryopreservation: A systematic review and meta-analysis. *Sci. Rep.* **2017**, *7*, 8538. [CrossRef] [PubMed]
47. Silber, S. Unifying theory of adult resting follicle recruitment and fetal oocyte arrest. *Reprod. Biomed. Online* **2015**, *31*, 472–475. [CrossRef]
48. Hayashi, K.; Ogushi, S.; Kurimoto, K.; Shimamoto, S.; Ohta, H.; Saitou, M. Offspring from oocytes derived from in vitro primordial germ cell–like cells in mice. *Science* **2012**, *338*, 971–975. [CrossRef]
49. Donnez, J.; Dolmans, M.-M. The ovary: From conception to death. *Fertil. Steril.* **2017**, *108*, 594–595. [CrossRef]
50. Damásio, L.C.V.; Soares-Júnior, J.M.; Iavelberg, J.; Maciel, G.A.; de Jesus Simões, M.; dos Santos Simões, R.; da Motta, E.V.; Baracat, M.C.; Baracat, E.C. Heterotopic ovarian transplantation results in less apoptosis than orthotopic transplantation in a minipig model. *J. Ovarian Res.* **2016**, *9*, 14. [CrossRef]
51. Zhang, J.-M.; Sheng, Y.; Cao, Y.-Z.; Wang, H.-Y.; Chen, Z.-J. Cryopreservation of whole ovaries with vascular pedicles: Vitrification or conventional freezing? *J. Assist. Reprod. Genet.* **2011**, *28*, 445–452. [CrossRef]
52. Kawamura, K.; Cheng, Y.; Suzuki, N.; Deguchi, M.; Sato, Y.; Takae, S.; Ho, C.H.; Kawamura, N.; Tamura, M.; Hashimoto, S.; et al. Hippo signaling disruption and Akt stimulation of ovarian follicles for infertility treatment. *Proc. Natl. Acad. Sci. USA* **2013**, *110*, 17474–17479. [CrossRef]
53. Silber, S. How ovarian transplantation works and how resting follicle recruitment occurs: A review of results reported from one center. *Women's Health Lond* **2016**, *12*, 217–227. [CrossRef]
54. Wallace, W.H.B.; Kelsey, T.W. Human ovarian reserve from conception to the menopause. *PLoS ONE* **2010**, *5*, e8772. [CrossRef]
55. Tica, O.A.; Tica, O.; Antal, L.; Hatos, A.; Popescu, M.I.; Pantea Stoian, A.; Bratu, O.G.; Gaman, M.A.; Pituru, S.M.; Diaconu, C.C. Modern oral anticoagulant treatment in patients with atrial fibrillation and heart failure: Insights from the clinical practice. *Farmacia* **2018**, *66*, 972–976. [CrossRef]
56. Faddy, M. Follicle dynamics during ovarian ageing. *Mol. Cell. Endocrinol.* **2000**, *163*, 43–48. [CrossRef]
57. Ayuandari, S.; Winkler-Crepaz, K.; Paulitsch, M.; Wagner, C.; Zavadil, C.; Manzl, C.; Ziehr, S.C.; Wildt, L.; Hofer-Tollinger, S. Follicular growth after xenotransplantation of cryopreserved/thawed human ovarian tissue in SCID mice: Dynamics and molecular aspects. *J. Assist. Reprod. Genet.* **2016**, *33*, 1585–1593. [CrossRef]
58. Kawamura, K.; Kawamura, N.; Hsueh, A.J. Activation of dormant follicles: A new treatment for premature ovarian failure? *Curr. Opin. Obstet. Gynecol.* **2016**, *28*, 217–222. [CrossRef]
59. Gavish, Z.; Peer, G.; Hadassa, R.; Yoram, C.; Meirow, D. Follicle activation and 'burn-out' contribute to post-transplantation follicle loss in ovarian tissue grafts: The effect of graft thickness. *Hum. Reprod.* **2014**, *29*, 989–996. [CrossRef]
60. Meirow, D.; Roness, H.; Kristensen, S.G.; Andersen, C.Y. Optimizing outcomes from ovarian tissue cryopreservation and transplantation; activation versus preservation. *Hum. Reprod.* **2015**, *30*, 2453–2456. [CrossRef]
61. Celik, S.; Celikkan, F.T.; Ozkavukcu, S.; Can, A.; Celik-Ozenci, C. Expression of inhibitor proteins that control primordial follicle reserve decreases in cryopreserved ovaries after autotransplantation. *J. Assist. Reprod. Genet.* **2018**, *35*, 615–626. [CrossRef]
62. Dolmans, M.-M.; Cordier, F.; Amorim, C.A.; Donnez, J.; Vander Linden, C. In vitro activation prior to transplantation of human ovarian tissue: Is it truly effective? *Front. Endocrinol.* **2019**, *10*, 520. [CrossRef]
63. Suzuki, N.; Yoshioka, N.; Takae, S.; Sugishita, Y.; Tamura, M.; Hashimoto, S.; Morimoto, Y.; Kawamura, K. Successful fertility preservation following ovarian tissue vitrification in patients with primary ovarian insufficiency. *Hum. Reprod.* **2015**, *30*, 608–615. [CrossRef]
64. Donnez, J.; Dolmans, M.-M. Fertility preservation in women. *N. Engl. J. Med.* **2017**, *377*, 1657–1665. [CrossRef]
65. Xia, X.; Yin, T.; Yan, J.; Yan, L.; Jin, C.; Lu, C.; Wang, T.; Zhu, X.; Zhi, X.; Wang, J.; et al. Mesenchymal stem cells enhance angiogenesis and follicle survival in human cryopreserved ovarian cortex transplantation. *Cell Transplant.* **2015**, *24*, 1999–2010. [CrossRef]
66. Andersen, C.Y.; Silber, S.J.; Berghold, S.H.; Jorgensen, J.S.; Ernst, E. Long-term duration of function of ovarian tissue transplants. *Reprod. Biomed. Online* **2012**, *25*, 128–132. [CrossRef]

67. Jensen, A.; Rechnitzer, C.; Macklon, K.; Ifversen, M.; Birkebæk, N.; Clausen, N.; Sørensen, K.; Fedder, J.; Ernst, E.; Yding Andersen, C. Cryopreservation of ovarian tissue for fertility preservation in a large cohort of young girls: Focus on pubertal development. *Hum. Reprod.* **2016**, *32*, 154–164. [CrossRef]
68. Wilkosz, P.; Greggains, G.D.; Tanbo, T.G.; Fedorcsak, P. Female reproductive decline is determined by remaining ovarian reserve and age. *PLoS ONE* **2014**, *9*, e108343. [CrossRef]
69. Rosendahl, M.; Simonsen, M.; Kjer, J. The influence of unilateral oophorectomy on the age of menopause. *Climacteric* **2017**, *20*, 540–544. [CrossRef]
70. Andersen, C.Y.; Kristensen, S.G. Novel use of the ovarian follicular pool to postpone menopause and delay osteoporosis. *Reprod. Biomed. Online* **2015**, *31*, 128–131. [CrossRef]
71. Yasui, T.; Hayashi, K.; Mizunuma, H.; Kubota, T.; Aso, T.; Matsumura, Y.; Lee, J.S.; Suzuki, S. Factors associated with premature ovarian failure, early menopause and earlier onset of menopause in Japanese women. *Maturitas* **2012**, *72*, 249–255. [CrossRef]
72. Herraiz, S.; Romeu, M.; Buigues, A.; Martínez, S.; Díaz-García, C.; Gómez-Seguí, I.; Martinez, J.; Pellicer, N.; Pellicer, A. Autologous stem cell ovarian transplantation to increase reproductive potential in patients who are poor responders. *Fertil. Steril.* **2018**, *110*, 496–505. [CrossRef]
73. Akahori, T.; Woods, D.C.; Tilly, J.L. Female Fertility Preservation through Stem Cell-based Ovarian Tissue Reconstitution in Vitro and Ovarian Regeneration in Vivo. *Clin. Med. Insights Reprod. Health.* **2019**, *13*, 1179558119848007. [CrossRef]
74. Meng, Y.; Xu, Z.; Wu, F.; Chen, W.; Xie, S.; Liu, J.; Huang, X.; Zhou, Y. Sphingosine-1-phosphate suppresses cyclophosphamide induced follicle apoptosis in human fetal ovarian xenografts in nude mice. *Fertil. Steril.* **2014**, *102*, 871–877. [CrossRef]
75. Li, F.; Turan, V.; Lierman, S.; Cuvelier, C.; De Sutter, P.; Oktay, K. Sphingosine-1-phosphate prevents chemotherapy-induced human primordial follicle death. *Hum. Reprod.* **2013**, *29*, 107–113. [CrossRef]
76. Guzel, Y.; Bildik, G.; Dilege, E.; Oktem, O. Sphingosine-1-phosphate reduces atresia of primordial follicles occurring during slow-freezing and thawing of human ovarian cortical strips. *Mol. Reprod. Dev.* **2018**, *85*, 858–864. [CrossRef]
77. Bedaiwy, M.A.; Hussein, M.R.; Biscotti, C.; Falcone, T. Cryopreservation of intact human ovary with its vascular pedicle. *Hum. Reprod.* **2006**, *21*, 3258–3269. [CrossRef]
78. Nichols-Burns, S.M.; Lotz, L.; Schneider, H.; Adamek, E.; Daniel, C.; Stief, A.; Grigo, C.; Klump, D.; Hoffmann, I.; Beckmann, M.W.; et al. Preliminary observations on whole-ovary xenotransplantation as an experimental model for fertility preservation. *Reprod. Biomed. Online* **2014**, *29*, 621–626. [CrossRef]
79. Kara, M.; Daglioglu, Y.K.; Kuyucu, Y.; Tuli, A.; Tap, O. The effect of edaravone on ischemia–reperfusion injury in rat ovary. *Eur. J. Obstet. Gynecol. Reprod. Biol.* **2012**, *162*, 197–202. [CrossRef]
80. Brännström, M.; Milenkovic, M. Whole ovary cryopreservation with vascular transplantation–A future development in female oncofertility. *Middle East. Fertil. Soc. J.* **2010**, *15*, 125–138. [CrossRef]
81. Maiani, E.; Di Bartolomeo, C.; Klinger, F.G.; Cannata, S.M.; Bernardini, S.; Chateauvieux, S.; Mack, F.; Mattei, M.; De Felici, M.; Diederich, M.; et al. Reply to: Cisplatin-induced primordial follicle oocyte killing and loss of fertility are not prevented by imatinib. *Nat. Med.* **2012**, *18*, 1172–1174. [CrossRef]
82. Kerr, J.B.; Hutt, K.J.; Michalak, E.M.; Cook, M.; Vandenberg, C.J.; Liew, S.H.; Bouillet, P.; Mills, A.; Scott, C.L.; Findlay, J.K.; et al. DNA damage-induced primordial follicle oocyte apoptosis and loss of fertility require TAp63-mediated induction of Puma and Noxa. *Mol. Cell* **2012**, *48*, 343–352. [CrossRef]
83. Sonigo, C.; Beau, I.; Binart, N.; Grynberg, M. Anti-Müllerian hormone in fertility preservation: Clinical and therapeutic applications. *Clin. Med. Insights Reprod. Health* **2019**, *13*, 1179558119854755. [CrossRef]
84. Laronda, M.M.; Rutz, A.L.; Xiao, S.; Whelan, K.A.; Duncan, F.E.; Roth, E.W.; Woodruff, T.K.; Shah, R.N. A bioprosthetic ovary created using 3D printed microporous scaffolds restores ovarian function in sterilized mice. *Nat. Commun.* **2017**, *8*, 15261. [CrossRef]
85. Luyckx, V.; Dolmans, M.M.; Vanacker, J.; Legat, C.; Moya, C.F.; Donnez, J.; Amorim, C.A. A new step toward the artificial ovary: Survival and proliferation of isolated murine follicles after autologous transplantation in a fibrin scaffold. *Fertil. Steril.* **2014**, *101*, 1149–1156. [CrossRef]

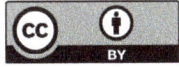

© 2020 by the authors. Licensee MDPI, Basel, Switzerland. This article is an open access article distributed under the terms and conditions of the Creative Commons Attribution (CC BY) license (http://creativecommons.org/licenses/by/4.0/).

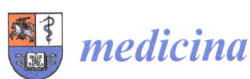

Article

Timing between Breast Reconstruction and Oncologic Mastectomy—One Center Experience

Adelaida Avino [1,2], Laura Răducu [1,2,*], Lăcrămioara Aurelia Brînduşe [3], Cristian-Radu Jecan [1,2] and Ioan Lascăr [2,4]

1. Department of Plastic and Reconstructive Surgery, "Prof. Dr. Agrippa Ionescu" Clinical Emergency Hospital, 011356 Bucharest, Romania; adelaida.avino@gmail.com (A.A.); jecan.radu@gmail.com (C.-R.J.)
2. Department of Plastic and Reconstructive Surgery, Faculty of Medicine "Carol Davila" University of Medicine and Pharmacy, 020021 Bucharest, Romania; ioan.lascar@gmail.com
3. Department of Public Health and Management, Faculty of Medicine, "Carol Davila" University of Medicine and Pharmacy, 020021 Bucharest, Romania; l.brinduse@yahoo.com
4. Department of Plastic and Reconstructive Surgery, Emergency Clinical Hospital of Bucharest, 014461 Bucharest, Romania
* Correspondence: raducu.laura@yahoo.com; Tel.: +40-723-511-985

Received: 28 December 2019; Accepted: 17 February 2020; Published: 20 February 2020

Abstract: *Background and objectives:* Breast cancer is the most common cancer in women. The immunohistochemical profile, but also the stage of the tumor determines the therapeutic management, which varies from conservative surgery to mastectomy associated with chemotherapy, hormonal and biological therapy and/or radiotherapy. Mastectomy remains one of the most radical surgical intervention for women, having great consequences on quality of life, which can be improved by realizing immediate or delayed breast reconstruction. The objective of the study was to evaluate the period of time between the mastectomy and the breast reconstruction. *Material and methods:* We performed a retrospective study on 57 female patients admitted to the Plastic Surgery Department of the Clinical Emergency Hospital "Prof. Dr. Agrippa Ionescu", Bucharest, Romania. All the patients underwent immediate or delayed breast reconstruction after mastectomy for confirmed breast cancer. Descriptive data analysis was realized with evaluation of type of breast reconstruction considering the staging of the tumor, the invaded lymph nodes, and the necessity of adjuvant chemoradiotherapy. Moreover, the median period between mastectomy and reconstruction was evaluated. *Results:* The immediate breast reconstruction was performed in patients with stage I, in patients with stage II, delayed reconstruction was performed after minimum six months, and the patients with stage III had the breast reconstructed with free flap (50%), 8–43 months post-mastectomy. Radiotherapy determines the type of breast reconstruction, in most of the cases the latissimus dorsi flap was used with implant (22.6%). *Conclusions:* Breast reconstruction is an important step in increasing the quality of life for women who underwent mastectomy after breast cancer. The proper timing for breast reconstruction must be settled by a team formed by the patient, the plastic surgeon, and the oncologist.

Keywords: breast reconstruction; timing; mastectomy; adjuvant therapy; quality of life

1. Introduction

Breast cancer is affecting nowadays millions of women worldwide [1]. Unfortunately, the incidence rate has an ascending trend [2]. It is considered to be a multifactorial disease, which is determined by numerous factors, from genetic to environmental ones [1]. The most important step of the treatment plan of breast cancer is surgery. Even if an increasing number of patients are diagnosed in early stages and can benefit of breast-conservatory surgery, total mastectomy is performed in the majority of cases [3]. It has been observed as an increasing tendency for immediate breast reconstruction, mostly in women in whom bilateral mastectomy was performed [4].

The breast represents a part of a woman's identity, symbolizing femininity, sexuality, beauty, and motherhood. The post-mastectomy scars may have great effect on the body and mind of the patients, especially in young women [5]. Breast reconstruction can be done using autologous tissue or implants. The options of the surgical intervention are established taking into consideration factors such as the type of mastectomy, adjuvant treatments, the body type of each individual, lifestyle, acceptance of possible risks [6]. Another important decisional factor is the patient's desire. The patient is advised by the plastic surgeon, who explains the options of breast reconstruction. Autologous reconstruction produces a more natural breast, which modifies with the variation of the body mass, being used also after radiotherapy. Implant-based reconstruction is preferred for being quicker, regarding the operating and recovery times [7]. The last method is considered to be the most performed breast reconstruction technique worldwide. In some cases, a tissue expander is utilized prior to the final implant [6]. The symmetry with the opposite breast is one of the final goals. Taking into account the oncological safety, a contralateral breast lift, breast reduction, or augmentation can be recommended to create a balanced result, increasing patient satisfaction [8]. The precise timing of the reconstructive procedure is decided by a multidisciplinary team composed by an oncologist, a radiotherapist, and a plastic surgeon.

In the last 10 years, many studies assessed the satisfaction and aesthetic outcome, in order to highlight the factors for a favorable surgical outcome [7]. Yueh et al.(2010), reported that autologous reconstructions are associated with higher patient satisfaction compared to prosthetic reconstruction [9], a result substantiated by Franco et al.(2018), in a recent publication [10].

The aim of the study was to evaluate the proper timing for the reconstructive procedure for the patients who underwent mastectomy.

2. Materials and Methods

We conducted a retrospective study on 57 patients admitted to the Plastic Surgery Department of the Clinical Emergency Hospital "Prof. Dr. Agrippa Ionescu", Bucharest, Romania, for breast reconstruction after mastectomy, within a period of 14 months (January 2018–February 2019). The inclusion criteria were: gender (female patients), patients who underwent mastectomy for confirmed breast cancer, immediate or delayed reconstructions. The patients who did not have available pathological data, those who presented local, post-radiotherapy trophic lesions, or metastases were excluded from the study. All data were taken from surgical operating files, medical letters, postoperative records. The preoperative data comprised demographic information, smoking history, but also comorbidities. The histopathological details of the tumor and adjuvant therapies were registered. The different surgical techniques and postoperative complications were analyzed.

Statistical analysis was performed using the SPSS software, version 23.0 and statistical significance was defined as $p < 0.05$. The results were presented as the mean and standard deviations for quantitative variables and as numbers and frequencies for qualitative variables. In order to study the differences among different types of reconstruction techniques, the chi square test was analyzed for qualitative variables, and one-way ANOVA for quantitative variables, respectively. Multivariate analysis was constructed to identify factors associated with the length of time between mastectomy and reconstruction. Covariates for multivariate analysis were selected based on bivariate analyses and included stage of breast cancer, number of affected lymph nodes, and unilateral or bilateral breast cancer.

Local ethical agreement and informed consent of the patient were obtained.

3. Results

Fifty-seven cases of immediate or delayed breast reconstructions were performed throughout the period of the study. The average age at primary surgery was 46.74 years (range 37–56 years).

From all the patients, 52 were living in an urban area and 16 were smokers. Regarding the breast tumors, in 28 cases ductal carcinoma was discovered, in 21 patients lobular carcinomas, and other types of cancer in eight patients. Twenty-two patients presented stage II cancer, stage III appeared in 18 cases, and stage IV was described for one patient. Axillary lymph node dissection was done in 44 cases, lymph nodes being invaded in 31 individuals (Table 1). Chemotherapy was recommended for 48 patients and radiotherapy for 31 patients. Hormone therapy was indicated in 32 cases. From 57 patients, unilateral breast reconstruction was performed in 46 patients, 10 underwent autologous tissue reconstruction (DIEP free flap). The remaining 48 patients experienced implant-based breast reconstruction: 11 latissimus dorsi flap with implant, 13 expander and implant, five expander Becker, and in 18 cases only implants were used.

Table 1. Variables of the study group.

Variable.	N (%)
Axillary Lymphadenectomy	44 (77,2)
Invaded lymph nodes	
0	26 (45,6)
1–3	13 (22,9)
4–9	17 (29,7)
>10	1 (1,8)
Chemotherapy	48 (84,2)
Radiotherapy	31 (54,4)
Hormonal therapy	32 (56,1)
Unilateral	46 (80,7)
Bilateral	11 (19,3)
Type of reconstruction	
Implant	18 (31.6)
Expander-implant	13 (22.8)
Latissimus dorsi flap + Implant	11 (19.3)
Free flap	10 (17.5)
Latissimus dorsi flap + Becker Expander	5 (8.8)
Complications	15 (26,3)
Period of time between mastectomy and reconstruction (median±SD) (months)	11,89 ± 9,11

There was a statistically significant association between unilateral mastectomy and implant-based reconstruction ($p = 0.003$). The least used was expandable breast implant insertion (10.9%). Moreover, there was an association between bilateral mastectomy and immediate breast reconstruction (Table 2).

In addition, there was a statistically significant association between the stage of the tumor and the type of breast reconstruction ($p < 0.001$). The implant-based breast reconstruction was used in all the patients with stage I, immediate reconstruction being decided in eight cases (50%). In stage II, delayed reconstruction was performed after minimum six months and the most common intervention was latissimus dorsi flap with implant (36.4%). The patients with stage III had the breast reconstructed with free flap (50%), 8–43 months post-mastectomy. The timing between mastectomy and breast reconstruction was determined also by the histological type of the tumor, 17.07 months in case of ductal carcinoma and 7.524 months in case of lobular carcinoma.

Radiotherapy influenced the type of breast reconstruction, a significant correlation between them ($p = 0.001$) being discovered; latissimus dorsi flap with implant was used most frequently (22.6%). Furthermore, the mean duration of hospitalization was strongly associated with the reconstructive intervention ($p = 0.003$). A significant association between postoperative complications and the type of the reconstructive procedure was noticed ($p = 0.001$). The complications were observed in patients with latissimus dorsi flap (46.7%), but also in those with free flap (33.3%). Wound dressings were used to heal the lesions.

There was a significant correlation between chemotherapy and breast reconstruction ($p = 0.049$), but there was not a significant correlation between smoking and type of reconstructive procedure ($p = 0.077$).

Table 2. Type of reconstruction depending on different variables.

	Type of Reconstruction					
	Implant N (%)	Expander + Implant N (%)	Latissimus Dorsi + Implant N (%)	Free Flap N (%)	Latissimus + Expander Becker N (%)	p Value
Unilateral	9 (19.6)	12 (26.1)	10 (21.7)	10 (21.7)	5 (10.9)	0.003
Bilateral	9 (81.8)	1 (9.1)	1 (9.1)	0 (0.0)	0 (0.0)	
Complications	1 (6.7)	0 (0.0)	7 (46.7)	5 (33.3)	2 (13.3)	0.001
Stage						
I	13 (81.2)	3 (18.8)	0 (0.0)	0 (0.0)	0 (0.0)	
II	4 (18.2)	6 (27.3)	8 (36.4)	1 (4.5)	3 (13.6)	<0.001
III	1 (5.6)	4 (22.2)	3 (16.7)	9 (50.0)	1 (5.6)	
IV	0 (0.0)	0 (0.0)	0 (0.0)	0 (0.0)	1 (100.0)	
Radiotherapy	4 (12.9)	6 (19.4)	7 (22.6)	1 (32.3)	4 (12.9)	0.001
Chemotherapy	12 (25.0)	10 (20.8)	11 (22.9)	10 (20.8)	5 (10.4)	0.049
Smoking	4 (25.0)	4 (25.0)	5 (31.2)	0 (0.0)	3 (18.8)	0.077
Hospital days (mean ± SD)	8.6 ± 4.6	10.1 ± 3.6	15.5 ± 5.6	13.7 ± 4.9	12.6 ± 4.2	0.003

4. Discussion

Breast cancer is one of the most frequent types of malignancies in women, among lung and colorectal cancer. Thirty percent of all new discovered tumors are breast cancer. Breast reconstruction methods are increasingly performed all over the world. From 2000 to 2016 their number increased with 39%. The most common procedure was the implant-based breast reconstruction. Less than 25% of the patients have immediate reconstruction after mastectomy [11].

In our study, 16 patients were diagnosed with stage I breast cancer and half of them had immediate breast reconstruction with implants (Figure 1). Nipple-sparing mastectomy (NSM) was performed in eight women using a surgical incision in the inframammary fold, five of them had contralateral prophylactic mastectomy, with positive BRCA genes. In three patients, delayed reconstruction with expander was decided. The others had delayed intervention with implants. The reconstructions were performed 3–12 months after mastectomy. None of the patients had radiotherapy. Seven patients had chemotherapy and two of them received also hormonal therapy. One patient presented a minor complication, a seroma.

In patients with stage I breast cancer, the surgical steps have changed over the years, from radical to nipple-sparing mastectomy, increasing the reconstructive and aesthetic results. Even though NSM was considered to have a high oncologic risk, it has been accepted as a reconstructive option in selected patients [12]. This technique is used in younger patients with early breast cancer stages or after prophylactic mastectomy [13].It can be done in one or two surgical steps, but most of the surgeons prefer the one-stage method due to its low overall costs, outstanding outcomes, and low revision rates [12]. Regarding complications, initially, skin and nipple necrosis were considered to be too high, but after being used worldwide, it was emphasized that these two complications have a rate up to 10% and can be treated conservatively, saving the nipple. The most important steps to avoid complications are to make the incisions far from the nipple and to use the inframammary fold, this being demonstrated by Garwood et al. (2009), but also by Colwell et al.(2014) in their studies [13]. In our clinic, this intervention is starting to be used with high frequency due to the fact the patients are presenting in early stages of the disease. Moreover, acellular dermal matrix can be used in immediate reconstruction, to guarantee an optimal placement of the implant [14].

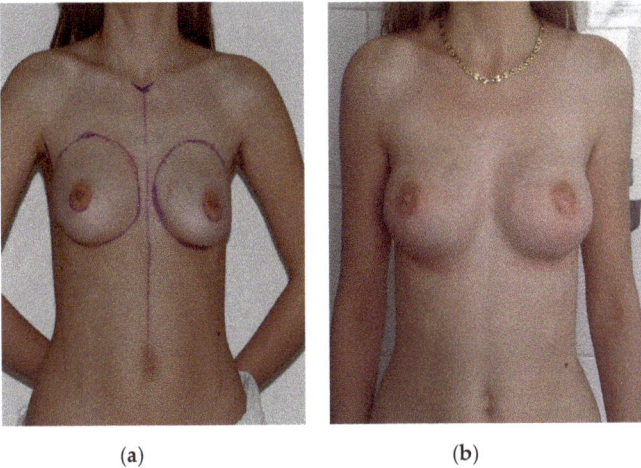

Figure 1. Patient with right breast cancer, stage I who underwent bilateral nipple sparing mastectomy with immediate reconstruction. (**a**) Preoperative photo. (**b**) Four months postoperative photo.

Twenty-two patients had stage II breast cancer and half of them had invasion of three axillary lymph nodes. The reconstruction was indicated after minimum six months after mastectomy, only one patient presented after 26 months. The reconstruction was performed using all five methods described in the study, depending on the surgeon's decision, but also patient's desire: One case of free flap, four cases of delayed reconstruction with implants, eight interventions combining autogenous tissue (pedicled latissimus dorsi flap) with implants (Figure 2), and nine were based on expanders, out of which five were with Becker expander. Postoperative complications, wound dehiscences, were observed in patients with latissimus dorsi flap. Special dressings with silver were used to accelerate the healing [15]; fortunately, nowadays there are a lot of modern dressings that aid the cure, reducing pain and local discomfort [16].

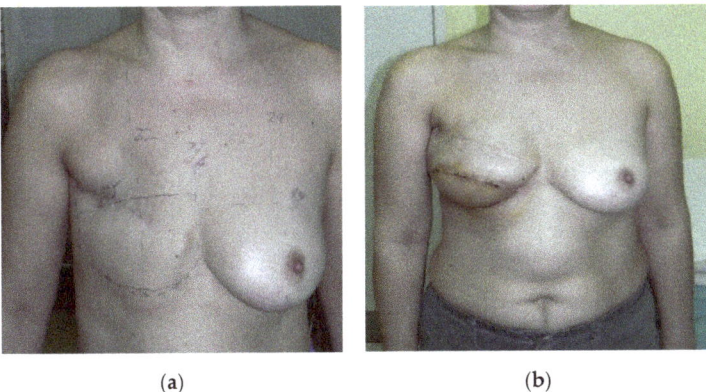

Figure 2. Patient with right breast cancer, stage II who underwent mastectomy. (**a**) Post-mastectomy photo. (**b**) Outcome of delay breast reconstruction with pedicled latissimus dorsi flap and implant shown four months postoperatively.

Concerning the 18 patients with stage III, the reconstructive procedure was performed 8–43 months post-mastectomy, using free flaps in half of the cases (Figure 3). All the patients presented invasive ductal carcinoma, with at least three invaded lymph nodes. All had chemoradiotherapy. From all

18 patients, the youngest was 30 years old and the eldest 63 years old. In four cases, the breast reconstruction was performed with an expander and in three cases with latissimus dorsi flap and implant. Taking into consideration the complications, we encountered a partial necrosis of one DIEP flap, which was excised early and the defect was covered with a local skin flap.

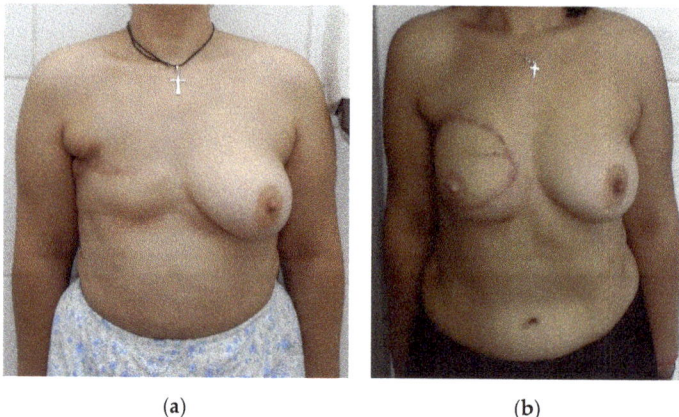

Figure 3. (a) Preoperative photo of patient with previous right mastectomy and subsequent radiation treatment. There is inadequate skin surface area to cover a reconstructed right breast. (b) Outcome of delayed right breast reconstruction with deep inferior epigastric perforator (DIEP) flap shown eight months postoperatively.

The patients with stage IV breast cancer do not consider reconstruction after mastectomy as an option, even if new modern therapies against metastasis are available. Their appreciation is that the reconstruction does not have value. However, systemic metastasis is not a contraindication to reconstruct the breast. A proper therapeutic management must be done [17,18]. In our clinic, we had one patient with stage IV breast cancer, with bone metastasis, who had chemoradiotherapy prior to the reconstruction. Her response to the adjuvant therapy was favorable and due to the fact that she was only 42 years old she asked for reconstruction. In her case, the decision was to use latissimus dorsi myocutaneous flap associated with a Becker expander implant. The intervention was performed 32 months post-mastectomy. No complications were observed postoperatively.

Another factor taken into consideration in our study was smoking. Due to the fact that smoking is a contraindication for immediate breast reconstruction, determining skin necrosis and infection [19], none of the smokers had this type of reconstructive procedure.

Another important factor in breast reconstruction is the proper timing after mastectomy. In our study, only 17 patients underwent the reconstruction procedure in the first six months. They had no invaded lymph nodes. In a study made by Lee et al. in 2015, it was demonstrated that the moment of the reconstructive procedure is settled mainly by patient preference, the plastic surgeons taking the responsibility for the best aesthetic result [20], but also by the necessity of postmastectomy radiotherapy [21]. Moreover, the decision of this intervention must be taken after consulting the oncologist [20]. In our study, none of the patients had postmastectomy radiotherapy. According to the stage of breast cancer, immediate reconstruction can be indicated for patients with stage O, I, or IIA. Those with early stage malignancy represent up to 70% of women who go through mastectomy. The new technique of nipple-sparing mastectomy gives an improved outcome and an excellent feedback from the patients. The diagnosis of breast cancer can be overwhelming, especially when the patients are diagnosed in stage IIB or III. Initially, patients focus on adjuvant therapies and lately they take into consideration post-mastectomy reconstruction, so, in these cases the procedure is delayed [21].

In our study, we highlight that it is possible to accurately predict the duration between mastectomy and reconstruction based on the stage of the disease, the number of affected lymph nodes, and the unilateral or bilateral breast involvement. The most important predictor is the stage of the disease (50%), followed by the number of lymph nodes (25%) and the unilateral or bilateral involvement (24%) (Figure 4).

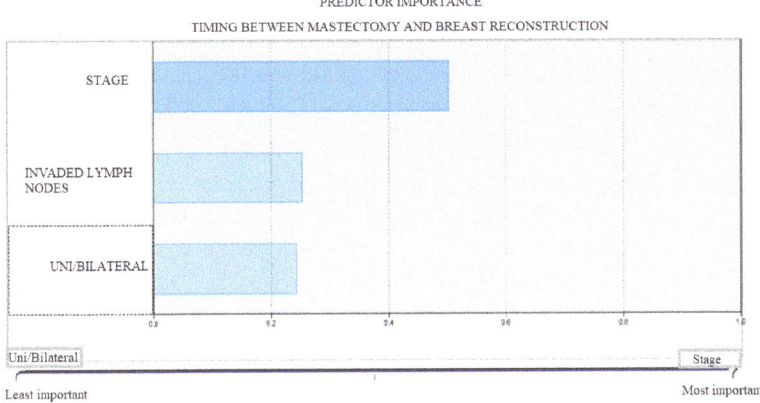

Figure 4. Predictor importance—Timing between mastectomy and breast reconstruction.

For plastic surgeons, breast reconstruction is a main step in the management of treatment, due to its benefits and impact on the quality of life of patients diagnosed with breast cancer. Worldwide, there are many countries with a low rate of this intervention, even if there are national programs to promote it. Regarding the geographic location, the patients from the rural area are associated with poor chances of having breast reconstruction [22]. In our study, only five patients were from a rural area. In Romania, there is a national program for breast reconstruction after oncologic surgery that covers the prosthesis. The surgical intervention is viewed as a reconstructive procedure, so it is covered by the national health insurance. Unfortunately, breast symmetry is considered to be an aesthetic procedure and it can be performed only in private hospitals.

5. Conclusions

Breast cancer is affecting more and more young women. New interdisciplinary protocols are developing for the best therapeutic management, maximizing the outcomes. The timing for breast reconstruction is important, but the decision must be taken after a strong collaboration between the patient, the oncologist, the radiotherapist, and the plastic surgeon.

Author Contributions: Conceptualization, L.R.; methodology, L.R., software, L.A.B., validation, I.L.; formal analysis, L.A.B; investigation, A.A.; resources, C.-R.J.; data curation, A.A.; writing—original draft, A.A.; supervision, I.L.; project administration, C.-R.J. All authors have read and agreed to the published version of the manuscript. All authors have contributed equally to the present work and thus are main authors.

Funding: This research received no external funding.

Conflicts of Interest: The authors declare no conflict of interest.

References

1. Momenimovahed, Z.; Salehiniya, H. Epidemiological characteristics of and risk factors for breast cancer in the world. *Breast Cancer* **2019**, *11*, 151–164. [CrossRef]
2. Ghoncheh, M.; Pournamdar, Z.; Salehiniya, H. Incidence and Mortality and Epidemiology of Breast Cancer in the World. *Asian Pac. J. Cancer Prev.* **2016**, *17*, 43–46. [CrossRef] [PubMed]

3. Qin, Q.; Tan, Q.; Lian, B.; Mo, Q.; Huang, Z.; Wei, C. Postoperative outcomes of breast reconstruction after mastectomy: A retrospective study. *Medicine* **2018**, *97*, e9766. [CrossRef] [PubMed]
4. Olsen, M.A.; Nickel, K.B.; Fox, I.K.; Margenthaler, J.A.; Wallace, A.E.; Fraser, V.J. Comparison of Wound Complications After Immediate, Delayed, and Secondary Breast Reconstruction Procedures. *JAMA Surg.* **2017**, *152*, e172338. [CrossRef]
5. Koçan, S.; Gürsoy, A. Body Image of Women with Breast Cancer after Mastectomy: A Qualitative Research. *J. Breast Health* **2016**, *12*, 145–150. [CrossRef] [PubMed]
6. Lee, G.K.; Sheckter, C.C. Breast Reconstruction Following Breast Cancer Treatment-2018. *JAMA* **2018**, *320*, 1277–1278. [CrossRef]
7. Cohen, O.; Small, K.; Lee, C.; Petruolo, O.; Karp, N.; Choi, M. Is Unilateral Implant or Autologous Breast Reconstruction Better in Obtaining Breast Symmetry? *Breast J.* **2015**, *22*, 75–82. [CrossRef]
8. Rizki, H.; Nkonde, C.; Ching, R.C.; Kumiponjera, D.; Malata, C.M. Plastic surgical management of the contralateral breast in post-mastectomy breast reconstruction. *Int. J. Surg.* **2013**, *11*, 767–772. [CrossRef]
9. Yueh, J.H.; Slavin, S.A.; Adesiyun, T.; Nyame, T.T.; Gautam, S.; Morris, D.J.; Tobias, A.M.; Lee, B.T. Patient Satisfaction in Postmastectomy Breast Reconstruction: A Comparative Evaluation of DIEP, TRAM, Latissimus Flap, and Implant Techniques. *Plast. Reconstr. Surg.* **2010**, *125*, 1585–1595. [CrossRef]
10. Fracon, S.; Renzi, N.; Manara, M.; Ramella, V.; Papa, G.; Arnež, Z.M. Patient satisfaction after breast reconstruction: Implants vs. autologous tissues. *Acta Chir. Plast.* **2018**, *59*, 120–128.
11. Oliver, J.D.; Boczar, D.; Huayllani, M.T.; Restrepo, D.J.; Sisti, A.; Manrique, O.J.; Broer, P.N.; McLaughlin, S.; Rinker, B.D.; Forte, A.J. Postmastectomy Radiation Therapy (PMRT) before and after 2-Stage Expander-Implant Breast Reconstruction: A Systematic Review. *Medicina* **2019**, *55*, 226. [CrossRef] [PubMed]
12. Roh, T.S.; Kim, J.Y.; Jung, B.K.; Jeong, J.; Ahn, S.G.; Kim, Y.S. Comparison of Outcomes between Direct-to-Implant Breast Reconstruction Following Nipple-Sparing Mastectomy through Inframammary Fold Incision versus Noninframammary Fold Incision. *J. Breast Cancer* **2018**, *21*, 213–221. [CrossRef] [PubMed]
13. Ashikari, A.Y.; Kelemen, P.R.; Tastan, B.; Salzberg, C.A.; Ashikari, R.H. Nipple sparing mastectomy techniques: A literature review and an inframammary technique. *Gland Surg.* **2018**, *7*, 273–287. [CrossRef] [PubMed]
14. Filip, C.I.; Berbece, S.; Raducu, L.; Florescu, I.P.; Ardeleanu, V.; Jecan, C.R. The Prospects of Using Meshes in Imediate Implant-Based Breast Reconstructions. *Mater. Plast.* **2017**, *54*, 414–417. [CrossRef]
15. Avino, A.; Jecan, C.R.; Cozma, C.N.; BalcangiuStroescu, A.E.; Balan, D.G.; Ionescu, D.; Mihai, A.; Tanase, M.; Raducu, L. Negative Pressure Wound Therapy Using Polyurethane Foam in a Patient with Necrotizing Fasciitis. *Mater. Plast.* **2018**, *55*, 603–605. [CrossRef]
16. Răducu, L.; Cozma, C.N.; BalcangiuStroescu, A.E.; Avino, A.; Tănăsescu, M.D.; Balan, D.; Jecan, C.R. Our Experience in Chronic Wounds Care with Polyurethane Foam. *Rev. Chim.* **2018**, *69*, 585–586. [CrossRef]
17. Durrant, C.A.; Khatib, M.; Macneill, F.; James, S.; Harris, P. Mastectomy and reconstruction in stage IV breast cancer: A survey of UK breast and plastic surgeons. *Breast* **2011**, *20*, 373–379. [CrossRef] [PubMed]
18. Iorga, R.A.; Bratu, O.G.; Marcu, R.D.; Constantin, T.; Mischianu, D.L.D.; Socea, B.; Gaman, M.A.; Diaconu, C.C. Venous thromboembolism in cancer patients: Still looking for answers. *Exp. Ther. Med.* **2019**, *18*, 5026–5032. [CrossRef]
19. Filip, C.I.; Jecan, C.R.; Raducu, L.; Neagu, T.P.; Florescu, I.P. Immediate Versus Delayed Breast Reconstruction for Postmastectomy Patients. Controversiesand Solutions. *Chirurgia* **2017**, *112*, 378–386. [CrossRef]
20. Lee, M.; Reinertsen, E.; McClure, E.; Liu, S.; Kruper, L.; Tanna, N.; Boyd, J.B.; Granzow, J.W. Surgeon motivations behind the timing of breast reconstruction in patients requiring postmastectomy radiation therapy. *J. Plast. Reconstr. Aesthet. Surg.* **2015**, *68*, 1536–1542. [CrossRef]
21. Ananthakrishnan, P.; Lucas, A. Options and considerations in the timing of breast reconstruction after mastectomy. *Clevel. Clin. J. Med.* **2008**, *75*, 30–33. [CrossRef] [PubMed]
22. Retrouvey, H.; Solaja, O.; Gagliardi, A.R.; Webster, F.; Zhong, T. Barriers of Access to Breast Reconstruction: A Systematic Review. *Plast. Reconstr. Surg.* **2019**, *143*, 465e–476e. [CrossRef] [PubMed]

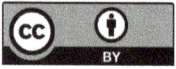

© 2020 by the authors. Licensee MDPI, Basel, Switzerland. This article is an open access article distributed under the terms and conditions of the Creative Commons Attribution (CC BY) license (http://creativecommons.org/licenses/by/4.0/).

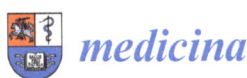

Article

Quality of Life in Patients with Surgically Removed Skin Tumors

Laura Răducu [1,2], Adelaida Avino [1,*], Raluca Purnichescu Purtan [3], Andra-Elena Balcangiu-Stroescu [4,5], Daniela Gabriela Bălan [5], Delia Timofte [4], Dorin Ionescu [6,7] and Cristian-Radu Jecan [1,2]

1. Department of Plastic and Reconstructive Surgery, Clinical Emergency Hospital "Prof. Dr. Agrippa Ionescu", 011356 Bucharest, Romania; raducu.laura@yahoo.com (L.R.); jecan.radu@gmail.com (C.-R.J.)
2. Department of Plastic and Reconstructive Surgery, Faculty of Medicine "Carol Davila" University of Medicine and Pharmacy, 020021 Bucharest, Romania
3. Department of Mathematical Methods and Models, Faculty of Applied Sciences, University Politehnica of Bucharest, 060042 Bucharest, Romania; raluca.purtan@gmail.com
4. Department of Dialysis, Emergency University Hospital Bucharest, 050098 Bucharest, Romania; stroescu_andra@yahoo.ro (A.-E.B.-S.); delia.timofte@gmail.com (D.T.)
5. Discipline of Physiology, Faculty of Dental Medicine, "Carol Davila" University of Medicine and Pharmacy, Bucharest, 020021 Bucharest, Romania; gdaniela.balan@yahoo.com
6. Discipline of Internal Medicine I and Nephrology, Faculty of Medicine, "Carol Davila" University of Medicine and Pharmacy, 020021 Bucharest, Romania; doriny27@gmail.com
7. Department of Nephrology, Emergency University Hospital Bucharest, 050098 Bucharest, Romania
* Correspondence: adelaida.avino@gmail.com; Tel.: +40-7711-7017-0545

Received: 30 December 2019; Accepted: 2 February 2020; Published: 9 February 2020

Abstract: *Background and Objectives*: Skin cancer is one of the most frequently diagnosed malignancies. The main goal of the therapeutic management is total excision with the prevention of recurrence and metastasis. The quality of life of the patients with skin cancer is affected by the morbidity risk, surgery, and cosmetic or functional aspects. The aim of this study was to evaluate the quality of life of patients with skin cancer prior to and post surgical intervention. *Material and methods*: We performed a prospective study on 247 patients with skin tumors. Quality of life was evaluated through an initial questionnaire that was given to all consenting patients. This was used to determine patients' mobility, selfcare, normal activities, pain, and despair, using a five-point Likert scale. The general autoperceived health state was also recorded using a 100-point scale. The study included the responses of all patients at hospital admission, after one month of surgery, and after one year of surgery. *Results*: In patients with squamous cell carcinoma (SCC), the general health state indicator statistically significantly decreased one month after surgery and increased at one-year follow-up. In malignant melanoma (MM) patients, mobility, selfcare, normal activities, and discomfort presented a decrease in values one year after surgery, compared to the values registered at hospital admission. In patients with basal cell carcinoma (BCC), all indicators of quality of life presented an impaired value one year after surgery, after a decreasing trend. The general health state indicator statistically significantly increased one month after surgery and after one year. *Conclusions*: Surgery is one of the main steps in treating skin cancer. It has a great impact on patients' quality of life because of pain andthe effect on mobility and normal activities. Skin cancers influence the quality of life of patients both psychologicallyand physically.

Keywords: skin cancer; squamous cell carcinoma; basal cell carcinoma; malignant melanoma; surgery; quality of life

1. Introduction

Skin cancer is considered to be an important public health issues worldwide. The most frequently diagnosed cancers are nonmelanoma skin cancer (NMSC) and cutaneous malignant melanoma (MM) [1]. NMSC represents a group of cutaneous lesions that do not derivefrom melanocytes. The most common forms of NMSC are squamous cell carcinoma (SCC) and basal cell carcinoma (BCC) [2]. In addition, it has been described the actinic keratosis (AK), which is a cutaneous lesion that can transform into SCC. It appears especially because of excessive ultraviolet exposure [3]. MM causes up to 80% of deaths related to cutaneous malignancy, representing 16% of the diagnosed neoplasia worldwide [4].

In recent decades, the cornerstone of the assessment of cancer treatment efficacy was the survival rate, as well as the recurrence or complication rates. Nowadays, the focus is also on the impact of the disease on patients' quality of life (QoL) [5]. The consequences of the malignancy on patients' psychosocial behavior can be assessed during three phases: at diagnosis, during treatment, and during long-term follow-up. Many factors, such as emotional, physical, aesthetic, or functional concerns regarding treatment, can significantly affect morbidity, mortality, survival rates, or prognoses. Both NMSC and MM are related to high levels of distress or behavioral alteration [6], from the impact of the scars to the diagnosis of malignancy. All these can affect patients' ability to leada fulfilling life. Moreover, up to 25% of newly diagnosed individuals with neoplasia present symptoms of depression [7].

The aim of this study was to evaluate the impact on the QoL of the patients with skin cancer prior to and post surgical intervention using the health-outcome questionnaireEQ-5D-5L (EuroQol 5 dimensions 5 levels).

2. Materials and Methods

We conducted a prospective study on 247 patients admitted in the Plastic Surgery Department of the Clinical Emergency Hospital "Prof. Dr. Agrippa Ionescu," Bucharest, Romania, with skin cancer, over a period of 24 months (January 2017 to December 2018). The inclusion criteria were age >18 years, and a current diagnosis of BCC, SCC, MM, or AK, which was considered a precancerous lesion. The preoperative data comprised demographic information, smoking history, and comorbidities. The histopathological details of the tumor and adjuvant therapies were registered. All patients filled out the EQ-5D-5L questionnaire to describe their perceived QoL.

Statistical analyses were performed using the SPSS software version 19.0 (SPSS Inc., Chicago, IL, USA). For all continuous data, a preliminary statistical analysis was performed in order to test the normality (Smirnov-Kolmogorov test). For nonnormally-distributed variables and noncontinuous data, the comparisons between groups were performed using nonparametric tests (Fisher's Exact Test, Chi-square Test, and Mann-Whitney U test), while for the normally-distributed data, Student's t-test and pairedsamples t-test were used. In addition, correlations between different measurements were determined using the Spearman correlation coefficient. Multilinear regression models were constructed with log-transformed variables. All differences and associations were considered statistically significant if the two-sided p-value was less than 0.05 (95% confidence intervals (CI)).

Local ethical agreement and informed consent of the patients were obtained. The number of the document from the Ethical Commission of Clinical Emergency Hospital "Prof. Dr. Agrippa Ionescu" is 1736615, 05.08.2014.

3. Results

The age of the 247 enrolled patients ranged between 26 and 96 years, with amean of 68 ± 13 years. Among the enrolled patients, 142 (58%) were men and 105 (42%) were women. Moreover, 161 (65%) were from urban areas, and 86 (35%) from rural areas. For the statistical analyses, we considered the following subgroups based on the types of skin cancer: SCC group, MM group, BCC group, and AK group (Table 1).

Table 1. Comparative demographic data of the subgroups.

	Squamous Cell Carcinoma (SCC) Group (n = 38)	Malignant Melanoma (MM) Group (n = 20)	Basal Cell Carcinoma (BCC) Group (n = 168)	Actinic Keratosis (AK) Group (n = 21)
Age (mean ± SD)	74.47 ± 13.24	56.50 ± 18.53	68.67 ± 11.02	67.90 ± 16.20
Gender				
Male	26 (68%)	12 (60%)	91 (54%)	13 (62%)
Female	12 (32%)	8 (40%)	77 (46%)	8 (38%)
Residence				
Urban area	21 (55%)	18 (90%)	105 (62%)	17 (81%)
Rural area	17 (45%)	2 (10%)	63 (38%)	4 (19%)

The mean age of the patients in the MM group was statistically significantly lower than that in all the other groups (t-test, $p < 0.05$ for all comparisons). There was no statistically-significant difference between the subgroups regarding gender structure (Fisher's Exact Test, $p > 0.05$). Regarding the residence area, the structures of the MM group and the AK group were significantly different from the other two groups: the patients in those groups were mostly from urban areas (Fisher's Exact Test, $p = 0.008$ and $p = 0.003$ for MM compared to SCC and BCC, $p = 0.014$ and $p = 0.034$ for AK compared to SCC and BCC).

We also compared the localization of the tumor, the maximum tumor diameter, solar exposure, and the skin type between the four groups. Because the maximum tumor diameter does not follow a normal distribution, median and range are reported (Table 2). The maximum tumor diameter was significantly lower in BCC and AK groups, compared to SCC and MM groups (Mann-Whitney Test, $p < 0.001$), and there was no significant difference between BCC and AKgroups (Mann-Whitney Test, $p = 0.377$). The distribution of the sun exposure in SCC, BCC, and AK groups was similar, with prevalence in the "frequent" category. The amount of sun exposure in the MM group was particularly different, with equal prevalence in both categories. Skin type distribution among the patients in the four groups presented no significant differences (Chi-square Test, all p-values > 0.05); skin types 2 and 3 were most prevalent in all groups.

Table 2. Maximum tumor diameter, solar exposure, and skin type between the subgroups.

	SCC Group (n = 38)	MM Group (n = 20)	BCC Group (n = 168)	AK Group (n = 21)
Maximum tumor diameter (median and range)	2.25 (0.7–4.5) cm	2.25 (0.6–9.5) cm	1.45 (0.3–6) cm	1.8 (0.3–3.8) cm
Sun exposure				
frequent	33 (87%)	10 (50%)	109 (65%)	17 (81%)
less frequent	5 (13%)	10 (50%)	59 (35%)	4 (19%)
Skin type				
1	2 (5%)	0 (0%)	3 (2%)	1 (5%)
2	15 (40%)	13 (65%)	98 (58%)	13 (62%)
3	17 (45%)	6 (30%)	66 (39%)	6 (28%)
4	4 (10%)	1 (5%)	1 (1%)	1 (5%)

In our study, the QoL was assessed using a five-point Likert scale (from 1 to 5, 1 indicating no impairment, and 5 indicating the most severe state) for mobility, selfcare, normal activities, pain (discomfort), and despair (Table 3). The general autoperceived health state was also recorded using a 100-point scale (100 representing the best health state). The study includes the responses of all patients at hospital admission, after one month of surgery, and one year after surgery. In order to determine the parameters that affect the indicators of the QoL, we considered the correlations between several variables, such as age, gender, skin type, diabetes, chronic heart failure, tumor localization, tumor diameter, type of surgery, and the presence of other tumors. Only the statistically-significant correlations are presented.

Table 3. Comparison of quality of life between groups.

	SCC Group (n = 38)	MM Group (n = 20)	BCC Group (n = 168)	AK Group (n = 21)
Mobility				
Hospital admission	1.26 ± 0.6	1.60 ± 0.38	1.14 ± 0.35	1.10 ± 0.34
After one month	1.16 ± 0.37	1.75 ± 0.58	1.10 ± 0.3	1.08 ± 0.27
After one year	1 ± 0.00	1.35 ± 0.58	1 ± 0.00	1 ± 0.00
Selfcare				
Hospital admission	2.45 ± 0.5	2 ± 0.91	2.10 ± 0.62	2.10 ± 0.39
After one month	1.97 ± 0.54	2.05 ± 0.6	1.43 ± 0.5	1.39 ± 0.5
After one year	1.05 ± 0.22	1.40 ± 0.59	1.05 ± 0.21	1 ± 0.00
Normal activities				
Hospital admission	2.68 ± 0.62	2.05 ± 0.99	2.38 ± 0.66	2.29 ± 0.46
After one month	2.11 ± 0.55	2.20 ± 0.61	1.67 ± 0.73	1.46 ± 0.52
After one year	1.05 ± 0.22	1.70 ± 0.65	1 ± 0.00	1.01 ± 0.07
Pain/discomfort				
Hospital admission	2.58 ± 0.55	2.05 ± 0.94	2.43 ± 0.5	2.26 ± 0.47
After one month	1.87 ± 0.34	2 ± 0.45	1.57 ± 0.5	1.41 ± 0.49
After one year	1 ± 0.00	1.55 ± 0.60	1 ± 0.00	1 ± 0.00
Despair				
Hospital admission	2.89 ± 0.69	2.10 ± 0.71	4 ± 0.77	4.23 ± 0.63
After one month	3.95 ± 0.92	4.70 ± 0.57	2.14 ± 0.57	2.10 ± 0.44
After one year	1.58 ± 0.5	2.75 ± 0.44	1 ± 0.00	1 ± 0.00
General health state				
Hospital admission	48.95 ± 9.25	78 ± 12.8	31.9 ± 7.49	29.20 ± 6.64
After one month	30.13 ± 10.55	21.5 ± 8.75	57.14 ± 9.56	59.35 ± 7.02
After one year	83.16 ± 7.74	59 ± 9.67	91.9 ± 7.49	94.46 ± 6.63

We analyzed the QoL between the groups as follows.

Mobility: There were no significant differences between the groups.

Selfcare: After one month of surgery, there wasa statistically-significant difference between SCC and MM groups and BCC and AK groups (t-test, $p < 0.001$). The values in BCC and AK groups were significantly lower than those in SCC and MM groups. After one year of surgery, the value in the MM group wassignificantly lowerthanthose in the other groups (t-test, $p = 0.003$, $p = 0.021$, and $p = 0.034$).

Normal activities: At hospital admission, the value in the MM group was significantly lower than those in theother groups (t-test, $p < 0.001$). After one month of surgery, the SCC and MM groups had significantly higher values than those in BCC and AK groups (t-test, $p = 0.013$). After one year of surgery, the value in the MM group was still significantly higher than those in the other groups ($p < 0.001$).

Pain/discomfort: After one month of surgery, there was a statistically-significant difference between SCC and MM groups and BCC and AK groups (t-test, $p = 0.012$). After one year of surgery, the value in the MM group was still significantly higher than those in the other groups ($p < 0.001$).

In the SCC group, all indicators of the QoL presented impaired values one year after surgery, after a decreasing trend (from the values registered at hospital admission), with statistically-significant differences (paired samples t-tests, all p-values < 0.05). The despair indicator slightly increased after one month of surgery, due to the impact of the histopathological result as well as the scars. The general health state indicator statistically significantly decreased after one month of surgery, and statistically significantly increased after one year (paired samples t-tests, $p = 0.021$ and $p < 0.001$, respectively).

In the MM group, the mobility, selfcare, normal activities, and pain/discomfort presented a decrease in values one year after surgery, compared to the values registered at hospital admission, with statistically-significant differences in selfcare (paired samples t-tests, $p = 0.007$). The despair indicator statistically significantly increased after one month of surgery (paired samples t-test, $p = 0.005$), and remained significantly higher than at hospital admission after one year (paired samples t-test, $p = 0.006$), due to the impact of being diagnosed with MM. Also, the general health state significantly decreased after one month of surgery (paired samples t-test, $p < 0.001$), and remained lower after one year, compared to the hospital admission value (paired samples t-test, $p < 0.001$).

In the BCC group, all indicators of the QoL presented impaired values one year after surgery, after a decreasing trend (from the values registered at hospital admission), with statistically-significant differences, except for mobility (paired samples t-tests, all p-values < 0.05). The general health state indicator statistically significantly increased one month after surgery and after one year (paired samples t-tests, $p < 0.001$).

In the AK group, all indicators of the QoL presented impaired values (1 or very close to 1) one year after surgery, after a decreasing trend (from the values registered at hospital admission), with statistically-significant differences, except for mobility (paired samples t-tests, all p-values < 0.05). The general health state indicator statistically significantly increased after one month of surgery and after one year (paired samples t-tests, $p < 0.001$).

4. Discussion

The incidence of MM and NMSC is increasing worldwide, becoming an issue for the healthcare systems due to treatment costs and morbidity [8]. The increased rate is related to the fact that in recent years, awareness of this disease has increased among patients and physicians. The number of surgical excisions of the skin tumors with confirmed histopathology has grown. Protocols have been created for the management of skin cancer for proper treatment and to prevent the disease [9]. Moreover, new studies are assessing the QoL of the patients diagnosed with skin cancer [10].

The factors that influence the QOL in patients with skin cancer are the diagnosis of the disease, surgical intervention, and scars. It must be highlighted that most of the NMSC appear on sun-exposed areas, such as the face, neck, and upper limbs [11]. These locations can lead to difficulties in the oncologic surgical excision with the best functional and aesthetic outcome [8]. In addition, the lesions can lead topain and pruritus, causing functional limitations [10]. In the case of MM, the main step of the treatment is the surgical excision, followed by the sentinel lymph node, depending on the staging of the disease [12]. Thus, the majority of skin cancers are surgically excised. In the case of positive surgical margins or recurrence, the patients must undergo a new surgical procedure. These facts change the daily routine and also have a financial impact. Postoperatively, more and more patients are complaining about scarring [10,13].

In our study, 38 patients presented SCC. The lesions appeared especially in elderly patients. In older individuals, comorbidities were associated, such as arterial hypertension and chronic heart failure [14,15]. The surgical excision was done with 0.6 cm safety margins, and the defects were covered with skin grafts or local flaps. A total of 10 patients had the lesion on the lower lip. The defects were covered with advanced flaps for a good functional result. Even if SCC of the lower lip is an invasion lesion, it does not have the same rate of metastasis as the Merkel cell carcinoma of the lower lip [16]. The QoL was affected one monthafter surgery, mostly because of the histopathological results as well asthe aesthetic and functional outcome.

In the 168 patients who were diagnosed with BCC, the excision was performed with 0.4 cm oncologic margins. Depending on the dimension of the tumor, a primary suture was preferred, followed by local flaps and skin grafting. In patients who presented wound dehiscence, a gel with polyhexanidine was used, due to its antiseptic properties [17]. Our patients reported an excellent QoL one year aftersurgery, without local recurrence.

A study conducted by Rhee et al. (2014) on 121 patients demonstrated that the QoL of patients with SCC is more affected in comparison to those with BCC, due to the fact that SCC is a more aggressive lesion that can lead to metastasis, and has a more invasive treatment [18].

A total of 21 patients had AK, with good reports of the QoL after one year. Philipp-Dormston et al. (2018) demonstrated that the progression from AK to SCC is associated with a significant reduction in QoL [2]. In our study, none of the patients with AK presented SCC after one year.

In the MM group, the QoL showed a significant decrease, with no additional increase, even after one year. The general health state had a very strong decrease after one month, and remained lower after one year, compared to the hospital admission value. The excision was performed with 0.5 cm at diagnosis, and reexcision was made with 1- or 2-cm oncologic margins, depending on the Breslow depth. The defects were covered with local flaps. Chernyshov et al. (2019) in their QoL report highlighted thatpatients with MM showed an increased physical functioning and bodily pain [19]. In addition, Newton-Bishop et al. (2014) demonstrated that the excision of the MM with more than 2 cm had a significant impact on the QoL, mostly in young patients and women [20]. The impact is higher if the melanoma is on the face, due to the scars resulting from the surgical excisionand the lymph node dissection.

5. Conclusions

Skin cancer is one of the most common types of malignancies, with a rapidly increasing incidence every year, affecting patients' QoL. Questionnaires evaluating the QoL are important and should be used by physicians as an outcome measure.

Author Contributions: Conceptualization, L.R.; methodology, D.T., software, R.P.P., validation, L.R. and C.-R.J.; formal analysis, R.P.P.; investigation, A.A. and A.-E.B.-S.; resources, D.G.B.; data curation, A.-E.B.-S. and D.G.B.; writing—original draft preparation, A.A.; visualization, D.T. and D.I.; supervision, C.-R.J.; project administration, D.I. All authors have read and agreed to the published version of the manuscript.

Funding: This research received no external funding.

Conflicts of Interest: The authors declare no conflict of interest.

References

1. Gordon, R. Skin cancer: An overview of epidemiology and risk factors. *Semin. Oncol. Nurs.* **2013**, *29*, 160–169. [CrossRef] [PubMed]
2. Philipp-Dormston, W.G.; Müller, K.; Novak, B.; Strömer, K.; Termeer, C.; Hammann, U.; Glutsch, J.W.; Krähn-Senftleben, G.; Lübbert, H.; Koller, M.; et al. Patient-reported health outcomes in patients with non-melanoma skin cancer and actinic keratosis: Results from a large-scale observational study analysing effects of diagnoses and disease progression. *JEADV* **2018**, *32*, 1138–1146. [CrossRef] [PubMed]
3. Dodds, A.; Chia, A.; Shumack, S. Actinic keratosis: Rationale and management. *Dermatol. Ther.* **2014**, *4*, 11–31. [CrossRef] [PubMed]
4. Avilés Izquierdo, J.A.; Molina López, I.; Sobrini Morillo, P.; Márquez Rodas, I.; Mercader Cidoncha, E. Utility of PET/CT in patients with stage I–III melanoma. *Clin. Transl. Oncol.* **2019**. [CrossRef] [PubMed]
5. Peisker, A.; Raschke, G.F.; Guentsch, A.; Roshanghias, K.; Eichmann, F.; Schultze-Mosgau, S. Longterm quality of life after oncologic surgery and microvascular free flap reconstruction in patients with oral squamous cell carcinoma. *Med. Oral Patol. Oral Cir. Bucal* **2016**, *21*, e420–e424. [CrossRef] [PubMed]
6. Vogel, R.I.; Strayer, L.G.; Engelman, L.; Nelson, H.H.; Blaes, A.H.; Anderson, K.E.; Lazovich, D. Comparison of quality of life among long-term melanoma survivors and non-melanoma controls: A cross-sectional study. *Qual. Life Res.* **2017**, *26*, 1761–1766. [CrossRef] [PubMed]
7. Abedini, R.; Nasimi, M.; Noormohammad Pour, P.; Moghtadaie, A.; Tohidinik, H.R. Quality of life in patients with non-melanoma skin cancer: Implications for healthcare education services and supports. *J. Cancer Educ.* **2019**, *34*, 755–759. [CrossRef] [PubMed]
8. Linos, E.; Katz, K.A.; Colditz, G.A. Skin Cancer-The Importance of Prevention. *JAMA Intern. Med.* **2016**, *176*, 1435–1436. [CrossRef] [PubMed]

9. Fahradyan, A.; Howell, A.C.; Wolfswinkel, E.M.; Tsuha, M.; Sheth, P.; Wong, A.K. Updates on the Management of Non-Melanoma Skin Cancer (NMSC). *Healthcare* **2017**, *5*, 82. [CrossRef] [PubMed]
10. Gaulin, C.; Sebaratnam, D.F.; Fernández-Peñas, P. Quality of life in non-melanoma skin cancer. *Australas. J. Dermatol.* **2015**, *56*, 70–76. [CrossRef] [PubMed]
11. Fessa, C.K.; Man Ying Tsang, V.; Fenández-Peñas, P. Relationship between visibility of skin condition and quality of life. *Australas. J. Dermatol.* **2011**, *52*, 11.
12. Essner, R. Surgical treatment of malignant melanoma. *Surg. Clin. N. Am.* **2003**, *83*, 109–156. [CrossRef]
13. Tiglis, M.; Neagu, T.P.; Elfara, M.; Diaconu, C.C.; Bratu, O.G.; Vacaroiu, I.A.; Grintescu, I.M. Nefopam and its role in modulating acute and chronic pain. *Rev. Chim. (Bucharest)* **2018**, *69*, 2877–2880. [CrossRef]
14. Diaconu, C.C.; Dragoi, C.M.; Bratu, O.G.; Neagu, T.P.; Stoian, P.; Cobelschi, P.C.; Nicolae, A.C.; Iancu, M.A.; Hainarosie, R.; Ana Maria Alexandra Stanescu, A.M.A.; et al. New approaches and perspectives for the pharmacological treatment of arterial hypertension. *Farmacia* **2018**, *66*, 408–415. [CrossRef]
15. Balcangiu-Stroescu, A.E.; Tanasescu, M.D.; Diaconescu, A.; Raducu, L.; Balan, D.G.; Mihai, A.; Tanase, M.; Stanescu, I.I.; Ionescu, D. Diabetic nephropathy: A concise assessment of the causes, risk factors and implications in diabetic patients. *Rev. Chim. (Bucharest)* **2018**, *69*, 3118–3121. [CrossRef]
16. Raducu, L.; Cozma, C.N.; BalcangiuStroescu, A.E.; Panduru, M.; Avino, A.; Tanasescu, M.D.; Badita, D.G.; Jecan, C.R. A rare case of a lower lip merkel cell carcinoma diagnosis and treatment. *Rev. Chim. (Bucharest)* **2018**, *69*, 354–357. [CrossRef]
17. Raducu, L.; Balcangiu-Stroescu, A.E.; Stanescu, I.I.; Tanasescu, M.D.; Cozma, C.N.; Jecan, C.R.; Badita, D.G. Use of polyhexanidine in treating chronic wounds. *Rev. Chim. (Bucharest)* **2017**, *68*, 2112–2113.
18. Rhee, J.S.; Matthews, B.A.; Neuburg, M.; Smith, T.L.; Burzynski, M.; Nattinger, A.B. Skin cancer and quality of life: Assessment with the dermatology life quality index. *Dermatol. Surg.* **2004**, *30*, 525–529. [CrossRef] [PubMed]
19. Chernyshov, P.V.; Lallas, A.; Tomas-Aragones, L.; Arenbergerova, M.; Samimi, M.; Manolache, L.; Svensson, A.; Marron, S.E.; Sampogna, F.; Spillekom-vanKoulil, S.; et al. Quality of life measurement in skin cancer patients: Literature review and position paper of the european academy of dermatology and venereology task forces on quality of life and patient oriented outcomes, melanoma and non-melanoma skin cancer. *J. Eur. Acad. Dermatol. Venereol.* **2019**, *33*, 816–827. [CrossRef] [PubMed]
20. Newton-Bishop, J.A.; Nolan, C.; Turner, F.; McCabe, M.; Boxer, C.; Thomas, J.M.; Coombes, G.; A'Hern, R.P.; Barrett, J.H. A quality-of-life study in high-risk (thickness ≥ 2 mm) cutaneous melanoma patients in a randomized trial of 1-cm versus 3-cm surgical excision margins. *J. Investig. Dermatol. Symp. Proc.* **2004**, *9*, 152–159. [CrossRef] [PubMed]

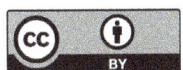

© 2020 by the authors. Licensee MDPI, Basel, Switzerland. This article is an open access article distributed under the terms and conditions of the Creative Commons Attribution (CC BY) license (http://creativecommons.org/licenses/by/4.0/).

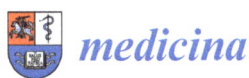

Case Report

Total Exenteration En Bloc with a Nephrectomy for Locally Advanced Cervical Cancer Invading a Pelvic Kidney—A Case Report and Literature Review

Nicolae Bacalbasa [1,2,3,†], Irina Balescu [4,*], Mihaela Vilcu [1,5], Simona Dima [3], Camelia Diaconu [1,6,†], Laura Iliescu [1,7,†], Alexandru Filipescu [1,8,†] and Iulian Brezean [1,5]

1. "Carol Davila" University of Medicine and Pharmacy, 020021 Bucharest, Romania; nicolae_bacalbasa@yahoo.ro (N.B.); mihaela.vilcu@gmail.ro (M.V.); drcameliadiaconu@gmail.com (C.D.); laurailiescu@gmail.ro (L.I.); iulianbrezean@gmail.ro (I.B.)
2. Department of Obstetrics and Gynecology, "I. Cantacuzino" Clinical Hospital, 030167 Bucharest, Romania
3. Department of Visceral Surgery, "Fundeni" Clinical Institute, 022328 Bucharest, Romania; simonadima@gmail.ro
4. Department of Surgery, "Ponderas" Academic Hospital, 021188 Bucharest, Romania
5. Department of Visceral Surgery, "I. Cantacuzino" Clinical Hospital, 030167 Bucharest, Romania
6. Department of Internal Medicine, Clinical Emergency Hospital of Bucharest, 105402 Bucharest, Romania
7. Department of Internal Medicine, "Fundeni" Clinical Institute, 022328 Bucharest, Romania
8. Department of Obstetrics and Gynecology, "Elias" Emergency University Hospital, 011461 Bucharest, Romania; alexandrufilipescu@gmail.ro
* Correspondence: irina.balescu@ponderas-ah.ro; Tel.: +40-72-407-7709
† Authors with equal contribution.

Received: 26 November 2019; Accepted: 10 January 2020; Published: 15 January 2020

Abstract: *Introduction*: Extended pelvic resection might be the option of choice in patients presenting locally advanced cervical cancer. However, the possibility of a co-existence of an ectopic, pelvic kidney that is invaded by such a tumor is extremely rare. *Case Presentation*: A 54-year-old female patient, diagnosed with locally advanced cervical cancer in the presence of a pelvic kidney, was submitted to surgery with curative intent. A large, abscessed cervical tumor invading the urinary bladder and the rectum was found, so a total exenteration was planned. Intraoperatively, tumor invasion of the left kidney, which was found in an ectopic, pelvic position was also encountered; therefore, total pelvic exenteration in association with a left nephrectomy was successfully performed. *Conclusions*: The presence of an ectopic, pelvic disposition of the kidney makes it susceptible to be invaded by locally advanced pelvic tumors; in such cases, a nephrectomy might also be needed.

Keywords: ectopic kidney; locally advanced cervical cancer; nephrectomy

1. Introduction

An ectopic kidney refers to the situation in which developmental arrest of the renal ascent is encountered, leading to the location of this viscus in the pelvic, iliac or abdominal area [1]. Most often, a pelvic kidney is situated opposite to the sacrum bone and below the aortic bifurcation and presents an incomplete rotation [2]. Such cases also present certain modifications with regard to the length and disposition of the ureter and vascular supply: In up to half of these patients, a certain degree of hydronephrosis can be encountered, while the renal arteries can arise from the distal aorta, aortic bifurcation, common or external iliac arteries or even from the inferior mesenteric artery [1,2]. Therefore, its pelvic location makes it susceptible to be invaded by all the tumoral processes of pelvic origin, while the surgical approach can be significantly influenced. The incidence of this anatomical particularity is estimated to be one in 2100 to 3000 cases [3].

2. Case Presentation

This study was approved by the hospital ethical committee (the ethical code number was 93/21.8.2019). A 54-year-old postmenopausal female patient was investigated for diffuse pelvic pain, vaginal bleeding and fever, and was diagnosed with a large cervical tumor invading the rectum and the urinary bladder, in association with a massive peritumoral abscess. In the meantime, a left pelvic kidney, with no demarcation line with the tumoral process, was described during the preoperative computed tomography scan. At the time of presentation, the patient presented constant vesperal fever in association with biological inflammatory syndrome. Due to the finding of a large pelvic abscess in association with the clinical–biological condition of the patient, surgery as the first therapeutic intention was decided. Intraoperatively, a large pelvic tumor invading the rectum and the urinary bladder, in association with local perforation and a secondary abscess, was found. In the meantime, invasion of the upper renal pole was also certified (Figures 1–4).

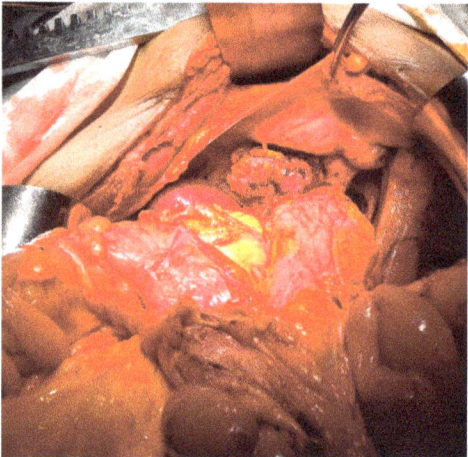

Figure 1. Initial intraoperative aspect: Large pelvic tumor invading the left kidney with a pelvic location.

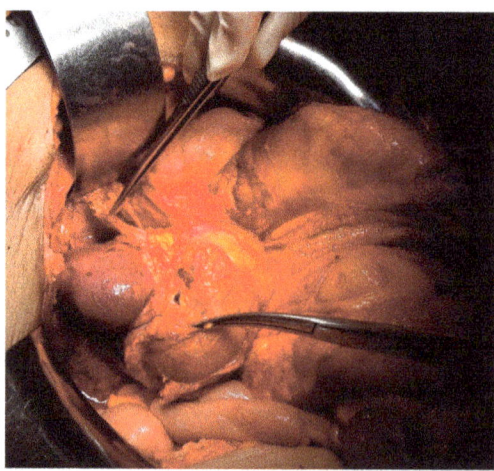

Figure 2. The aspect after tumoral mobilization—presence of ureteral invasion as well as renal invasion.

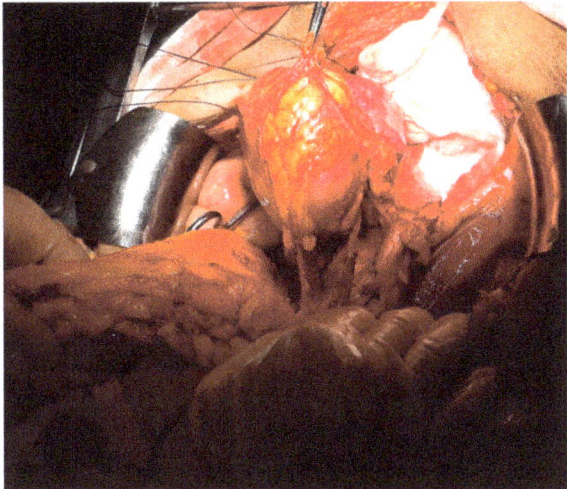

Figure 3. The aspect after rectal sectioning and posterior dissection of the tumor.

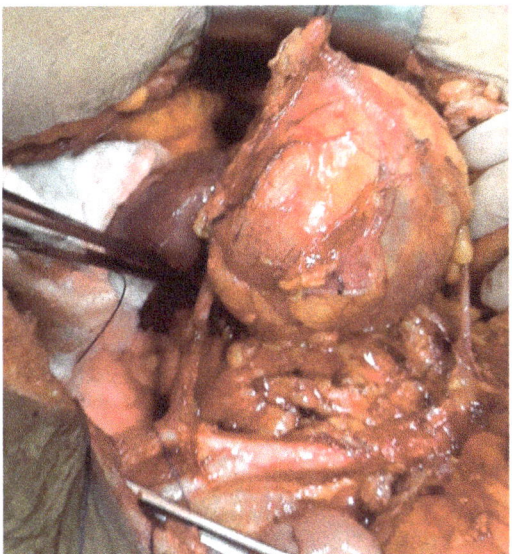

Figure 4. The final aspect after mobilization of the tumor en bloc with the left kidney and lymph node dissection.

Therefore, total exenteration en bloc with a nephrectomy, as well as pelvic and para-aortic lymph node dissection was performed. The right ureter was exteriorized in a right terminal cutaneous ostomy, while the terminal end of the sigmoidian loop was exteriorized in a left cutaneous colostomy. The decision of not re-establishing the continuity of the digestive or urinary tract was taken due to the association of the tumoral perforation with a secondary pelvic abscess. The postoperative outcome was uneventful, the patient being discharged in the 14th postoperative day. The histopathological studies confirmed the presence of a moderately differentiated squamous cell carcinoma originating from the uterine cervix. At the one-month follow-up, the patient was referred to the oncology service in order to be submitted to adjuvant therapy and presented a satisfactory urinary function, with a mean level of creatinine of 1.2 mg/dL.

3. Discussion

Patients presenting ectopic kidneys with pelvic localization usually are at risk of developing hydronephrosis; therefore, in such cases, association of a pelvic malignancy can pose serious problems in terms of establishing whether the ureteral dilatation is induced by tumoral invasion or is the consequence of the pelvic disposition of the kidney [1,4]. So, clarification between the two situations should be carried out in order to correctly classify and stage the patient before deciding the therapeutic strategy [5,6]. In the case presented, the invasion was evident and affected the parenchymal area of the kidney and not the ureter, therefore a nephrectomy was needed. However, this circumstance of a pelvic kidney in association with cervical cancer has been rarely reported so far, with only a few case reports having been published. The most relevant ones are summarized in Table 1.

Interestingly, in the case reported by Ripley et al., the patient presented a pelvic kidney as the result of a previous kidney transplant; in this case, the radiation field could be established in a manner which avoided the renal involvement [7]. Similarly, in Abouna's case report the patient also had been submitted nine years previously for a kidney transplantation, but in this case the therapeutic strategy when the cervical cancer was encountered was different and consisted of a renal replacement in the upper abdomen and revascularization by the use of a splenic artery followed by radiation therapy [8].

Another important issue that should be underlined in such cases is the one related to irradiation; patients presenting an association of a pelvic kidney and a locally advanced cervical tumor cannot be submitted to radiotherapy without risking injury to the kidney [9,10]; therefore, in such cases, including the kidney into the radiation field increases the risk of developing malignant hypertension and increases the chances to necessitate a therapeutic nephrectomy [9–13]. In such cases, certain authors proposed performing radical surgery followed by repositioning the kidney out of the pelvic area, in order to allow the patient to be further on submitted to the adjuvant treatment [14]. The first case of a patient presenting a pelvic kidney in association with cervical cancer, in whom the authors decided for a radical hysterectomy and kidney fixation in an extrapelvic area, followed by radiotherapy, was reported in 1980 by Rosenheim et al. [4]. However, in our case, due to the presence of a parenchymatous invasion of the kidney, nephrectomy was also imposed in order to achieve radical surgery.

Interestingly, in the case reported by Roth et al., published in 2004, both kidneys were found to have an ectopic location at the level of the pelvic area; moreover, the ureteral length was 9 cm in both ureters, making kidney fixation out of the pelvic area impossible, followed by radiation therapy. Therefore, the authors opted for per primam surgery, consisting of pelvic exenteration [5].

Recently, the American study group conducted by Lataifeh et al. reported the successful chemo-radiation of a patient with a stage IIB cervical tumor (IIB - Cervical carcinoma invades beyond the uterus, but not to the lower third of the vagina or to the pelvic wall with parametrial invasion) and ectopic kidney. The chemo-radiation protocol was applied with curative intent, with good oncological outcomes, but with the disadvantage of involving the pelvic kidney into the radiation field. However, the initial workup had revealed the fact that the left kidney was only partially functional; therefore, pelvic irradiation did not induce the development of renal insufficiency or malignant hypertension [6].

However, if surgery with radical intent is proposed, attention should be focused on the anatomical particularities of patients presenting a pelvic kidney [15,16]. Therefore, in such cases, the renal pedicle as well as the ureter can be situated in close contact with the iliac vessels, particular attention being needed in order to perform the pelvic lymph node dissection [17–19].

Table 1. Relevant studies presenting a pelvic kidney in association with cervical cancer.

Name, Year	Age of the Patient (Years)	Presumed FIGO Stage—Preoperatively	Histopathological Type	Therapeutic Strategy	Follow-up
Bakri, 1993 [1]	65	IIB	Squamous cell carcinoma	Per primam surgery—radical abdominal hysterectomy en bloc with left parametrectomy, left ureteral resection and reimplantation into the urinary bladder using a Boari flap technique Followed by adjuvant chemotherapy—Cisplatinum 100 mg/m^2 3 weeks, 3 courses	Alive without recurrence at 6 years after surgery
Roth, 2003 [5]	48	IIB	Squamous cell carcinoma	Per primam surgery—anterior exenteration without vaginal reconstruction and distal ileal conduit	No evidence of disease at 14 months follow-up
Lataifeh, 2007 [6]	50	IIB	Adenocarcinoma	Definitive radio-chemotherapy—4500 cGy and cisplatin with curative intent for 9 weeks	Disease free at two years follow-up, normal renal function
Ripley, 1995 [7]	NR	IB	Adenocarcinoma of the cervix in a previously kidney transplanted patient	Definitive external radiotherapy—4000 cGy and intracavitary radiotherapy with curative intent for 6.5 weeks	NR

FIGO, International Federation of Obstetrics and Gynecology; IIB, Cervical carcinoma invades beyond the uterus, but not to the lower third of the vagina or to the pelvic wall with parametrial invasion; IB, Invasive carcinoma with measured deepest invasion ≥5.0 mm, limited to the cervix uteri; NR, not reported.

The single case series that has been published so far on this theme originates from India and included three such cases. The first case was initially diagnosed with a FIGO (International Federation of Obstetrics and Gynecology) stage IIB (Cervical carcinoma invades beyond the uterus, but not to the lower third of the vagina or to the pelvic wall with parametrial invasion) tumor and a right pelvic kidney and was submitted to external beam radiotherapy with a total dose of 500 Gy followed by a radical hysterectomy with bilateral adnexectomy and pelvic lymph node dissection, the ectopic kidney being successfully preserved. The second case was diagnosed with a stage IB1 cervical tumor and left pelvic kidney and was submitted to a total radical hysterectomy with bilateral adnexectomy and pelvic lymph node dissection. The third case was per primam submitted for a radical hysterectomy followed by adjuvant radiotherapy with a total dose of 500 Gy. In all cases, good oncological and renal long-term outcomes were obtained [2].

4. Conclusions

The association between pelvic kidneys and cervical cancer represents a scarce eventuality, only few cases being reported so far. In such patients, the therapeutic strategy should be carefully analyzed, with multiple dilemmas being reported so far. Moreover, the association between advanced cervical cancer and an ectopic kidney is even rarer, a single case which was finally submitted for anterior pelvic exenteration being reported so far. When it comes to the necessity of an association of total pelvic exenteration with a nephrectomy, to the best of our knowledge, this is the first case reported so far. The presence of a massive local invasion in the surrounding viscera, as well as renal invasion in association with the presence of a massive peritumoral abscess, enabled us to consider that total pelvic exenteration en bloc with a nephrectomy represent the best option for this case.

Author Contributions: N.B., performed surgery; I.B., prepared the manuscript; M.V. and A.F., part of the surgical team; C.D. and L.I., advised about the nephrological outcome; S.D., produced figures; I.B. and C.D., finally reviewed the manuscript and advised about the surgical procedure; all the authors agreed with the final version of the manuscript. All authors have read and agreed to the published version of the manuscript.

Funding: This research received no external funding.

Acknowledgments: This work was supported by the project entitled "Multidisciplinary Consortium for Supporting the Research Skills in Diagnosing, Treating and Identifying Predictive Factors of Malignant Gynecologic Disorders", project number PN-III-P1-1.2-PCCDI2017-0833.

Conflicts of Interest: The authors declare no conflict of interest.

References

1. Bakri, Y.N.; Mansi, M.; Sundin, T. Stage IIB carcinoma of the cervix complicated by an ectopic pelvic kidney. *Int. J. Gynaecol. Obstet.* **1993**, *42*, 174–176. [CrossRef]
2. Ramamurthy, R.; Muthusamy, V.; Hussain, S.A. Approach to carcinoma cervix with pelvic kidney. *Indian J. Surg. Oncol.* **2010**, *1*, 323–327. [CrossRef] [PubMed]
3. Dretler, S.P.; Olsson, C.; Pfister, R.C. The anatomic, radiologic and clinical characteristics of the pelvic kidney: An analysis of 86 cases. *J. Urol.* **1971**, *105*, 623–627. [CrossRef]
4. Rosenshein, N.B.; Lichter, A.S.; Walsh, P.C. Cervical cancer complicated by a pelvic kidney. *J. Urol.* **1980**, *123*, 766–767. [CrossRef]
5. Roth, T.M.; Woodring, C.T.; McGehee, R.P. Stage II-B carcinoma of the cervix complicated by bilateral pelvic kidneys. *Gynecol. Oncol.* **2004**, *92*, 376–379. [CrossRef] [PubMed]
6. Lataifeh, I.; Amarin, Z.; Jaradat, I. Stage IIB carcinoma of the cervix that is associated with pelvic kidney: A therapeutic dilemma. *Am. J. Obstet. Gynecol.* **2007**, *197*, e8–e10. [CrossRef] [PubMed]
7. Ripley, D.; Levenback, C.; Eifel, P.; Lewis, R.M. Adenocarcinoma of the cervix in a renal transplant patient. *Gynecol. Oncol.* **1995**, *59*, 151–155. [CrossRef] [PubMed]
8. Abouna, G.M.; Micaily, B.; Lee, D.J.; Kumar, M.S.; Jahshan, A.E.; Lyons, P. Salvage of a kidney graft in a patient with advanced carcinoma of the cervix by reimplantation of the graft from the pelvis to the upper abdomen in preparation for radiation therapy. *Transplantation* **1994**, *58*, 520–522. [CrossRef] [PubMed]

9. Kunkler, P.B.; Farr, R.F.; Luxton, R.W. The limit of renal tolerance to x-rays; an investigation into renal damage occurring following the treatment of tumours of the testis by abdominal baths. *Br. J. Radiol.* **1952**, *25*, 192–201. [PubMed]
10. Crummy, A.B., Jr.; Hellman, S.; Stansel, H.C., Jr.; Hukill, P.B. Renal hypertension secondary to unilateral radiation damage relieved by nephrectomy. *Radiology* **1965**, *84*, 108–111. [CrossRef] [PubMed]
11. Iliescu, L.; Herlea, V.; Toma, L.; Orban, C. Association between chronic HCV hepatitis, membranoproliferative glomerulopathy and cutaneous sarcoidosis. *J. Gastrointest. Liver Dis.* **2015**, *24*, 8.
12. Iliescu, L.; Mercan-Stanciu, A.; Toma, L.; Ioanitescu, E.S. A severe case of hyperglycemia in a kidney transplant recipient undergoing interferon-free therapy for chronic hepatitis C. *Acta Endocrinol. Buchar* **2018**, *14*, 533–538. [CrossRef] [PubMed]
13. Iliescu, L.; Ioanitescu, S.; Toma, L.; Orban, C. Spontaneous portohepatic venous shunt: Ultrasonographic aspect. *Ultrasound Q.* **2015**, *31*, 141–144. [CrossRef]
14. Koff, S.A.; Hayden, L.J.; Wise, H.A. Anomalies of the kidney. In *Adult and Pediatric Urology*; Doody, D.G., Gillenwater, J.Y., Eds.; Yearbook Medical Publishers: Chicago, IL, USA, 1987; Chapter 47; p. 1604.
15. Bodean, O.; Bratu, O.; Munteanu, O.; Marcu, D.; Spinu, D.A.; Socea, B.; Diaconu, C.; Cirstoiu, M. Iatrogenic injury of the low urinary tract in women undergoing pelvic surgical interventions. *Arch. Balk. Med. Union* **2018**, *53*, 281–284. [CrossRef]
16. Bumbu, A.; Nacer, K.; Bratu, O.; Berechet, M.; Bumbu, G.; Bumbu, B. Ureteral lesions in gynecological pathology. In Proceedings of the 14th National Congress of Urogynecology and the National Conference of the Romanian Asociation for the Study of Pain, Bucharest, Romania, 26–27 October 2017; pp. 82–89.
17. Rusu, M.C.; Ilie, A.C.; Brezean, I. Human anatomic variations: Common, external iliac, origin of the obturator, inferior epigastric and medial circumflex femoral arteries and deep femoral artery course on the medial side of the femoral vessels. *Surg. Radiol. Anat.* **2017**, *39*, 1285–1288. [CrossRef]
18. Brezean, I.; Aldoescu, S.; Catrina, E.; Valcu, M.; Ionut, I.; Predescu, G.; Degeratu, D.; Pantea, I. Pelvic and abdominal-wall actinomycotic infection by uterus gateway without genital lesions. *Chirurgia* **2010**, *105*, 123–125.
19. Balescu, I.; Bacalbasa, N.; Vilcu, M.; Brasoveanu, V.; Brezean, I. Sentinel lymph node in early stage ovarian cancer; a literature review. *J. Mind Med. Sci.* **2018**, *5*, 184–188. [CrossRef]

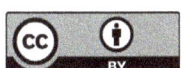

© 2020 by the authors. Licensee MDPI, Basel, Switzerland. This article is an open access article distributed under the terms and conditions of the Creative Commons Attribution (CC BY) license (http://creativecommons.org/licenses/by/4.0/).

MDPI
St. Alban-Anlage 66
4052 Basel
Switzerland
Tel. +41 61 683 77 34
Fax +41 61 302 89 18
www.mdpi.com

Medicina Editorial Office
E-mail: medicina@mdpi.com
www.mdpi.com/journal/medicina